T0348554

HIV

Editor

PAUL E. SAX

INFECTIOUS DISEASE CLINICS OF NORTH AMERICA

www.id.theclinics.com

Consulting Editor
HELEN W. BOUCHER

September 2019 • Volume 33 • Number 3

ELSEVIER

1600 John F. Kennedy Boulevard • Suite 1800 • Philadelphia, Pennsylvania, 19103-2899.

http://www.theclinics.com

INFECTIOUS DISEASE CLINICS OF NORTH AMERICA Volume 33, Number 3
September 2019 ISSN 0891–5520, ISBN-13: 978-0-323-68232-9

Editor: Kerry Holland
Developmental Editor: Donald Mumford

© **2019 Elsevier Inc. All rights reserved.**

This periodical and the individual contributions contained in it are protected under copyright by Elsevier, and the following terms and conditions apply to their use:

Photocopying

Single photocopies of single articles may be made for personal use as allowed by national copyright laws. Permission of the Publisher and payment of a fee is required for all other photocopying, including multiple or systematic copying, copying for advertising or promotional purposes, resale, and all forms of document delivery. Special rates are available for educational institutions that wish to make photocopies for non-profit educational classroom use. For information on how to seek permission visit www.elsevier.com/permissions or call: (+44) 1865 843830 (UK)/(+1) 215 239 3804 (USA).

Derivative Works

Subscribers may reproduce tables of contents or prepare lists of articles including abstracts for internal circulation within their institutions. Permission of the Publisher is required for resale or distribution outside the institution. Permission of the Publisher is required for all other derivative works, including compilations and translations (please consult www.elsevier.com/permissions).

Electronic Storage or Usage

Permission of the Publisher is required to store or use electronically any material contained in this periodical, including any article or part of an article (please consult www.elsevier.com/permissions). Except as outlined above, no part of this publication may be reproduced, stored in a retrieval system or transmitted in any form or by any means, electronic, mechanical, photocopying, recording or otherwise, without prior written permission of the Publisher.

Notice

No responsibility is assumed by the Publisher for any injury and/or damage to persons or property as a matter of products liability, negligence or otherwise, or from any use or operation of any methods, products, instructions or ideas contained in the material herein. Because of rapid advances in the medical sciences, in particular, independent verification of diagnoses and drug dosages should be made.

Although all advertising material is expected to conform to ethical (medical) standards, inclusion in this publication does not constitute a guarantee or endorsement of the quality or value of such product or of the claims made of it by its manufacturer.

Infectious Disease Clinics of North America (ISSN 0891–5520) is published in March, June, September, and December by Elsevier Inc., 360 Park Avenue South, New York, NY 10010-1710. Periodicals postage paid at New York, NY and additional mailing offices. Subscription prices are $330.00 per year for US individuals, $660.00 per year for US institutions, $100.00 per year for US students, $396.00 per year for Canadian individuals, $824.00 per year for Canadian institutions, $432.00 per year for international individuals, $824.00 per year for international institutions, and $200.00 per year for Canadian and international students. To receive student rate, orders must be accompanied by name of affiliated institution, date of term, and the *signature* of program/ residency coordinator on institution letterhead. Orders will be billed at individual rate until proof of status is received. Foreign air speed delivery is included in all *Clinics* subscription prices. All prices are subject to change without notice. **POSTMASTER**: Send address changes to *Infectious Disease Clinics of North America,* Elsevier Health Sciences Division, Subcription Customer Service, 3251 Riverport Lane, Maryland Heights, MO 63043. **Customer Service: 1-800-654-2452 (US). From outside of the US and Canada, call 1-314-447-8871. Fax: 1-314-447-8029. E-mail: JournalsCustomerService-usa@elsevier.com (print support) or JournalsOnlineSupport-usa@elsevier.com (online support).**

Infectious Disease Clinics of North America is also published in Spanish by Editorial Inter-Médica, Junin 917, 1er A 1113, Buenos Aires, Argentina.

Reprints. For copies of 100 or more, of articles in this publication, please contact the Commercial Reprints Department, Elsevier Inc., 360 Park Avenue South, New York, New York 10010-1710. Tel. 212-633-3874, Fax: 212-633-3820, E-mail: reprints@elsevier.com.

Infectious Disease Clinics of North America is covered in *MEDLINE/PubMed (Index Medicus), Current Contents/ Clinical Medicine, Science Citation Alert, SCISEARCH,* and *Research Alert.*

Printed in the United States of America.

Contributors

CONSULTING EDITOR

HELEN W. BOUCHER, MD, FIDSA, FACP
Director, Infectious Diseases Fellowship Program, Division of Geographic Medicine and Infectious Diseases, Tufts Medical Center, Associate Professor of Medicine, Tufts University School of Medicine, Boston, Massachusetts, USA

EDITOR

PAUL E. SAX, MD
Clinical Director, Division of Infectious Diseases, Brigham and Women's Hospital, Professor of Medicine, Harvard Medical School, Boston, Massachusetts, USA

AUTHORS

WENDY S. ARMSTRONG, MD
Professor, Department of Medicine, Division of Infectious Diseases, Emory University School of Medicine, Atlanta, Georgia, USA

SABA BERHIE, MD
Department of Obstetrics and Gynecology, Division of Maternal Fetal Medicine, Northwestern University Feinberg School of Medicine, Chicago, Illinois, USA

ISAAC I. BOGOCH, MD
Associate Professor, Department of Medicine, Division of Infectious Diseases, University of Toronto, Canada

CHRISTOPHER M. BOSITIS, MD, AAHIVS
Assistant Professor, Department of Family Medicine, Tufts University School of Medicine, Clinical Program Director, HIV and Viral Hepatitis, Greater Lawrence Family Health Center, Lawrence, Massachusetts, USA

BERNARD M. BRANSON, MD
Principal Consultant, Scientific Affairs LLC, Atlanta, Georgia, USA

ANN M. DENNIS, MD, MS
Assistant Professor, Division of Infectious Diseases, University of North Carolina at Chapel Hill, Chapel Hill, North Carolina, USA

BRANDON DIONNE, PharmD
Assistant Clinical Professor, Department of Pharmacy and Health System Sciences, Northeastern University, Clinical Pharmacist, Infectious Diseases, Pharmacy Department, Brigham and Women's Hospital, Boston, Massachusetts, USA

KRISTINE M. ERLANDSON, MD, MS
Associate Professor of Medicine, University of Colorado, Aurora, Colorado, USA

CLAIRE E. FAREL, MD, MPH
Assistant Professor, Division of Infectious Diseases, University of North Carolina at Chapel Hill, Chapel Hill, North Carolina, USA

AMILA HEENDENIYA, MD
Clinical Fellow, Department of Medicine, Division of Infectious Diseases, University of Toronto, Canada

JENNIFER JAO, MD, MPH
Associate Professor, Department of Pediatrics, Department of Medicine, Division of Infectious Diseases, Northwestern University Feinberg School of Medicine, Chicago, Illinois, USA

NIKOLAUS JILG, MD, PhD
Instructor, Division of Infectious Diseases, Massachusetts General Hospital, Harvard Medical School, Boston, Massachusetts, USA

MAILE Y. KARRIS, MD
Associate Professor of Medicine, University of California San Diego, San Diego, California, USA

SEAN G. KELLY, MD
Assistant Professor of Medicine, Division of Infectious Diseases, Vanderbilt University Medical Center, Nashville, Tennessee, USA

JONATHAN Z. LI, MD, MMSc
Assistant Professor, Division of Infectious Diseases, Brigham and Women's Hospital, Harvard Medical School, Boston, Massachusetts, USA

VINCENT C. MARCONI, MD
Professor, Division of Infectious Diseases, Department of Global Health, Emory University School of Medicine, Rollins School of Public Health, Atlanta, Georgia, USA

MARY CLARE MASTERS, MD
Clinical Fellow, Infectious Diseases, Division of Infectious Diseases, Northwestern University Feinberg School of Medicine, Chicago, Illinois, USA

SUZANNE M. McCLUSKEY, MD
Instructor, Division of Infectious Diseases, Harvard Medical School, Massachusetts General Hospital, Boston, Massachusetts, USA

MICHAEL J. MUGAVERO, MD
Professor, Department of Medicine, Division of Infectious Diseases, University of Alabama at Birmingham, Birmingham, Alabama, USA

AADIA I. RANA, MD
Associate Professor, Department of Medicine, Division of Infectious Diseases, University of Alabama at Birmingham, Birmingham, Alabama, USA

MARK J. SIEDNER, MD, MPH
Associate Professor, Division of Infectious Diseases, Harvard Medical School, Massachusetts General Hospital, Boston, Massachusetts, USA

DANIEL A. SOLOMON, MD
Instructor, Division of Infectious Diseases, Harvard Medical School, Brigham and Women's Hospital, Boston, Massachusetts, USA

JOSHUA ST. LOUIS, MD, MPH, AAHIVS
Assistant Professor, Department of Family Medicine, Tufts University School of Medicine, Adult Inpatient Medicine Coordinator, Lawrence Family Medicine Residency, Lawrence, Massachusetts, USA

NATHAN A. SUMMERS, MD
Fellow, Department of Medicine, Division of Infectious Diseases, Emory University School of Medicine, Atlanta, Georgia, USA

BABAFEMI O. TAIWO, MBBS
Professor of Medicine, Division of Infectious Diseases, Northwestern University Feinberg School of Medicine, Chicago, Illinois, USA

BRIAN R. WOOD, MD
Associate Professor of Medicine, Division of Allergy and Infectious Diseases, University of Washington, Mountain West AIDS Education and Training Center, Seattle, Washington, USA

LYNN YEE, MD, MPH
Assistant Professor, Department of Obstetrics and Gynecology, Division of Maternal Fetal Medicine, Northwestern University Feinberg School of Medicine, Chicago, Illinois

DANIEL A. SOLOMON, MD
Instructor, Division of Infectious Diseases, Harvard Medical School, Brigham and Women's Hospital, Boston, Massachusetts, USA

JOSHUA ST. LOUIS, MD, MPH, AAHIVS
Assistant Professor, Department of Family Medicine, Tufts University School of Medicine; Adult Inpatient Medicine Coordinator, Lawrence Family Medicine Residency, Lawrence, Massachusetts, USA

NATHAN A. SUMMERS, MD
Fellow, Department of Medicine, Division of Infectious Diseases, Emory University School of Medicine, Atlanta, Georgia, USA

BABAFEMI O. TAIWO, MBBS
Professor of Medicine, Division of Infectious Diseases, Northwestern University Feinberg School of Medicine, Chicago, Illinois, USA

BRIAN R. WOOD, MD
Associate Professor of Medicine, Division of Allergy and Infectious Diseases, University of Washington, Mountain West AIDS Education and Training Center, Seattle, Washington, USA

LYNN YEE, MD, MPH
Assistant Professor, Department of Obstetrics and Gynecology, Division of Maternal-Fetal Medicine, Northwestern University Feinberg School of Medicine, Chicago, Illinois

Contents

> Profound changes in technology have revolutionized laboratory testing for human immunodeficiency virus (HIV) since the first laboratory enzyme immunoassays that detected only immunoglobulin G (IgG) antibodies. Instrumented fourth-generation random-access chemiluminescent assays are now recommended for initial screening because they become reactive in as little as 2 weeks after infection. Using HIV-1 RNA viral load assays after a reactive initial test could confirm infection and provide useful clinical information. Early initiation of antiretroviral therapy and use of preexposure prophylaxis can alter the evolution of biomarkers and assay reactivity, leading to ambiguous test results.

> Preventing new human immunodeficiency virus (HIV) infections is essential to halting the global pandemic. HIV prevention strategies include integrating both nonpharmacologic (eg, safe sexual counseling, circumcision) and pharmacologic approaches. Several pharmacologic HIV prevention strategies are increasingly used globally and include postexposure prophylaxis, preexposure prophylaxis, and treatment as prevention. These prevention modalities have enormous clinical and public health appeal, as they effectively reduce HIV acquisition in individuals and also may lower HIV incidence in communities when integrated and implemented broadly. Efforts are now underway to scale HIV prevention programs using these techniques in both high- and low-resource settings.

> Laboratory tests are an important tool in the care of patients with human immunodeficiency virus. An organized approach to laboratory ordering helps clinicians to understand the utility of each test, ensure a comprehensive evaluation, and decrease use of unnecessary tests. Tests are organized around the following goals of care: confirm the diagnosis, assess for immune suppression, guide antiretroviral therapy, screen for coinfections and latent infections, monitor response to therapy, and provide preventative care. This article reviews appropriate testing for patients with human immunodeficiency virus to accomplish these goals with a focus on how each test is useful in clinical practice.

Since 2014, a consensus of landmark studies has justified starting antiretroviral therapy (ART) regardless of CD4 count. The evidence for immediate and universal ART is strong, clearly showing individual and population-level benefits, and is supported by all major guidelines groups. Altogether, improvements in ART and recognition of its clinical and epidemiologic benefits justify near-universal ART, preferably as soon after the diagnosis of human immunodeficiency virus (HIV) as possible. Case-based discussions provide a framework to explore the evidence behind the current recommendation for ART for all HIV-positive persons and specific scenarios are discussed in which ART initiation may be delayed.

With the second-generation integrase inhibitors (dolutegravir and bictegravir) extending the attributes of earlier integrase inhibitors, three-drug regimens containing integrase inhibitors plus two nucleos(t)ide reverse transcriptase inhibitors are now widely recommended for first-line (initial) treatment of human immunodeficiency virus-1 infection. Led by dolutegravir plus lamivudine, two-drug therapy is emerging as a way to reduce antiretroviral therapy cost and adverse effects without compromising treatment options should virologic failure occur. Initial two-drug therapy has limitations, including the relative incompatibility with the coemerging concept of same-day antiretroviral therapy initiation.

This review provides a synopsis of key clinical considerations for switching antiretroviral therapy (ART) for individuals with human immunodeficiency virus who have maintained a routinely suppressed viral load. There may be benefits but also risks involved in every ART regimen change, so strategies for prioritizing individuals for a switch based on the specific antiretroviral agents in the regimen are discussed, along with approaches to ensure maintenance of viral suppression after treatment modifications. Controversial and evolving questions in the area of ART switches and simplifications are also considered.

Approximately 20% of people with HIV in the United States prescribed antiretroviral therapy are not virally suppressed. Thus, optimal management of virologic failure has a critical role in the ability to improve viral suppression rates to improve long-term health outcomes for those infected and to achieve epidemic control. This article discusses the causes of virologic failure, the use of resistance testing to guide management after failure, interpretation and relevance of HIV drug resistance patterns, considerations for selection of second-line and salvage therapies, and management of virologic failure in special populations.

Nathan A. Summers and Wendy S. Armstrong

Great progress has been made in caring for persons with human immuno-deficiency virus. However, a significant proportion of individuals still present to care with advanced disease and a low CD4 count. Careful considerations for selection of antiretroviral therapy as well as close monitoring for opportunistic infections and immune reconstitution inflammatory syndrome are vitally important in providing care for such individuals.

Kristine M. Erlandson and Maile Y. Karris

Health care for older adults with human immunodeficiency virus can be highly complex, resource intensive, and carry a high administrative burden. Data from aging longitudinal cohorts and feedback from the human immunodeficiency virus community suggest that the current model is not meeting the needs of these older adults. We introduce the 6 Ms approach, which acknowledges the multicomplexity of older adults with human immunodeficiency virus, simplifies geriatric principles for non–geriatrics-trained providers, and minimizes extensive training and specialized screening tests or tools. Implementing novel approaches to care requires support at local/national levels.

Brandon Dionne

Antiretroviral therapy has advanced significantly since zidovudine was first approved. Although 31 antiretrovirals have been approved by the FDA, only about half of those are commonly used. Newer, more tolerable agents have made human immunodeficiency virus into a chronic condition, which can be managed with medication. The most common antiretroviral regimens consist of 2 nucleoside reverse transcriptase inhibitors plus a third agent, often an integrase inhibitor because of better tolerability and fewer drug interactions than other regimens. Understanding the dosage forms, adverse effects, and drug interactions of antiretrovirals allow clinicians to choose the most appropriate regimen for their patient. New developments, such as branded generic regimens and long-acting intramuscular injections, may play a larger role in the future.

Aadia I. Rana and Michael J. Mugavero

Ending the HIV Epidemic: A Plan for America" (EtHE), launched by the Department of Health and Human Services (DHHS), is predicated on actionable data systems to monitor progress toward ambitious goals and to guide human immunodeficiency virus (HIV) testing, prevention, and treatment services. Situated on a status-neutral continuum of HIV prevention and care, EtHE relies on coordination across DHHS agencies and utilization of data systems established for

INFECTIOUS DISEASE CLINICS
OF NORTH AMERICA

THE CLINICS ARE AVAILABLE ONLINE!
Access your subscription at:
www.theclinics.com

Preface

Nearly Two Decades Later, Exciting Progress in HIV, But Challenges Remain

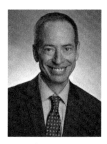

Paul E. Sax, MD
Editor

In 2001, I wrote an article for *Infectious Disease Clinics of North America* on human immunodeficiency virus (HIV)-related opportunistic infections (OIs). Entitled, "Opportunistic Infections in Human Immunodeficiency Virus Disease: Down But not Out," the review focused on specific strategies for prevention, diagnosis, and treatment of these potentially life-threatening infections. While citing the dramatic reduction in OIs since the introduction of effective antiretroviral therapy (ART), I also noted that such treatment had just become widely adopted in the late 1990s, hence experience with OIs in the "ART era" was relatively limited. As a result, there were several remaining areas of uncertainty. These included risk factors for and management of the immune reconstitution inflammatory syndrome, alterations in the "natural history" of OIs with ART, and the concern about OI risk among those on failing ART regimens.

Fast forward to our current issue of *Infectious Disease Clinics of North America*, and today, we clinicians and researchers engaged in HIV care are in a very different place. Substantial advances in ART since 2001 include numerous coformulations and, more importantly, new drug classes, in particular, the integrase strand transfer inhibitors, which have assumed a central role in both treatment-naive and treatment-experienced patients. Indeed, the potency and tolerability of ART have so vastly improved that essentially all patients adherent to their regimens achieve and maintain viral suppression, with its consequent improvement in immune function. As a result, OI management occupies a relatively small component of HIV care, mostly limited to those either not receiving or having just started ART.

With these advances, the priorities of HIV care have shifted from management of OIs and achieving viral suppression to how to maximize the health of those living, and aging, with HIV. In addition, the entire field of HIV prevention has undergone

Infect Dis Clin N Am 33 (2019) xiii–xiv
https://doi.org/10.1016/j.idc.2019.05.010
0891-5520/19/© 2019 Published by Elsevier Inc.

transformation, with both the introduction of preexposure prophylaxis and the growing data on treatment as prevention. The reviews assembled here probe more deeply into the critical issues and remaining challenges arising in HIV diagnosis, prevention, and treatment in the current ART era. The experts invited to review these topics outline how HIV care can be further improved, until we ultimately have a cure – indeed, research on HIV cure fittingly closes this volume.

Paul E. Sax, MD
Division of Infectious Diseases
Brigham and Women's Hospital
Harvard Medical School
75 Francis Street
Boston, MA 02115, USA

E-mail address:
psax@bwh.harvard.edu

HIV Diagnostics
Current Recommendations and Opportunities for Improvement

Bernard M. Branson, MD

KEYWORDS

- HIV testing • HIV antibody test • HIV diagnosis • HIV testing algorithm
- HIV viral load

KEY POINTS

- Instrumented laboratory human immunodeficiency virus (HIV) tests detect immunoglobulin G (IgG) and IgM antibodies and HIV-1 p24 antigen and are more sensitive during early infection.
- Rapid point-of-care HIV tests detect IgG antibodies and can be used with whole blood or oral fluid but are less sensitive during early infection.
- Recommended HIV testing begins with a sensitive p24 antigen-HIV-1/HIV-2 antibody combination immunoassay that can detect HIV as soon as 2 weeks after infection.
- An HIV-1 viral load test might be used after an initially reactive immunoassay to confirm infection and provide more clinically useful information than the recommended second antibody test.
- Early initiation of antiretroviral therapy and taking preexposure prophylaxis can alter the evolution of HIV biomarkers and reactivity of immunoassays and lead to ambiguous results.

INTRODUCTION

According to the Centers for Disease Control and Prevention (CDC), an estimated 1.1 million persons aged ≥13 years in the United States were living with human immunodeficiency virus (HIV) infection at the end of 2015, an estimate that has remained consistent since 2003.[1,2] The percentage unaware of their infection decreased from 25% in 2003 to 14.5% in 2015, where it has been relatively stable. The benefits of early diagnosis and immediate antiretroviral therapy (ART) for both improving health and preventing transmission are compelling. The CDC, the US Preventive Services Task Force, and professional medical associations recommend routine HIV screening

Disclosure Statement: Dr B.M. Branson has served as a consultant to Chembio Diagnostic Systems Inc and Gilead Sciences, Inc. From 2003 to 2014, Dr. Branson was Associate Director for Laboratory Diagnostics in the Division of HIV/AIDS Prevention, Centers for Disease Control and Prevention.
Scientific Affairs LLC, 2175 Eldorado Drive, Atlanta, GA 30345, USA
E-mail address: BBRANSON@SCIENTIFICAFFAIRS.US

Infect Dis Clin N Am 33 (2019) 611–628
https://doi.org/10.1016/j.idc.2019.04.001
0891-5520/19/© 2019 Elsevier Inc. All rights reserved.

id.theclinics.com

and selective, periodic retesting, but as of 2017, only 46% of persons 18 to 64 reported ever having had an HIV test.[3–6]

HIV diagnostics are essential for both diagnosis and management of HIV infection. The laboratory diagnosis of HIV employs a sequence of tests with an algorithm for resolving discordant test results to maximize overall sensitivity and specificity.[7] In June 2014, the CDC issued updated testing recommendations for the diagnosis of HIV infection.[8] This update marked the first time tests recommended for HIV diagnosis diverged completely from those used for screening blood donations: none of the tests in the diagnostic algorithm are licensed for donor screening. Although clinicians often do not know which specific assays will be used when they order an HIV test, the tests differ in subtle ways with different implications depending on the reasons for testing. This article provides a brief review and history of HIV test development, describes technologies currently in use, current recommendations for which tests to use, discusses options for the choice of confirmatory tests, and mentions the potential effects of early antiretroviral treatment and PrEP on HIV test results.

VIROLOGY

HIV exists as 2 major viral species. HIV type 1 (HIV-1), identified first, is the more virulent of the 2 and responsible for most AIDS cases worldwide. HIV-2, first isolated in 1986, has properties similar to those of HIV-1, but is less pathogenic, differs in some of its antigenic components, and has a more limited geographic distribution.[9] The mature HIV virion consists of 2 copies of single-stranded RNA surrounded by structural proteins, a matrix shell, and lipid envelope. The RNA genome contains the *env*, *gag*, and *pol* genes, which encode envelope glycoproteins, structural proteins, and viral enzymes, respectively. The Western blot technique was used to separate the HIV-1 viral proteins by their molecular weight (**Fig. 1**). These proteins were later

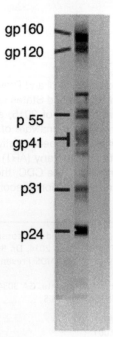

gp160
gp120

p 55
gp41

p31

p24

Fig. 1. Positive HIV-1 Western blot result.

related to HIV morphology (**Fig. 2**). The nomenclature of viral proteins indicates "gp" for glycoprotein or "p" for protein followed by a number representing its molecular weight. The major components of diagnostic utility for HIV-1 include envelope proteins (gp41, gp120, and their precursor, gp160), the core gene proteins (p55, p24, p17), and the polymerase (*pol*) gene proteins (p66, p51, p31). HIV-2 proteins are similar but differ somewhat in the molecular weight of the individual gene products (eg, p26 corresponds to p24; gp36 and gp105 correspond to gp41 and gp120).

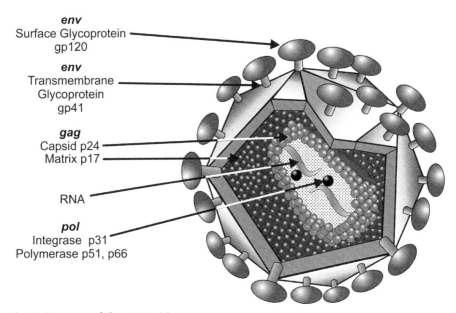

env
Surface Glycoprotein
gp120

env
Transmembrane
Glycoprotein
gp41

gag
Capsid p24
Matrix p17

RNA

pol
Integrase p31
Polymerase p51, p66

Fig. 2. Structure of the HIV-1 virion.

EVOLUTION OF HUMAN IMMUNODEFICIENCY VIRUS DIAGNOSTICS

After HIV-1 infection, HIV-1-specific markers appear in the blood in the following chronologic order: HIV-1 RNA, p24 antigen, HIV-1 immunoglobulin M (IgM) antibody, and HIV-1 IgG antibody (**Fig. 3**). Time from HIV acquisition to reactivity for an assay depends on which target is being detected, when that target can be detected after infection, concentration of the target in the specimen, the volume of specimen tested, and the test's analytical sensitivity. Understanding how these variables affect test results is essential for understanding the advantages and limitations of different types of tests for specific clinical situations.

Serologic tests for HIV have been grouped informally into generations based on the test's principle. Each subsequent generation led to a shorter false-negative window period between infection and detection. As tests other than enzyme immunoassays (EIAs) emerged, including point-of-care rapid tests, classification by generation became less clear cut, and an alternative taxonomy has been suggested.[10] This article refers to tests by generation as described in CDC's 2014 HIV laboratory testing recommendations (**Box 1**).[8]

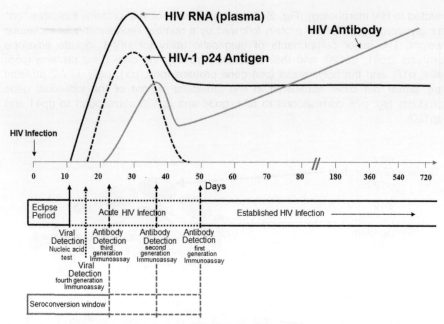

Fig. 3. Sequence of appearance of laboratory markers for HIV-1 infection. Units for vertical axis are not noted because their magnitude differs for RNA, p24 antigen, and antibody. (*Data from* Refs.[22,23,30])

Box 1
Human immunodeficiency virus immunoassay techniques
First generation
Antigens used to bind anti-HIV antibodies: lysate of whole HIV-1 viruses grown in cell culture
Format: indirect immunoassay using labeled anti-human IgG
Detects: IgG anti-HIV antibodies
Second generation
Antigens used to bind anti-HIV antibodies: synthetic peptide or recombinant viral proteins
Format: indirect immunoassay using labeled anti-human IgG or, in rapid tests, protein A, which binds to human IgG with high affinity
Detects: IgG anti-HIV antibodies
Advantages: eliminating cellular contaminants from viral lysates improves specificity by eliminating cross-reactivity with cellular proteins; design of specific antigenic epitopes improves sensitivity for HIV-1, group O, and HIV-2
Third generation
Antigens used to bind anti-HIV antibodies: synthetic peptide or recombinant viral proteins
Format: antigen sandwich (HIV antibodies in the specimen bind to HIV antigens on the assay substrate and then to HIV antigens conjugated to indicator molecules)
Detects: IgG and also IgM anti-HIV antibodies, which develop sooner
Advantage: becomes reactive earlier during seroconversion

Fourth generation

Antigens used to bind anti-HIV antibodies: synthetic peptide or recombinant viral proteins; also, contain monoclonal anti-p24 antibodies

Format: antigen sandwich

Detects: IgG and IgM anti-HIV antibodies, HIV-1 p24 antigen

Advantage: becomes reactive shortly before HIV-1 seroconversion

The earliest HIV EIAs used lysate of whole HIV-1 purified from cell cultures as the source of antigens to bind antibodies to HIV-1. Anti-human IgG conjugated to an enzyme would bind to HIV-1 antibodies, if present, and produce a color change when the enzyme's substrate was added. The viral lysate EIAs had high empirical sensitivity for HIV IgG antibodies but could remain negative for up to 12 weeks after infection before antibodies developed.[11] False-positive test results also occurred, associated with other infections, pregnancy, autoimmune disease, and unspecified conditions. Concerns about the potential for false-positive results from screening with a test with uncertain implications[12] led public health officials to endorse a 2-test strategy to maximize specificity. The HIV-1 Western blot also uses first-generation principles: whole viral lysate as the source of antigens and anti-IgG conjugated to an enzyme to bind to individual HIV proteins. In 1989, the Public Health Service established minimum criteria for a positive Western blot interpretation (presence of any 2 of the p24, gp41, and gp120/gp160 bands) and recommended that no positive HIV result be given until after a repeatedly reactive antibody EIA was confirmed by a positive Western blot.[13] Thus, a specimen was obtained at the initial visit and sent to a laboratory for testing, and a second in-person visit was necessary to obtain test results, both positive and negative. In the late 1990s, second-generation EIAs incorporated synthetic HIV-1 protein and recombinant peptide antigens instead of whole viral lysate and added specific antigens to detect HIV-2. These modifications improved the sensitivity and specificity of the assays, but also added HIV-2 tests to the recommended confirmatory sequence after negative or indeterminate Western blot results.[14] Second-generation EIAs still detected only IgG antibody, but shortened the antibody-negative window period by about 9 days compared with first-generation tests.[15]

Tables 1 and **2** list immunoassays approved by the Food and Drug Administration (FDA) for HIV diagnosis as of May 2019. Profound changes in testing technology have revolutionized laboratory testing for HIV, starting with the introduction of rapid HIV antibody assays beginning in 2002[16] and their subsequent eligibility for waived status under the Clinical Laboratory Improvement Amendments of 1988 (CLIA).[17] CLIA-waived tests can be used in outreach settings and other venues by persons with no previous laboratory training, but only with unprocessed specimens, venous or finger-stick whole blood or oral fluid. (When the same tests are used with serum or plasma, they are classified as moderate complexity and are subject to personnel requirements and more regulatory oversight.) Point-of-care rapid tests dramatically improved receipt of test results by obviating a return visit to obtain them.[18]

RAPID HUMAN IMMUNODEFICIENCY VIRUS ANTIBODY TESTS

At the time rapid HIV tests were introduced 10 to 15 years ago, their performance was equivalent to or better than that of the second-generation conventional HIV assays in widespread use.[19] Most single-use rapid HIV tests are based on second-generation principles, using HIV antigens embedded either on a lateral flow strip

Table 1
Food and Drug Administration–approved rapid and point-of-care human immunodeficiency virus tests

Test[a]	Specimen Types	Antigenic Markers Used for Detection	Principle	Generation
OraQuick Advance Rapid HIV-1/2 Antibody Test	Oral fluid, whole blood; plasma	gp41, gp36	Lateral flow	Second
Reveal G4 Rapid HIV-1 Antibody Test	Whole blood, serum, plasma	gp41, gp120	Flow through	Second
Uni-Gold Recombigen HIV-1/2	Whole blood; serum, plasma	gp41, gp120, gp36	Lateral flow	Third
Multispot HIV-1/HIV-2 Rapid Test	Serum, plasma	gp41, gp36	Flow through	Second
Chembio HIV 1/2 Stat Pak Assay	Whole blood; serum, plasma	gp41, gp120, gp36	Lateral flow	Second
Chembio Sure Check HIV 1/2 Assay	Whole blood; serum, plasma	gp41, gp120, gp36	Lateral flow	Second
INSTI HIV-1 Antibody Test Kit	Whole blood; serum, plasma	gp41, gp36	Flow through	Second
Chembio DPP HIV 1/2 Assay	Oral fluid, whole blood, serum, plasma	gp41, gp120, gp36	Dual path platform	Second
Alere Determine HIV 1/2 Ag/Ab Combo	Whole blood, serum, plasma	gp41, gp120, gp36; p24 antibodies	Lateral flow	Fourth
Geenius HIV 1/2 Supplemental Assay	Whole blood, serum, plasma	p24, p31, gp41, gp160, gp36, gp140	Dual path platform	Second

[a] Tests are listed in the order in which they received FDA approval.

(immunochromatography) or in a flow-through membrane (immunoconcentration) to capture antibodies. Antibody detection is accomplished by colloidal gold conjugated to protein A, which binds with high affinity to IgG antibodies[20] and produces a visible colored line or spot when antibodies bind to the HIV antigens or anti-IgG control.[21] Experiments with panels of specimens collected before and during seroconversion demonstrate lateral flow rapid antibody tests become reactive a few days before or at the same time as the HIV-1 Western blot.[22,23] Flow-through rapid assays detect antibodies several days sooner.[24] The dual path platform is another rapid test technique in which specimen is added to a sample pathway that flows toward the long edge of a test strip, onto which one or more antigens have been applied. Buffer is then added that flows across the test strip in a perpendicular direction, activating the detection reagent (colloidal gold conjugated to protein A) that then binds to anti-HIV antibodies, if present. The dual path principle appears to be especially useful for multiplex testing for different antibodies on the same strip, as used by the FDA-approved HIV-1/2 differentiation assay.

THIRD-GENERATION ANTIBODY ASSAYS

An EIA based on novel technology received FDA approval in 1992. This third-generation EIA also used synthetic and recombinant antigens to bind anti-HIV

Table 2
Food and Drug Administration–approved instrumented human immunodeficiency virus immunoassays

Test	Antigenic Markers Used for Detection	Analytes Detected	Generation
EIAs			
Avioq HIV-1 Microelisa System	Viral lysate, gp160	IgG antibodies	Second
Bio-Rad GS HIV-1/2 *PLUS* O	Recombinant p24, gp160, HIV-2 gp36, synthetic group O peptide	IgG & IgM antibodies	Third
Bio-Rad GS HIV Combo Ag/Ab EIA	Synthetic gp41, recombinant gp160, HIV-2 gp36, synthetic group O peptide, p24 monoclonal antibodies	IgG & IgM antibodies p24 antigen	Fourth
CIAs			
Abbott Architect HIV Ag/Ab Combo	Synthetic and recombinant gp41 and HIV-2 gp36, group O peptide, anti-p24 monoclonal antibodies	IgG & IgM antibodies P24 antigen	Fourth
Ortho Vitros Anti-HIV 1 + 2	Recombinant p24, gp41, gp41/120, HIV-2 gp36	IgG & IgM antibodies	Third
Siemens Advia Centaur HIV 1/O/2	Recombinant gp41/120, p24, HIV-2 gp36, group O peptide	IgG & IgM antibodies	Third
Siemens Advia Centaur HIV Ag/Ab combo	Recombinant gp41/120, HIV-2 gp36, group O peptide, anti-p24 monoclonal antibodies	IgG & IgM antibodies p24 antigen	Fourth
Roche Elecsys Combi PT	Recombinant gp41, HIV-2 gp36, HIV-1 RT, HIV-2 RT	IgG & IgM antibodies p24 antigen	Fourth
Ortho Vitros Combi	Recombinant gp41/120, HIV-2 gp36, group O peptide, anti-p24 monoclonal antibodies		Fourth
Multiplex flow immunoassay			
BioRad Bioplex 2200 HIV Ag-Ab	Recombinant gp160, HIV-2 gp36, group O peptide, anti-p24 monoclonal antibodies	IgG & IgM antibodies p24 antigen (detection and differentiation)	Fourth

antibodies, but for detection, used enzymes conjugated to HIV antigens instead of anti-IgG. This "sandwich" principle (antibodies sandwiched between 2 antigens) allowed binding to and detection of both IgM and IgG antibodies and shortened the time from HIV acquisition to detection to 20 to 25 days. The third-generation assay was adopted for screening blood donors but did not come into routine clinical use until the remaining first-generation test was withdrawn from the market in 2007.[25] At about that same time, manufacturers began to replace EIAs with chemiluminescent immunoassays (CIAs), also based on third-generation sandwich principles, that use particles coated with HIV antigen to capture HIV antibodies.[26–28] HIV antigen conjugated to a luminescent chemical adheres to both IgG and IgM anti-HIV antibodies, and reaction with the luminescent marker emits light, measured as relative light units. Advantages of CIAs include shorter incubation and reaction times than EIAs, which can reduce testing time to as little as 30 to 60 minutes, and their suitability for random access analyzers that can run specimens either one at a time or in batches and thus deliver rapid results from instruments designed for automation and high throughput. Third-generation EIAs and CIAs incorporate specific antigens to detect antibodies against HIV-1, HIV-2, and HIV-1 group O (see **Table 2**).

FOURTH-GENERATION ANTIGEN/ANTIBODY COMBINATION ASSAYS

Fourth-generation EIAs and CIAs, termed antigen/antibody (Ag/Ab) combination assays, add monoclonal anti-p24 antibodies to the recombinant viral antigens to simultaneously detect viral p24 antigen in addition to HIV-1 and HIV-2 antibodies. p24 antigen can be detected directly because each HIV-1 virion contains approximately 2000 to 3000 copies of the p24 molecule, compared with 2 RNA molecules. Detection thresholds for p24 antigen during acute infection correspond to approximately 30,000 viral RNA copies per milliliter.[29] p24 antigen becomes detectable by HIV Ag/Ab combination assays about 5 days after plasma viral RNA,[30] but only transiently. Once anti-p24 antibodies develop, they form immune complexes with p24 antigen and block its detection. Most Ag/Ab combination assays produce a binary positive/negative result and do not identify which component (antigen or antibody) caused the reactivity, with 2 exceptions. The Alere Determine HIV-1/2 Combo Ag/Ab (Abbott Diagnostics, Waltham, MA, USA) is a CLIA-waived lateral-flow rapid test that uses the antigen sandwich technique with a colloidal selenium conjugate to detect IgG and IgM antibodies at 1 location on the test strip and p24 antigen at a separate location.[31] In 2015, the FDA approved the Bio-Plex 2200 (Bio-Rad Laboratories, Hercules, CA, USA), an instrument based on a bead multiplexing technique that uses magnetic beads coated with antigen or antibody and different fluorescent markers. When exposed to lasers (in a manner analogous to flow cytometry), identification of specific beads allows the test to differentiate which component (HIV-1 antibody, HIV-2 antibody, or p24 antigen) caused reactivity.[32]

DURATION OF THE WINDOW PERIOD

Each newer generation of immunoassays improved sensitivity for early HIV-1 infection and narrowed the interval between the time of HIV acquisition and its detection (see **Fig. 3**). A recent analysis used modeling to estimate the eclipse period between infection and first detection of RNA (median duration 11.5 days, 99th percentile 33 days) and combined these estimates with test results from plasma seroconversion panels to estimate the median window period and the 99th percentile for each class of immunoassays (**Table 3**).[33] (These window periods are estimates for testing plasma specimens. Testing finger-stick whole blood or oral fluid adds an additional delay in time to detection of 1–3 weeks.[34–36]) The 99th percentile estimate helps to select an appropriate interval for retesting after a possible exposure to be certain infection has not occurred. The CDC recommends retesting serum or plasma at least 45 days after a negative Ag/Ab combination test or after at least 90 days for all other HIV tests.[37]

CURRENT RECOMMENDATIONS FOR LABORATORY TESTING AND RECENT UPDATES

HIV-1 Western blot had long been the gold standard for confirmation after a reactive initial immunoassay,[13] but its shortcomings became increasingly apparent. Numerous

Table 3
Window periods between human immunodeficiency virus acquisition and detection by different test technologies

Type of Test	Median Window Period, d	99th Percentile, d
Instrumented fourth-generation laboratory assay	17.8	44.3
Instrumented third-generation laboratory assay	23.1	49.5
Single-use rapid antibody test	31.1	56.7
HIV-1/HIV-2 differentiation assay	33.4	58.2
Western blot	36.5	64.8

Data from Delaney KP, Hanson DL, Masciotra S, et al. Time Until Emergence of HIV Test Reactivity Following Infection With HIV-1: Implications for Interpreting Test Results and Retesting After Exposure. Clin Infect Dis. 2017;64:53–59.

studies documented high levels of HIV-1 RNA in persons who were reactive by sensitive immunoassays but negative or indeterminate by Western blot.[38,39] In addition, because of cross-reactivity, the Western blot was interpreted as positive for HIV-1 in 46% to 85% of specimens from persons found to be infected with HIV-2, resulting in incorrect or delayed diagnosis. The 2014 updated CDC testing algorithm sought to improve diagnosis of early infections, reduce indeterminate results, accurately diagnose HIV-2 infection, and determine its prevalence. The recommended testing sequence, updated as of January 2018, is shown in **Fig. 4**: initial testing with an Ag/Ab combination assay, reflexing reactive specimens to a second-generation HIV-1/HIV-2 antibody differentiation assay.[8] Reactive results on these two tests identify most HIV infections (those that are positive for HIV-1 IgG antibodies) and reduces turnaround time for confirmation compared with Western blot because the FDA-approved HIV-1/HIV-2 differentiation assay is a rapid test. The key feature of the updated algorithm is the third step: HIV-1 RNA testing for those specimens negative

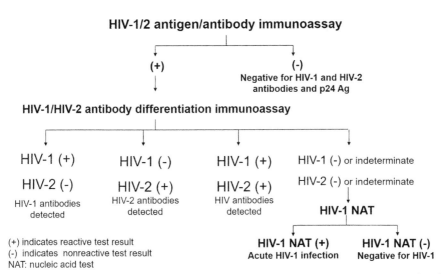

Fig. 4. Recommended laboratory testing algorithm for serum or plasma specimens. Updated January 2018. (*From* 2018 Quick reference guide: recommended laboratory HIV testing algorithm for serum or plasma specimens. Available at: https://stacks.cdc.gov/view/cdc/50872.)

for anti-HIV IgG antibodies. However, only 1 differentiation assay, the Multispot HIV-1/HIV-2 rapid test (Bio-Rad Laboratories), and 1 HIV-1 RNA assay, the APTIMA HIV-1 RNA Qualitative assay (Hologic Inc, San Diego, CA, USA), were FDA approved for diagnosis.

In 2016, Multispot was withdrawn from the market and replaced by the Geenius HIV-1/2 supplemental assay (Bio-Rad Laboratories, Redmond, WA, USA). The Geenius test strip incorporates 4 separate HIV-1 antigens (p24, p31, gp41, and gp160) and 2 HIV-2 antigens (gp36 and gp140) to differentiate HIV-1 from HIV-2 antibodies. The rapid test cartridge uses an automated reader and software that provides 8 possible interpretations according to a proprietary algorithm based on the presence and intensity of the bands (**Table 4**). These interpretations include 2 results not generated before: HIV-2 indeterminate and HIV indeterminate. For either of these test results, CDC recommends repeating the test, and if still reactive, conducting an HIV-1 RNA test to exclude acute HIV-1 infection. If the HIV-1 RNA is negative, supplemental HIV-2 testing (antibody or RNA testing, not FDA approved but available from some commercial laboratories, public health laboratories, and CDC) should be performed, or the testing sequence should be repeated in 2 to 4 weeks.[40]

Since CDC issued the 2014 recommendations, evidence accumulated to show that, with serum or plasma, the Determine Combo rapid test became reactive earlier in seroconversion than instrumented antibody-only third-generation tests, but later than instrumented fourth-generation assays. In a 2017 technical update, CDC reiterated that instrumented Ag/Ab combination tests are preferred for initial testing because of their superior sensitivity, but for laboratories in which instrumented Ag/Ab testing is not feasible, the Determine HIV-1/2 Combo Ag/Ab rapid test can be used with serum or plasma as the first step in the testing algorithm.[41] In contrast, evidence suggests that when used with whole blood, the Determine Combo rapid test showed a significant delay in reactivity compared with plasma and rarely detects p24 antigen during acute infection.[34,42] With finger-stick whole blood, its sensitivity during early infection is similar to that of flow-through rapid HIV antibody tests.

Table 4
Interpretations of the results of the Geenius human immunodeficiency virus-1/2 supplemental assay

HIV-1 Result	HIV-2 Result	Assay Interpretation
Negative	Negative	HIV negative
Indeterminate	Negative	HIV-1 indeterminate[a]
Negative	Indeterminate	HIV-2 indeterminate[b]
Indeterminate	Indeterminate	HIV indeterminate[c]
Positive	Negative	HIV-1 positive
Positive	Indeterminate	HIV-1 positive
Negative	Positive	HIV-2 positive
Indeterminate	Positive	HIV-2 positive
Positive	Positive	HIV-2 positive with HIV-1 cross-reactivity
Positive	Positive	HIV positive untypeable (undifferentiated)

[a] HIV-1 bands detected but did not meet the criteria for HIV-1 positive.
[b] HIV-2 bands detected but did not meet the criteria for HIV-2 positive.
[c] HIV bands detected but did not meet the criteria for HIV-1 positive or HIV-2 positive.

CHALLENGES AND OPPORTUNITIES FOR IMPROVEMENT

Testing with Ag/Ab combination assays has succeeded in identifying acute HIV infections in routine HIV screening programs,[43] and in high-risk populations, they identified 82% of the antibody-negative infections otherwise detectable only by RNA.[44] False-positive results are rare: fewer than 2 per 10,000 test with assays currently in use. This high specificity calls into question the diagnostic value added by a second, corroborating HIV-1 antibody test, and with few reports of HIV-2 infections, it no longer appears warranted to test all fourth-generation reactive specimens for HIV-2 antibodies.[45]

With current technology, it would be more efficient to reverse the current confirmatory testing sequence and, after a reactive Ag/Ab combination assay, perform a quantitative HIV-1 RNA viral load test to both confirm the diagnosis and contribute to immediate clinical management. Based on the specificity of fourth-generation tests, a viral load would be clinically recommended as a next step for the 99.6% of those with a reactive result who are HIV-1 positive, with either a new or previous diagnosis. The US Department of Health and Human Services Panel on Antiretroviral Therapy Guidelines recommends initiation of ART for all persons with HIV-1 infection immediately upon diagnosis to reduce the risk of disease progression and to prevent HIV transmission.[46] Treatment of HIV infection in the earliest stages of acute infection preserves gut-associated immune responses and limits seeding of the long-lived viral reservoir, suggesting that very early ART may help reduce inflammation and HIV-related comorbidities over the long term.[47,48] Early treatment also quickly and substantially reduces transmission.[49] ART is therefore considered urgent in acute HIV, and optimally, initiated on the same day of diagnosis, before HIV resistance genotyping results.[50] Performing an immediate viral load test without an intervening antibody test could facilitate earlier initiation of ART and other aspects of HIV care.

Six HIV-1 RNA viral load tests are available for clinical laboratories with sensitive limits of detection that can establish the presence of HIV-1 RNA (**Table 5**), but so far they are FDA approved only to assess prognosis and monitor response to ART.

Table 5
Food and Drug Administration –approved quantitative viral load assays and specimen requirements

Test and Manufacturer	Amplification Method; Target	Range (Copies/mL)
Amplicor HIV-1 Monitor version 1.5 (Roche Diagnostics, Indianapolis, IN, USA)	RT-PCR; *gag* gene	
Standard		400–750,000
Ultrasensitive		50–100,000
Cobas AmpliPrep/Cobas TaqMan HIV-1 Version 2.0 (Roche Diagnostics)	Real-time RT-PCR; *LTR, gag* gene	20–10,000,000
RealTime HIV-1 (Abbott Molecular, Des Plaines, IL, USA)	Real-time RT-PCR; integrase gene	40–10,000,000
Versant HIV-1 RNA 3.0 (bDNA) (Siemens Healthcare Diagnostics, Tarrytown, NY, USA)	bDNA; *pol* gene	75–500,000
NucliSens HIV-1 QT (BioMérieux, Inc, Durham, NC, USA)	NASBA; *gag* gene	176–3,470,000
APTIMA HIV-1 Quant (Hologic Inc)	TMA; LTR, *pol* gene	30–10,000,000

The qualitative HIV-1 RNA assay, available at far fewer laboratories, is FDA approved for diagnosis,[51] but confirming with the qualitative test adds expense with little additional clinical utility. Without a diagnostic indication, laboratories cannot reflexively conduct a viral load test after a reactive Ag/Ab combination assay, but clinicians can order one until such time that a manufacturer obtains a diagnostic indication, as recently happened with the hepatitis C viral load test.[52]

Current HIV-1 RNA assays are expensive, time-consuming, and require a sophisticated laboratory, but technologic advancements may expand opportunities to use HIV-1 RNA assays for HIV diagnosis. Two simplified rapid HIV-1 RNA tests with short (1–2 hour) turnaround times are now commercially available outside the United States: one is qualitative or semiquantitative[53] and the other is a quantitative viral load assay.[54] Both are suitable for near-patient diagnosis and could add timely and actionable information during the same clinic visit. Neither has yet been submitted for FDA approval.

An undetectable HIV-1 RNA result is not sufficient to rule out HIV infection after a reactive fourth-generation assay. HIV-1 RNA was undetectable in 2% to 4% of specimens that were immunoassay reactive and positive on HIV-1 Western blot.[22,39,55] Some percentage of these might have been from persons on ART, but to achieve final resolution of the testing algorithm, specimens negative for HIV-1 RNA should be tested with the HIV-1/HIV-2 antibody differentiation assay to identify any specimens positive for HIV-1 antibodies or the occasional HIV-2 infection.

THE NEXT FRONTIER: THE EFFECT OF EARLY TREATMENT AND PREEXPOSURE PROPHYLAXIS ON DIAGNOSTIC TEST RESULTS

The new emphasis on rapid, even same-day treatment initiation, especially during acute infection, promises to pose challenges for HIV diagnostics.[56] Early initiation of ART profoundly alters the evolution of HIV biomarkers and the reactivity of immunoassays as depicted in **Fig. 5**, compared with the more predictable sequence in **Fig. 3**.[57] The performance of second-, third-, and fourth-generation screening immunoassays and Western blots were recently rigorously characterized in a large cohort of participants who initiated ART during acute HIV infection.[58] Suppressing viremia during early phases of infection altered the maturation of antibody responses against different HIV-specific antibodies, especially when treatment was started when RNA but not p24 antigen was detectable. Antibody seroconversion did not fully evolve, and seroreversion occurred due to viral suppression. Among 96 participants who were started on ART before any antibody was detectable, 46%, 7%, and 29% were nonreactive on second-generation, third-generation, and fourth-generation immunoassays, respectively, after 26 weeks of treatment. The lower frequency of nonreactive results obtained with the third-generation immunoassays was attributed to the greater breadth of antigens (gp41, p24, gp160) versus gp41 only in the fourth-generation immunoassay, as is the case with FDA-approved third- and fourth-generation assays. Although this study did not report changes in the concentrations of antibodies to specific antigens, 1 study in HIV-infected subjects with a rapid test that detects gp41 antibody only reported gp41 reversion and false-negative results in participants initiating ART early after HIV diagnosis.[59]

These findings likely have ramifications for persons who might become infected with HIV while taking antiretrovirals for preexposure prophylaxis (PrEP). During clinical trials, persons who became infected while taking PrEP demonstrated attenuated seroconversion, with elongation of the intervals between the appearance of each of the laboratory markers and longer delays before infection was detected by rapid tests than persons who became infected while taking placebo.[60] In another trial,

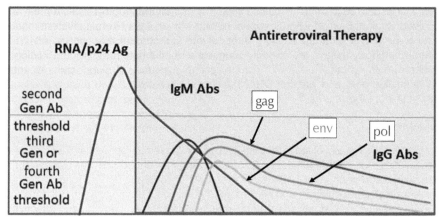

Fig. 5. Effect of ART during acute HIV infection on laboratory markers of HIV-1 infection. After HIV infection, p24 antigen (Ag; *red line*), IgM (*blue line*), and IgG (*green lines*) antibody (Ab) seroconversion occur, which are progressively detected by fourth-, third-, or second-generation assays over the weeks after infection. Diverse Ag-specific IgG responses can be differentially detected during this period by Western blot and other confirmatory assays (indicated by gag, pol, and env *green lines*). Sustained antigenic stimulation is required for maturation and maintenance of these Ab responses. Early treatment with ART aborts the development of antibodies if treatment is initiated very early, and subsequent seroreversion may occur if treatment is initiated shortly following seroconversion, making it difficult to detect or confirm HIV infection by standard diagnostic tests. (*From* Keating SM, Pilcher CD, Busch MP. Editorial commentary: timing is everything: shortcomings of current HIV diagnostics in the early treatment era. Clin Infect Dis 2016;63:562–4; with permission.)

participants who became infected while receiving tenofovir took longer to develop a reactive oral fluid rapid test result than those receiving placebo, suggesting a blunted antibody response.[61]

Four cases of indeterminate or ambiguous HIV test results from recommended testing algorithms have been reported recently in persons who acquired HIV infection while adherent to daily doses of PrEP.[62] These patients tested reactive with Ag/Ab combination assays, but supplemental tests, including HIV-1/2 differentiation assays, Western blot, and HIV RNA tests, when done, were inconsistently positive. In 1 case, findings included a reactive Ag/Ab combination assay, persistently negative Multispot HIV-1/2 supplemental tests, and detectable but not quantifiable HIV-1 RNA, consistent with low-level HIV-1 viremia and immune system preservation without seroconversion.[63] A third drug was added to the PrEP regimen, and the ambiguous test results persisted. RNA viral load remained extremely low, but coding regions were eventually amplified from HIV-1 DNA extracted from isolated CD4+ lymphocytes. In a second case, the Ag/Ab combination assay was reactive, and only gp160 antibodies were present on Western blot. Plasma RNA was undetectable, and neither HIV RNA nor DNA could be isolated from mononuclear cells. PrEP was suspended, and HIV-1 RNA became detectable 17 days later, after which the full antibody response evolved on the Western blot. Although breakthrough infections on PrEP are expected to be few, those that do occur might present dilemmas for diagnosis. Repeated false-positive Ag/Ab combination assay results are rare but especially problematic in the context of PrEP.[64]

If recommended tests produce ambiguous results, repeat testing a few days to weeks later may resolve them if the ambiguities were due to very early infection or technical issues, such as a mislabeled specimen. If the ambiguous results remain unresolved, it might be useful first to repeat testing with an assay from a different manufacturer or with a different antigen composition. Concordant reactive results on 2 different antibody assays are strongly suggestive of infection. Further investigation if results remain ambiguous would include testing plasma and CD4[+] cells for total HIV-1 nucleic acid and proviral DNA, but these are research use assays available only at select laboratories.[62]

SUMMARY

HIV diagnostics have evolved in tandem with a changing social context and advances in therapeutics since 1985, when the first EIA for anti-HIV antibodies was approved for screening blood donations. In that same year, the Public Health Service funded alternative test sites where persons who wanted an HIV test could obtain one without donating blood to do so,[65] making available anonymous HIV testing on demand and effectively removing much of HIV testing from health care settings. Before effective therapy and with potential for substantial stigma, recommendations for diagnostic testing emphasized specificity, requiring confirmation of a highly accurate antibody test with a second, more specific antibody test. Once effective therapy became available, the benefits from an early and accurate HIV diagnosis became increasingly apparent. Rapid tests that detect IgG anti-HIV antibodies in finger-stick blood and oral fluid specimens were introduced, allowing HIV testing to expand to even more nonclinical settings, increasing the number of people aware of their HIV status and allaying many fears about adverse consequences from preliminary false-positive results.

Rapid test technology has seen minimal change since the tests were introduced, but instrumented laboratory assays have evolved considerably in the last 10 years. New immunoassay techniques that detect both IgM and IgG antibodies identify HIV infections sooner, and the ability to directly detect viral p24 antigen allows routine serologic screening to detect HIV-1 infection at just about 2 weeks after acquisition, 5 to 6 days after RNA first appears. Current testing recommendations specify an initial Ag/Ab combination assay, followed, if reactive, by an HIV-1/HIV-2 antibody differentiation assay. If those antibody test results are negative or indeterminate, an HIV-1 RNA assay is performed to identify acute HIV infections.

The new emphasis on rapid treatment initiation suggests performing an HIV-1 RNA viral load assay as the next step after a reactive Ag/Ab combination assay might confirm infection and facilitate earlier ART initiation. The HIV-1/HIV-2 differentiation assay would be reserved for specimens that were negative for HIV-1 RNA. Earlier initiation of ART and administration of PrEP are likely to complicate HIV diagnostics because lack of antigenic stimulation alters the evolution of biomarkers, affecting the reactivity of immunoassays. Technologic advancements promise to expand opportunities to use rapid, easy-to-use HIV-1 RNA assays that can help foster the transition from diagnostic testing to treatment for persons with either newly identified or previously diagnosed HIV infection.

REFERENCES

1. Glynn M, Rhodes P. Estimated HIV prevalence in the United States at the end of 2003. Abstract from National HIV Prevention Conference. Atlanta, GA, June 12–15, 2005.
2. CDC. Estimated HIV incidence and prevalence in the United States, 2010–2015. HIV Surveillance Supplemental Report 2018;23(1):17–9. Available at: http://www.cdc.gov/hiv/library/reports/hiv-surveillance.html. Accessed November 14, 2018.

3. Branson BM, Handsfield HH, Lampe MA, et al. Revised recommendations for HIV testing of adults, adolescents, and pregnant women in health-care settings. MMWR Recomm Rep 2006;55(RR-14):1–17. Available at: https://www.cdc.gov/mmwr/preview/mmwrhtml/rr5514a1.htm.

4. Moyer VA. Screening for HIV: U.S. preventive services task force recommendation statement. Ann Intern Med 2013;159:51–60.

5. Qaseem A, Snow V, Shekelle P, et al, Clinical Efficacy Assessment Subcommittee, American College of Physicians. Screening for HIV in health care settings: a guidance statement from the American College of Physicians and HIV Medicine Association. Ann Intern Med 2009;150:125–31.

6. Kaiser Family Foundation. Percentage of persons aged 18-64 who reported ever receiving an HIV test, 2017. State Health Facts 2018. Available at: https://www.kff.org/other/state-indicator/hiv-testing-rate-ever-tested/. Accessed Deccember 12, 2018.

7. Albritton WL, Vittinghoff E, Padian NS. Human immunodeficiency virus testing for patient-based and population-based diagnosis. J Infect Dis 1996;174(suppl 2): S176–81.

8. Centers for Disease Control and Prevention, Association of Public Health Laboratories. Laboratory testing for the diagnosis of HIV infection: updated recommendations 2014. p. 1–66. Available at: http://stacks.cdc.gov/view/cdc/23447. Accessed September 20, 2018.

9. Clavel F, Guétard D, Brun-Vézinet F, et al. Isolation of a new human retrovirus from West African patients with AIDS. Science 1986;233:343–6.

10. Delaney KP, Wesolowski LG, Owen SM. The evolution of HIV testing continues. Sex Transm Dis 2017;44:747–9.

11. Petersen LR, Satten GA, Dodd R, et al. Duration of time from onset of human immunodeficiency virus type 1 infectiousness to development of detectable antibody. The HIV Seroconversion Study Group. Transfusion 1994;34:283–9.

12. Meyer KB, Pauker SG. Screening for HIV: can we afford the false positive rate? N Engl J Med 1987;317:238–41.

13. Centers for Disase Control (CDC). Interpretation and use of the Western blot assay for serodiagnosis of human immunodeficiency virus type 1 infections. MMWR Morb Mortal Wkly Rep 1989;38:1–7.

14. O'Brien TR, George JR, Epstein JS, et al. Testing for antibodies to human immunodeficiency virus type 2 in the United States. MMWR Recomm Rep 1992;41:1–9.

15. Busch MP, Lee LL, Satten GA, et al. Time course of detection of viral and serologic markers preceeding human immunodeficiency virus type 1 seroconversion: implications for screening of blood and tissue donors. Transfusion 1995;35:91–7.

16. Centers for Disease Control and Prevention. Notice to readers: approval of a new rapid test for HIV antibody. MMWR Morb Mortal Wkly Rep 2002;51:1051–2.

17. O'Rourke M, Branson B, del Rio C, et al. Rapid fingerstick testing: a new era in HIV diagnostics. AIDS Clin Care 2003;15:19–23, 30.

18. Hutchinson AB, Branson BM, Kim A, et al. A meta-analysis of the effectiveness of alternative HIV counseling and testing methods to increase knowledge of HIV status. AIDS 2006;20:1597–604.

19. CDC. Protocols for confirmation of rapid HIV tests. MMWR Morb Mortal Wkly Rep 2004;53:221–2.

20. Forsgren A, Nordstrom K. Protein A from Staphylococcus aureus: the biological significance of its reaction with IgG. Ann N Y Acad Sci 1974;236:252–66.

21. Branson BM. Rapid tests for HIV antibody. AIDS Rev 2000;2:76–83.

22. Owen SM, Yang C, Spira T, et al. Alternative algorithms for human immunodeficiency virus infection diagnosis using tests that are licensed in the United States. J Clin Microbiol 2008;46:1588–95.

23. Masciotra S, McDougal JS, Feldman J, et al. Evaluation of an alternative HIV diagnostic algorithm using specimens from seroconversion panels and persons with established HIV infections. J Clin Virol 2011;52(Suppl 1):S17–22. Available at: https://www.ncbi.nlm.nih.gov/pubmed/21981983.

24. Adams S, Luo W, Wesolowski L, et al. Performance evaluation of the point-of-care INSTI HIV-1/2 antibody test in early and established HIV infections. J Clin Virol 2017;91:90–4.

25. Association of Public Health Laboratories. HIV: 2009 HIV diagnostic survey 2010. Available at: https://www.aphl.org/programs/infectious_disease/Documents/ID_2010March_HIV-2009-Survey-Issue-Brief.pdf. Accessed October 17, 2018.

26. Shah D, Chang C, Cheng K, et al. Combined HIV antigen and antibody assay on a fully automated chemiluminescence based analyzer. 11th International Symposium on Bioluminescence and chemiluminescence. Pacific Grove, CA: World Scientific Publishing Co. Pte. Ltd.; 2000:365–368.

27. Siemens Healthcare. HIV 1/O/2 Enhanced (EHIV) [product insert] 2006. Available at: http://www.fda.gov/downloads/Biologicsbloodvaccines/Bloodbloodproducts/Approvedproducts/PremarketApprovalsPMAs/UCM091286.pdf. Accessed July 12, 2013.

28. Ortho diagnostics. VITROS Immunodiagnostic products, Anti-HIV 1+2 Reagent Pack [product insert]. Available at: http://www.fda.gov/downloads/BiologicsBloodVaccines/BloodBloodProducts/ApprovedProducts/PremarketApprovalsPMAs/ucm092018.pdf. Accessed July 14, 2013.

29. Brennan CA, Yamaguchi J, Vallari A, et al. ARCHITECT(R) HIV Ag/Ab Combo assay: correlation of HIV-1 p24 antigen sensitivity and RNA viral load using genetically diverse virus isolates. J Clin Virol 2013;57:169–72.

30. Fiebig EW, Wright DJ, Rawal BD, et al. Dynamics of HIV viremia and antibody seroconversion in plasma donors: implications for diagnosis and staging of primary HIV infection. AIDS 2003;17:1871–9. Available at: https://journals.lww.com/aidsonline/Fulltext/2003/09050/Dynamics_of_HIV_viremia_and_antibody.5.aspx.

31. Alere Inc. Alere Determine HIV 1/2 Ag/Ab Combo [product insert] 2013. Available at: http://www.alere.com/content/alere/us/en/product-details/determine-1-2-ag-ab-combo-us.html.html. Accessed October 30, 2014.

32. Salmona M, Delarue S, Delaugerre C, et al. Clinical evaluation of Bioplex 2200 HIV Ag-Ab, an automated screening method providing discrete detection of HIV-1 p24 antigen, HIV-1 antibody, and HIV-2 antibody. J Clin Microbiol 2014; 52:103–7.

33. Delaney KP, Hanson DL, Masciotra S, et al. Time until emergence of HIV test reactivity following infection with HIV-1: implications for interpreting test results and retesting after exposure. Clin Infect Dis 2017;64:53–9. Available at: https://www.ncbi.nlm.nih.gov/pubmed/27737954.

34. Masciotra S, Luo W, Westheimer E, et al. Performance evaluation of the FDA-approved Determine HIV-1/2 Ag/Ab Combo assay using plasma and whole blood specimens. J Clin Virol 2017;91:95–100. Available at: https://www.ncbi.nlm.nih.gov/pubmed/28372891.

35. Luo W, Masciotra S, Delaney KP, et al. Comparison of HIV oral fluid and plasma antibody results during early infection in a longitudinal Nigerian cohort. J Clin Virol 2013;58(Suppl 1):e113–8.

36. Delaney K, Violette L, Ure G, et al. Estimated time from HIV infection to earliest detection for 4 FDA-approved point-of-care tests. Conference on retroviruses and opportunistic infections 2018. Available at: http://www.croiconference.org/sites/default/files/posters-2018/1430_Stekler_565.pdf. Accessed December 16, 2018.

37. CDC. How soon after an exposure to HIV can a test detect if I have HIV? 2017. Available at: https://www.cdc.gov/hiv/basics/testing.html. Accessed December 10, 2018.

38. Pandori MW, Hackett J Jr, Louie B, et al. Assessment of the ability of a fourth-generation immunoassay for human immunodeficiency virus (HIV) antibody and p24 antigen to detect both acute and recent HIV infections in a high-risk setting. J Clin Microbiol 2009;47:2639–42.

39. Patel P, Mackellar D, Simmons P, et al. Detecting acute human immunodeficiency virus infection using 3 different screening immunoassays and nucleic acid amplification testing for human immunodeficiency virus RNA, 2006-2008. Arch Intern Med 2010;170:66–74.

40. CDC. Technical update on HIV-1/2 differentiation assays 2016. Available at: https://stacks.cdc.gov/view/cdc/40790. Accessed November 14, 2018.

41. CDC. Technical update: use of the determine HIV 1/2 Ag/Ab combo test with serum or plasma in the laboratory algorithm for HIV diagnosis 2017. Available at: https://stacks.cdc.gov/view/cdc/48472. Accessed December 14, 2018.

42. Rosenberg NE, Kamanga G, Phiri S, et al. Detection of acute HIV infection: a field evaluation of the Determine(R) HIV-1/2 Ag/Ab combo test. J Infect Dis 2012;205:528–34.

43. White DAE, Giordano TP, Pasalar S, et al. Acute HIV discovered during routine HIV screening with HIV antigen-antibody combination tests in 9 US emergency departments. Ann Emerg Med 2018;72:29–40.e2. Available at: https://www.ncbi.nlm.nih.gov/pubmed/29310870.

44. Peters PJ, Westheimer E, Cohen S, et al. Screening yield of HIV antigen/antibody combination and pooled HIV RNA testing for acute HIV infection in a high-prevalence population. JAMA 2016;315:682–90. Available at: https://www.ncbi.nlm.nih.gov/pubmed/26881371.

45. Perulski A. HIV-1/2 differentiation in the United States HIV testing algorithm: high burden, low yield. Presented at 2019 HIV Diagnostics Conference, March 26, 2019. Available at: http://hivtestingconference.org/wp-content/uploads/2019/04/B5_Anne-Peruski.pdf.

46. Panel on Antiretroviral Guidelines for Adults and Adolescents. Guidelines for the use of antiretroviral agents in adults and adolescents living with HIV 2018. Available at: https://aidsinfo.nih.gov/contentfiles/lvguidelines/adultandadolescentgl.pdf. Accessed November 20, 2018.

47. Ananworanich J, Schuetz A, Vandergeeten C, et al. Impact of multi-targeted antiretroviral treatment on gut T cell depletion and HIV reservoir seeding during acute HIV infection. PLoS One 2012;7:e33948.

48. Schuetz A, Deleage C, Sereti I, et al. Initiation of ART during early acute HIV infection preserves mucosal Th17 function and reverses HIV-related immune activation. PLoS Pathog 2014;10:e1004543.

49. Kroon E, Phanuphak N, Shattock AJ, et al. Acute HIV infection detection and immediate treatment estimated to reduce transmission by 89% among men who have sex with men in Bangkok. J Int AIDS Soc 2017;20:21708. Available at: https://onlinelibrary.wiley.com/doi/full/10.7448/IAS.20.1.21708.

50. Jacobson KR, Arora S, Walsh KB, et al. High feasibility of empiric HIV treatment for patients with suspected acute HIV in an emergency department. J Acquir Immune Defic Syndr 2016;72:242–5.
51. Hologic Inc. Aptima® HIV-1 RNA qualitative assay [product insert] 2015. Available at: https://www.hologic.com/sites/default/files/package-insert/501623-IFU-PI_001_01.pdf. Accessed December 8, 2018.
52. Roche Diagnostics. FDA approves expanded use of Roche hepatitis C virus RNA test as aid in diagnosis. Available at: https://diagnostics.roche.com/us/en/news-listing/2016/fda-approves-expanded-use-of-roche-hepatitis-c-virus-rna-test-as-aid-in-diagnosis.html. Accessed January 4, 2019.
53. Ritchie AV, Ushiro-Lumb I, Edemaga D, et al. SAMBA HIV semiquantitative test, a new point-of-care viral-load-monitoring assay for resource-limited settings. J Clin Microbiol 2014;52:3377–83.
54. Jordan JA, Plantier JC, Templeton K, et al. Multi-site clinical evaluation of the Xpert((R)) HIV-1 viral load assay. J Clin Virol 2016;80:27–32.
55. Linley L, Ethridge SF, Oraka E, et al. Evaluation of supplemental testing with the Multispot HIV-1/HIV-2 Rapid Test and APTIMA HIV-1 RNA Qualitative Assay to resolve specimens with indeterminate or negative HIV-1 Western blots. J Clin Virol 2013;58(Suppl 1):e108–12.
56. Pilcher CD, Ospina-Norvell C, Dasgupta A, et al. The effect of same-day observed initiation of antiretroviral therapy on HIV viral load and treatment outcomes in a US public health setting. J Acquir Immune Defic Syndr 2017;74:44–51.
57. Keating SM, Pilcher CD, Busch MP. Editorial commentary: timing is everything: shortcomings of current HIV diagnostics in the early treatment era. Clin Infect Dis 2016;63:562–4.
58. de Souza MS, Pinyakorn S, Akapirat S, et al. Initiation of antiretroviral therapy during acute HIV-1 infection leads to a high rate of nonreactive HIV serology. Clin Infect Dis 2016;63:555–61. Available at: https://academic.oup.com/cid/article/63/4/555/2566634.
59. O'Connell RJ, Merritt TM, Malia JA, et al. Performance of the OraQuick rapid antibody test for diagnosis of human immunodeficiency virus type 1 infection in patients with various levels of exposure to highly active antiretroviral therapy. J Clin Microbiol 2003;41:2153–5.
60. Donnell D, Ramos E, Celum C, et al. The effect of oral preexposure prophylaxis on the progression of HIV-1 seroconversion. AIDS 2017;31:2007–16.
61. Suntharasamai P, Martin M, Choopanya K, et al. Assessment of oral fluid HIV test performance in an HIV pre-exposure prophylaxis trial in Bangkok, Thailand. PLoS One 2015;10:e0145859.
62. Smith DK, Switzer WM, Peters P, et al. A strategy for PrEP clinicians to manage ambiguous HIV test results during follow-up visits. Open Forum Infect Dis 2018;5:ofy180. Available at: https://academic.oup.com/ofid/article/5/8/ofy180/5056925.
63. Markowitz M, Grossman H, Anderson PL, et al. Newly acquired infection with multidrug-resistant HIV-1 in a patient adherent to preexposure prophylaxis. J Acquir Immune Defic Syndr 2017;76:e104–6.
64. Stekler JD, Violette LR, Niemann L, et al. Repeated false-positive HIV test results in a patient taking HIV pre-exposure prophylaxis. Open Forum Infect Dis 2018;5:ofy197.
65. Public Health Service. Program announcement. alternate testing sites to perform human T-lymphotropic virus-type III (HTLVIII) antibody testing; availability of funds for fiscal year 1985. Fed Regist 1985;50(48):9909–10.

Antiretroviral Medications for the Prevention of HIV Infection

A Clinical Approach to Preexposure Prophylaxis, Postexposure Prophylaxis, and Treatment as Prevention

Amila Heendeniya, MD[a], Isaac I. Bogoch, MD[a,b,c],*

KEYWORDS

- HIV • Prevention • Preexposure prophylaxis • PrEP • Postexposure prophylaxis
- PEP • Treatment as prevention

KEY POINTS

- Effective human immunodeficiency virus (HIV) prevention strategies include both behavioral and pharmacologic methods.
- Antiretroviral drugs to prevent HIV may be used proactively (preexposure prophylaxis), retroactively (postexposure prophylaxis), and at a population level (treatment as prevention).
- HIV prevention clinic appointments are opportune times to address other common comorbidities that may influence HIV acquisition risk, such as mental health issues and abuse (eg, sexual, drug, or alcohol).

INTRODUCTION

The past 30 years have seen tremendous progress in both the care of human immunodeficiency virus (HIV)-positive individuals and HIV prevention techniques, and currently the pendulum is swinging toward strategies and policies that will enable an HIV-free world. In 2014, The Joint United Nations Programme on HIV/AIDS

Disclosures: Both authors have no conflicts of interest to declare.
[a] Division of Infectious Diseases, Toronto General Hospital, Toronto General Hospital, 200 Elizabeth Street, Toronto, Ontario M5G 2C4, Canada; [b] Department of Medicine, University of Toronto, 190 Elizabeth Street, R. Fraser Elliott Building, 3-805, Toronto, Ontario M5G 2C4, Canada; [c] Division of General Internal Medicine, Toronto General Hospital, University Health Network, Toronto, Ontario, Canada
* Corresponding author. Toronto General Hospital, 200 Elizabeth Street – 14EN – 209, Toronto, Ontario M5G 2C4, Canada.
E-mail address: isaac.bogoch@uhn.ca

Infect Dis Clin N Am 33 (2019) 629–646
https://doi.org/10.1016/j.idc.2019.04.002
0891-5520/19/© 2019 Elsevier Inc. All rights reserved.

id.theclinics.com

(UNAIDS) unveiled their ambitious "90-90-90" plan, with the goal that 90% of HIV-infected individuals will have a diagnosis (from 79%), treatment rates will increase to 90% (from 59%), and the rates of individuals with a suppressed viral load will increase to 90% (from 47%).[1] These targets were established with the ambition to vastly curb the HIV epidemic by 2020 and eliminate the disease by 2030.[1] Recent global data have demonstrated increasing HIV treatment coverage and decreasing HIV-related deaths, culminating in the highest prevalence of people with HIV, at an estimated 36.9 million people in 2017.[2] Such metrics demonstrate the success of current programs and also highlight the need to continue advocating for policies that ensure people affected with HIV have access to necessary care.

Ending the global HIV epidemic will involve intersectoral cooperation and coordination with several partners, including the public sector, industry, academia, and civic representation.[3] Several active areas of research and quality improvement initiatives are focused on curbing the epidemic and include (1) the implementation of current knowledge to enable better access to HIV and HIV-prevention care, (2) vaccine development, and (3) cure research. Although HIV prevention strategies are one piece of a much larger puzzle pointing tward the global eliination of HIV, such prevention strategies are now viewed as integral aspects in routine clinical and public health care by frontline health care providers and policy makers. Successful HIV prevention care involves the use of both pharmacologic and nonpharmacologic tools (often referred to as "biological" and "nonbiological"), and although the focus here is on pharmacologic mechanisms of HIV prevention, the authors believe nonpharmacologic principles should be seamlessly integrated into routine clinical practice. Such nonpharmacologic principles may include safe sexual counseling, access to harm-reduction strategies (eg, safe injection sites), addressing psychosocial determinants of health, and circumcision, for example.[4–6]

Pharmacologic methods for HIV prevention generally focus on 3 main areas: postexposure prophylaxis (PEP), preexposure prophylaxis (PrEP), and treatment as prevention (TasP). Here, the authors discuss the evidence driving these HIV prevention modalities and provide practical clinical advice for frontline health care providers seeing patients at risk for HIV infection.

POSTEXPOSURE PROPHYLAXIS
Introduction

Exposures to HIV are generally classified as either occupational (requiring occupational PEP [oPEP]) or nonoccupational (requiring nonoccupational PEP [nPEP]).[7,8] This distinction is important, as there are occasionally unique challenges when managing nonoccupational compared with occupational HIV exposures. Although confirmed or potential HIV exposures may cause emotional distress in both occupational and nonoccupational settings, cases of oPEP are typically easier to manage for several reasons. First, there are usually more opportunities for source-patient HIV testing in occupational settings, whereas this is often very challenging to coordinate in nonoccupational settings. Secondly, antiretroviral therapy (ART) can be initiated rather quickly in most occupational settings and is often started within a few hours of the exposure, whereas there are frequently major delays in accessing PEP care in nonoccupational settings. Finally, occupational exposures typically have less physical or emotional trauma compared with nPEP cases, where, for example, sexual assault, intoxication, or physical violence are common themes and may affect access and adherence to care. Still, with all types of PEP, addressing the patient's pharmacologic and nonpharmacologic needs is paramount to ensure that patients adhere to their 28-day ART regimen, return for follow-up testing, and access any additional support services that may be helpful.

PEP was first used following occupational exposures in the late 1980s,[9,10] and the US Center for Disease Control and Prevention (CDC) first introduced occupational guidelines for ART use in 1990.[11] An evaluation of risk factors for percutaneous HIV transmission and efficacy of PEP was first demonstrated in a large case-control study using zidovudine (AZT) monotherapy in health care workers with percutaneous exposures to HIV-positive patients. AZT monotherapy significantly reduced one's risk of HIV acquisition by about 80% in this landmark study.[12] Large cohort studies have also demonstrated PEP efficacy with 3 ART agents in nonoccupational settings; for example, one large cohort evaluating 702 individuals with nonoccupational HIV exposures demonstrated 7 seroconversions (1%) after PEP initiation and found that of these 7 seroconversions, several individuals may have not been adherent to their medications.[13] Currently 3-drug regimens are the norm for oPEP and nPEP, and most health care settings have protocolized the management of exposures, with evidence-based guidelines now widely available.[7,14–16]

PEP management involves addressing 5 key questions:

1. Did an HIV exposure occur?
2. If a confirmed or potential HIV exposure occurred, what is the risk of HIV transmission?
3. Should this patient initiate PEP and if so, with what drugs?
4. What other infectious and noninfectious disease issues should be addressed?
5. What is an appropriate follow-up strategy?

Did an exposure occur?

An exposure to HIV or bloodborne pathogens involves the source patient's blood, mucous membrane, or other potentially infectious bodily fluid coming into contact with a patient's blood or mucous membrane. Although this may seem obvious in the case of percutaneous injury (eg, needlestick injuries) or a history of condomless sexual activity, it is often challenging to confirm if an exposure occurred in nPEP cases involving intoxication or physical and psychological trauma. Many clinicians tend to treat "worst-case" scenarios and prescribe PEP in situations where there is uncertainty determining if an exposure occurred given the time-sensitive nature of initiating PEP (it must be initiated within 72 hours of the exposure), balanced with the relative tolerability of current PEP regimens.

What is the risk of human immunodeficiency virus transmission?

HIV exposures may be categorized by the type of exposure and the corresponding risk of HIV acquisition. Several factors should be considered when evaluating the risk of HIV transmission, including the following:

- The source patient:
  - Is the source patient known to be HIV-positive? If so,
    - Is the source patient currently on ART?
    - Does the source patient have a detectable viral load?
  - Does the source patient have an unknown HIV serostatus? If so,
    - Does the source patient belong to a cohort with a greater prevalence of HIV (eg, men who have sex with men [MSM], person who injects drugs [PWID], incarceration history, from a country with greater than 1% HIV seroprevalence, perpetrator of sexual assault or sexual partner of a member with one of the risk factors)[17]

o Is the source patient has very low risk for HIV? For example, does the source patient have a recent negative HIV test with no HIV risk factors? Is the source patient using and adherent to PrEP?

- Was this a mucosal or a percutaneous exposure?
- What was the type and volume of exposed body fluid?

The relative risks for HIV acquisition if exposed to a source patient with nonsuppressed HIV infection are outlined in **Table 1**.[17] Condomless sexual exposures with an HIV-positive individual who has a suppressed viral load (<200 copies/mL) for greater than 6 months have a zero-to-negligible risk for HIV transmission.[18] Although most PEP cases involve percutaneous or sexual exposures, occasionally there are exposures that fall outside of these traditional categories; however, such exposures are mostly very low-risk situations where PEP would have a negligible benefit.[19]

Should this patient initiate postexposure prophylaxis and if so, with what medications?

PEP should be initiated in a setting where there is greater than a negligible-to-low risk for HIV acquisition (see **Table 1**). PEP should be initiated as soon as possible and before 72 hours, following a potential or confirmed HIV exposure, and continued for 28 days.[7,14–16] Rarely, PEP can be initiated after the 72 hours window following an exposure; however, this is on a case-by-case basis and typically in cases of very high-risk exposures.

There are several options for PEP regimens, and **Fig. 1** highlights guideline-recommended approaches.[7,14–16] Dolutegravir was previously a common medication used in PEP regimens; however, it should be avoided in pregnant women and women of childbearing age, given the recent findings suggesting an increased risk of neural tube defects if a woman conceives while receiving this drug.[20,21] Although there are several drugs that may be used safely, certain drugs should be avoided, including abacavir, as there is the potential for hypersensitivity reactions and requires human leukocyte antigen testing before use, which may take several days to return.[22] In addition, efavirenz should be avoided due to short-term mental status changes and

Table 1
Human immunodeficiency virus transmission risks from exposure to an HIV-positive source with a nonsuppressive viral load

Risk Level	Exposure Category	HIV Transmission Risk from a Source with Nonsuppressed HIV Infection
High	Blood transfusion	92.5%
	Mother-to-child (vertical) transmission	22.6%
	Receptive anal intercourse	1.38%
	Needle sharing for injection drug use	0.63%
Moderate	Needlestick injury	0.23%
	Insertive anal intercourse	0.11%
	Vaginal intercourse (receptive)	0.08%
	Vaginal intercourse (insertive)	0.04%
Low	Insertive or receptive oral intercourse	No estimate
	Sharing sex toys	
	Blood on compromised skin	

Data from Tan DHS, Hull MW, Yoong D, et al. Canadian guideline on HIV pre-exposure prophylaxis and nonoccupational postexposure prophylaxis. Can Med Assoc J. 2017;189(47):E1448-E1458; and Patel P, Barkowf CB, Brooks JT, Lasry A, Lansky A, Mermin J. Estimating per-act HIV transmission risk: a systematic review. AIDS. 2014;28(10):1509-1519.

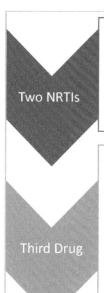

Two NRTIs
- Recommended:
  - Emtricitabine/tenofovir disoproxil fumarate (FTC/TDF) 300/200 mg PO once daily
- Alternative:
  - Zidovudine/lamivudine 300/150 mg PO twice daily
  - Tenofovir disoproxil fumarate (TDF) 300 mg PO once daily + lamivudine (3TC) 300 mg PO once daily

Third Drug
- Recommended:
  - Raltegravir 400 mg PO twice daily
  - Darunavir 800 mg PO once daily + ritonavir 100 mg PO once daily
  - Dolutegravir 50 mg PO once daily[a]
- Alternative:
  - Darunavir/cobicistat 800/150 mg PO once daily
  - Elvitegravir/cobicistat 150/150 mg (coformulated with TDF/FTC) PO once daily. Note that is a three-drug regimen that does not require additional medications
  - Lopinavir/ritonavir 800/200 mg PO once daily
  - Atazanavir 300 mg PO once daily + ritonavir 100 mg PO once daily

Fig. 1. Antiretroviral therapy options for PEP, favoring a 3-drug approach combining 2 NRTIs and an integrase inhibitor or a protease inhibitor. NRTIs, nucleoside reverse transcriptase inhibitors. [a] Dolutegravir should not be used in pregnant women and women of childbearing age, given the potential risk of neural tube defects.[20,21]. (*Data from* Refs. [7,14,16,24])

potential teratogenicity.[23,24] Older drugs that are no longer recommended for HIV treatment due to toxicity, such as indinavir, stavudine, and didanosine, should also not be used for PEP.[25,26]

What other infectious and noninfectious disease issues should be addressed?

The first point of health care contact following a potential HIV exposure is usually an emergency department or an outpatient clinical setting. Before initiating PEP, patients should have baseline investigations, including HIV testing (preferably with a fourth-generation assay that detects both HIV antibodies and p24 antigen), hepatitis B and C serology, in addition to a complete blood count, creatinine, electrolytes, liver enzyme testing, and a pregnancy test for female patients. Patients presenting after a sexual exposure should be screened for chlamydia and gonorrhea (with urine, pharyngeal, and rectal screening, using nucleic acid amplification tests, where available) and syphilis serology. Inquiry into concomitant medications (including nonprescribed "over-the-counter" medications) and allergies is important to limit the risk of potential drug interactions and adverse effects. If the patient is nonimmune to hepatitis B, consideration should be given to starting hepatitis B postexposure prophylaxis[27] as well as vaccination for hepatitis B and A where necessary.[28,29]

PEP visits are teachable moments and great opportunities for health promotion. Such clinic visits enable health care providers to explore concomitant syndemic health problems such as drug or alcohol abuse, other mental health issues, and physical and sexual abuse that may increase one's risk for HIV acquisition.[30–32] PEP visits are also an opportune time to liaise individuals with targeted resources to help mitigate these syndemic health issues.

During the consultation, patients should be counseled on the importance of PEP adherence and what an HIV seroconversion illness is, and that they should seek care should they have such symptoms. They should also be advised on taking necessary steps to prevent transmission to others until their follow-up HIV status is confirmed as negative, such as wearing barrier protection during intercourse and refraining from donating blood, plasma, semen, breast milk, or organs, in addition to refraining from sharing drug injection paraphernalia, razors, and tooth brushes.

What is an appropriate follow-up strategy?

Poor adherence to 28-day PEP regimens and to clinic appointments is a frequent issue.[33] PEP regimens containing integrase inhibitors are generally well tolerated, and PEP regimens may be changed to these if there are side effects with other ARV classes to help improve adherence.[34–37] Ensuring patients have a close friend, family member, or community support worker to help facilitate improved adherence to medications and clinic appointments is helpful.

A fourth-generation HIV assay and hepatitis C virus serology should be repeated at 3 to 4 months following the initial exposure. If hepatitis C was acquired from the exposure, HIV testing should be repeated at the 6-month mark as there may be delayed seroconversion in these instances.[7,16] Repeat testing for hepatitis B should be considered if the patient is hepatitis B nonimmune and did not receive HBV postexposure prophylaxis. Depending on the exposure, patients should be rescreened for other sexually transmitted infections (STIs) such as gonorrhea, chlamydia and syphilis. Female patients who require PEP for a sexual exposure should have a pregnancy test repeated at 6 to 12 weeks. Any baseline bloodwork that was noted to be abnormal will need ongoing monitoring while the patient is on PEP, typically at the 2-week mark, and this may include abnormal liver function tests, renal function tests, and glucose.[16] As with the initial PEP clinic appointment, follow-up appointments are also opportune times for health promotion and to screen for drug or alcohol abuse, conduct safe sexual counseling, and to connect patients with helpful resources. Many patients presenting for PEP may be good candidates for other HIV prevention modalities such as PrEP, and the final PEP appointment may be an appropriate time to transition from PEP to PrEP care in those with ongoing HIV risk factors.[38]

PREEXPOSURE PROPHYLAXIS
Introduction

Select populations remain at increased risk for HIV acquisition. For example, the risk of acquiring HIV is 27 times higher among MSM, 23 times higher among PWID, and 13 times higher among female commercial sex workers compared with the general public.[2] In 2016, MSM represented 64% of the population with HIV in the United States, and they accounted for 66% of new infections overall.[39,40] PWID accounted for an estimated 6% to 9% of new HIV diagnoses in the United States between 2010 and 2015.[39,40] Canadian statistics show similar estimates, with MSM and PWID accounting for 52.5% and 14.3% of HIV incidences, respectively.[41] Globally, Southern and Eastern Africa are home to more than half of the total number of people with HIV[42] and there continue to be several logistic, financial, cultural, and legal barriers that stand in the way of implementing widescale HIV prevention strategies in this region.[43,44] Harm-reduction counseling and education alone have not been able to reduce the rates of HIV in at-risk populations, and additional pharmacologic HIV prevention approaches are necessary to curb the epidemic.

PrEP is the proactive use of ART in HIV-negative individuals to mitigate the risk of HIV acquisition in those at greater risk for infection. This approach has gained ground quickly in the past few years as part of an integrated strategy to reduce the global burden of HIV. PrEP was first introduced into routine clinical practice in 2012, with the US Food and Drug Administration (FDA) approving combined emtricitabine/tenofovir disoproxil fumarate (FTC/TDF) for use in HIV-negative individuals[45] and then with the World Health Organization (WHO) releasing PrEP guidelines that same year.[46] To date, multiple public health organizations have released PrEP guidelines.[16,24,47–49] Although PrEP may reduce HIV acquisition at an individual level, it is also demonstrated to significantly reduce HIV transmission at a population level when implemented broadly,[50] and there are currently efforts to scale up PrEP use in both high- and low-resource settings outside of clinical trials and into routine clinical care.

Early Evidence for Preexposure Prophylaxis

The path toward the FDA and WHO's approval of PrEP involved decades of research beginning with nonhuman studies and culminating in large clinical trials. In 1995, Tsai and colleagues[51] were able to demonstrate reductions in Simian Immunodeficiency Virus transmission in macaques by using TDF before and shortly after inoculation. Multiple nonhuman primate studied followed, with sentinel human studies emerging in 2010 and outlined in **Table 2**.

The iPrEx study is an early landmark PrEP trial where 2499 HIV-negative MSM or transgender women received either FTC/TDF or placebo and were followed prospectively. This study demonstrated that those receiving FTC/TDF as PrEP had a 44% reduction in HIV incidence.[52] Several subsequent studies then evaluated the role of PrEP in heterosexual populations, notably women. The FEM-PrEP Study Group's trial in Kenya, South Africa, and Tanzania evaluated the effectiveness of PrEP for HIV-negative heterosexual women with HIV-positive partners but failed to show a reduction in HIV acquisition risk.[53] Similarly, the VOICE trial conducted in South Africa, Uganda, and Zimbabwe also failed to show a significant reduction in HIV acquisition with oral or vaginal PrEP in at-risk heterosexual women.[54] The lack of efficacy in these trials is attributed to the very low adherence to PrEP, measured at 12% in FEM-PrEP[53]

Table 2
Early landmark trials studying human immunodeficiency virus preexposure prophylaxis and their overall efficacies

Study Name (Year)	Population	PrEP Regimen	Overall HIV Reduction	HIV Reduction in Those Adhering to PrEP
iPrEx (2010)	MSM and transgender women	FTC/TDF daily	44%	92%
TDF2 (2012)	Heterosexual couples	TDF	62%	-
FEM-PrEP (2012)	Heterosexual women	FTC/TDF	0%[a]	-
Partners PrEP (2013)	Heterosexual serodiscordant couples	FTC/TDF TDF	75% 67%	86% 90%
Bangkok Tenofovir Study (2013)	People who use injection drugs	TDF	49%	70%
VOICE (2015)	Heterosexual women	FTC/TDF TDF	0%[a] 0%[a]	-
PROUD (2016)	MSM	FTC/TDF	86%	86%

[a] Low adherence was noted in these studies.

and between 25% and 30% of individuals in VOICE, despite a self-reported adherence rate of 90%.[54]

The Partners PrEP Study randomized serodiscordant heterosexual couples to once-daily TDF, FTC/TDF, or placebo in Kenya and Uganda. All participants were also educated on risk reduction and safe sexual practices. A reduction in HIV transmission was observed with the use of TDF or FTC/TDF, and although nonsignificant, FTC/TDF demonstrated a higher relative reduction in HIV incidence compared with TDF alone.[55] Unlike the FEM-PrEP and VOICE trials, the Partners PrEP Study reported better adherence (up to 92%) to prescribed medications.

The TDF2 trial attempted to demonstrate PrEP efficacy in heterosexual couples in Botswana with FTC/TDF; however, the study was not adequately powered for this purpose.[56] Although the trial was terminated early due to low retention rates, interim efficacy analyses demonstrated a 62.6% reduction in HIV infections, but these data must be interpreted in the appropriate context, given the early termination of the trial.

The PROUD study, published in 2016, was an open-label randomized trial conducted in England that looked to address the efficacy of PrEP in real-world settings.[57] Five hundred fourty-four individuals deemed to be at risk for HIV acquisition were randomized to receive FTC/TDF either immediately or a year later. The study reported an 86% relative reduction of HIV incidence in the early PrEP group compared with those in the delayed group.

Lastly, the Bangkok Tenofovir Study (BTS) evaluated PrEP with daily TDF (compared with placebo) in PWID in Bangkok, Thailand.[58] All participants received monthly HIV testing and individualized risk-reduction counseling and were offered condoms and methadone treatment. The study arm demonstrated a 48.9% reduction in HIV incidence without a significant difference in serious adverse outcomes. BTS highlights the efficacy of PrEP in PWID when used in combination with other harm-reduction strategies.

Outside of controlled trials, PrEP had demonstrated incredible efficacy in "real-world" situations with robust data emerging in Canada, United States, and Australia.[50,59–62]

Prescribing Preexposure Prophylaxis

The initial preexposure prophylaxis visit

Pragmatic, user-friendly PrEP Guidelines are now available from many public health bodies and outline routine PrEP care in clinical practice.[16,24,48,49] Patients presenting for PrEP may be referred to specialist clinics or present directly to primary care providers and occasionally nurse-led providers.[63] The initial visit should focus on evaluating a patient's current and near-future risk for HIV acquisition and other preventable infections, screening for syndemic health issues such as depression or drug and alcohol abuse, and reiterating education related to HIV risk reduction (Table 3).[64] The HIV Incidence Risk Index for Men who have Sex with Men is a tool to help identify MSM who may benefit from PrEP[16,65]; however, many clinicians do not use this in routine practice, as it may be time consuming in an otherwise busy clinic. Clinical appointments are an opportune time to link individuals with helpful resources, such as alcohol or drug abuse programs, or psychosocial support where necessary.

Baseline investigations should be obtained before PrEP initiation and include a complete blood count, liver enzyme tests, and creatinine. HIV screening should preferably use a fourth-generation assay. In the context of a potential acute HIV infection, testing for HIV RNA nucleic acid is preferable, and if it is not available, then repeat testing with another fourth-generation HIV screen 2 to 4 weeks later is

Table 3
Important aspects of the medical history specific to preexposure prophylaxis

Issues on Medical History	Relevance to PrEP
1. Past medical history including a focus on bone and renal health	Currently FTC/TDF is the only recommended PrEP medication, and this may reduce bone density and has the potential for nephrotoxicity[73,75]
2. Current medications	Prescribed and nonprescribed medication may interact with FTC/DTF
3. Allergies	Many STI treatments involve beta-lactam antibiotics (eg, ceftriaxone for gonorrhea treatment). Inquire about drug allergies, as many patients on PrEP are at increased risk for acquiring STIs.[89]

4. Risk of HIV acquisition	i. Sexual risk factors
	  a. Frequency of sexual encounters
	  b. Number of sexual partners
	  c. Number of known HIV-positive partners
	  d. Number of partners with known STI history
	  e. Patterns of barrier protection usage
	  f. Use of concomitant alcohol or drugs with sex or participation in chemsex[a]
	  g. Current or past history of sexual abuse or challenges with condom negotiation

5. Injection drug use	i. Frequency of injection drug use ii. Sharing of drug paraphernalia iii. Safety of drug use (eg, inject with partner supervision, use of safe injection sites, naloxone kit availability)

[a] Intercourse under the influence of psychoactive substances to enhance sexual arousal; often associated with geolocating mobile applications.

recommended.[16,49] HIV testing should ideally be negative within a week before starting PrEP. Other blood work should include hepatitis A, B, and C serology and then ensuring individuals are immune to hepatitis A and B.[16,66,67] Patient should be screened for STIs, such as chlamydia, gonorrhea (urine nucleic acid amplification test, rectal and pharyngeal culture, or nucleic acid amplification tests, if indicated by exposure), and syphilis, and treated as per local guidelines.

What should you prescribe and how should you follow the patient?
FTC/TDF is currently the only medication approved for PrEP; however, the DISCOVER trial recently demonstrated the noninferiority of combined emtricitabine/tenofovir alafenamide (FTC/TAF) compared with FTC/TDF in PrEP care and will likely be used more regularly in this setting given the favorable renal and bone toxicity profiles.[68] Although once-daily FTC/TDF is the more widely used PrEP regimen, "on-demand" (also referred to as "event-driven") PrEP is an alternative method. The ANRS IPERGAY evaluated on-demand PrEP in 414 MSM participants who were randomized to either using FTC/TDF or placebo before and shortly after sex.[69] FTC/TDF was prescribed as a fixed-dose combination (200 mg of FTC and 300 mg of TDF per pill) and participants administered a loading dose of 2 pills 2 to 24 hours before sex, followed by a third pill 24 hours after the first pill, and finally a fourth pill 24 hours later. Although 14 HIV infections were seen in the placebo group, the on-demand PrEP group only saw 2

infections for a relative risk reduction of 86%.[69] We present both daily and on-demand PrEP options to most patients and find that most individuals prefer daily PrEP due to the high frequency of condomless sexual activity and ease of a once-daily medication.

Patients taking PrEP are to follow-up in clinic every 3 months to screen for HIV, STIs, medication toxicity, and medication adherence. These are also opportune times to discuss other health promotion strategies (eg, seasonal influenza vaccination) and continue to screen and offer support for additional issues such as alcohol and drug abuse or mental health issues. The authors prescribe PrEP in 4-month increments and ask patients to follow-up in 3- to 3.5-month increments, as some patients may miss a scheduled appointment and the longer prescription time allows for such scheduling issues while ensuring patients do not go without PrEP.

The authors also screen patients at each follow-up visit to determine if PrEP is still indicated. Many individuals have some fluidity in their sexual risk and may start and stop PrEP based on their most current risk. At follow-up visits, repeat HIV testing and STI screening should be performed as outlined in the initial visit, and safety laboratories include a complete blood count, creatinine, and a urine protein-to-creatinine ratio to screen for possible adverse effects of FTC/TDF.[16,48,49]

Additional Preexposure Prophylaxis Considerations

Other human immunodeficiency virus prevention modalities

Some patients may request a pharmacologic HIV prevention modality but have very few condomless sexual exposures to warrant daily PrEP. In such cases, it is challenging to balance using daily medications to prevent very rare HIV exposures with the costs of medication and potential side effects such as renal and bone toxicity. In addition, there is some uncertainty in the efficacy of on-demand PrEP in individuals with very infrequent potential HIV exposures. In these circumstances, one may consider "on-demand PEP," also termed "PEP-in-pocket," (or "PIP"), where patients who have up to 4 potential HIV exposures per year are given a prescription for a 28-day supply of PEP (see **Fig. 1**). Patients are counseled to fill the prescription and only take the medications should they have a potential HIV exposure. Patients are counseled to follow-up in clinic within a week of their exposure if they started PEP for baseline investigations. Such an approach may enable timely access to HIV prevention, promote autonomy over one's care, and avoid emergency department visits.[70]

Pregnancy and lactation

The effect of FTC/TDF on fetal and infant growth is not well understood but thought to be relatively safe.[71] FTC/TDF did not demonstrate any significant effect on pregnancy outcomes in the Partners PrEP trial,[55] and data from HIV-positive women exposed to TDF also corroborate the relative safety in pregnancy.[72] Given the limited evidence in peripartum use of PrEP, patients should be counseled on potential benefits versus risks of PrEP during pregnancy and lactation.[48]

Adverse effects

Serious adverse effects are very infrequent in those on PrEP. Mild gastrointestinal symptoms are reported to be the most common adverse symptoms and are generally limited to the first month of PrEP use.[52,55] PrEP has also been associated with a decline in renal function. For example, the Partners PrEP Study demonstrated a decrease in estimated glomerular filtration rate (eGFR) starting at 1 month of PrEP use; however, this decline in GFR did not progress and is not thought to be clinically relevant in those with normal baseline eGFRs.[73] Also reassuring is that renal function recovered with discontinuation of PrEP[74]; however, because of the potential for nephrotoxicity, PrEP should only be used in those with a glomerular filtration rate of greater than or equal to 60 mL/min.[16,24,48,49] Several studies have demonstrated a mild but significant decrease in bone mineral density (BMD) on PrEP, even as early as 24 weeks after initiating FTC/TDF.[75] Although this is thought to be statistically significant, it has not demonstrated clinical significance in those with normal BMDs, and BMD returns to normal with discontinuation of PrEP. FTC/TAF has a favorable renal and bone toxicity profile compared with FTC/TDF.[68] With the recent noninferiority findings of this medication compared with FTC/TDF in PrEP care, we may see a reduced rate of adverse outcomes with scale-up of this drug; however, at the time of writing, this FTC/TAF has not been approved in HIV prevention guidelines.[68]

Change in sexual behavior and sexually transmitted infection risk while on preexposure prophylaxis

There are concerns for greater rates of condomless sexual activities and increasing rates of bacterial STIs with PrEP scale-up, especially in the context of emerging drug-resistant STIs.[76] Although behavioral data in real world settings are limited, several randomized controlled trials demonstrated decreasing rates of high-risk sexual behavior while on PrEP.[52,53,56,58] In contrast, the ANRS IPERGAY study demonstrated greater rates of condomless sex during the course of that study.[69] A recent systematic review looking at 16 studies demonstrated more condomless sexual acts and a significant increase in rectal chlamydia in those on PrEP,[77] but the utility of this review was limited by the heterogeneity of the included studies. Still this highlights the importance of safe sexual counseling and the need for frequent STI screening (and treatment if necessary) at 3-month intervals in those taking PrEP.

Antiviral resistance and human immunodeficiency virus acquisition

There is a risk of developing HIV resistant to FTC/TDF if HIV is acquired while on PrEP or if patients initiate PrEP with unrecognized HIV infection. For example, the FEM-PrEP trial reported antiretroviral resistance developing among 4 recently infected patients following PrEP initiation.[53] In addition, a man in Toronto acquired a multidrug-resistant HIV-1 strain despite using PrEP with biochemical data suggesting adequate drug adherence.[78] Hence, it is crucial to ensure patients are HIV-negative before initiating PrEP and to counsel those on PrEP to use barrier protection.

Treatment as Prevention

Treatment as Prevention (TasP) entails prescribing ART to everyone infected with HIV with the goal of reducing viral loads to non-detectable levels in individuals, and subsequently reducing HIV transmission in communities. Several studies over the past decade demonstrate that an individual's HIV transmission risk can theoretically be eliminated if their viral load is undetectable. Data published in 2011 demonstrated that the early initiation of ART significantly reduced transmission of HIV between serodiscordant couples.[79] In addition, a systematic review of HIV transmission in HIV-discordant heterosexual couples with viral load suppression less than 400 copies/mL showed a transmission rate of 1 per 79 person years.[80] Similarly, a prospective cohort analysis of HIV serodiscordant couples in 7 African nations demonstrated a 92% reduction in transmission in those on ART with suppressed viral loads.[81] A recent retrospective analysis of Taiwan's HIV surveillance data showed a 53% reduction in HIV transmission rates after providing free ART to all HIV-infected citizens,[82] and a similar population-based study in British Columbia demonstrated a 52% reduction in new HIV diagnoses with increasing financial coverage for ART.[83] Initiation of ART showed not only a significant impact on reduction of HIV transmission but also a reduction in tuberculosis transmission in highly endemic regions.[84]

The PARTNER study from 2016 and the PARTNER 2 study from 2019 provided recent and robust data supporting TasP.[18,85] These studies evaluated condomless sexual activity among serodiscordant couples when the HIV-positive partner had an undetectable viral load (<200 copies/mL) that did not result in HIV transmission to the HIV-negative partner.[18] This prospective, observational, multicenter study included serodiscordant heterosexual couples and MSM and prompted the Undetectable = Untransmittable (U = U) movement.[86] U = U promotes the notion that those HIV-positive individuals on suppressive ART with undetectable viral loads (<200 copies/mL for >6 months) cannot sexually transmit the virus to their partners, and this is now being accepted by major public health bodies and integrated into guidelines.[8,49,87] Other recent studies that support U = U include the "Opposites Attract" study, where there were no phylogenetically linked cases of HIV transmission between 343 serodiscordant male couples (where one was virologically suppressed) and 232.2 couple years of follow-up in a prospective international study.[88]

Although TasP and U = U have widescale public health implications, these concepts are also applicable at the clinical level. These concepts (and the primary data that drives them) are frequently discussed in routine clinical settings while counseling patients at risk for HIV acquisition. TasP and U = U can help frame the discussion related to whether a patient is a candidate for PEP, PrEP, or other HIV prevention modalities and is helpful for patient-level education of HIV transmission risk, especially for serodiscordant couples.

SUMMARY

PEP, PrEP, and TasP are very effective HIV prevention modalities that have the potential to benefit individuals at risk for HIV acquisition and decrease HIV transmission in populations. Although these tools are now becoming more firmly entrenched into routine clinical practice, there is room for scale in many low-resource settings, especially those that are most affected by the HIV pandemic. Increasing global implementation of these HIV prevention modalities will be integral in halting the pandemic.

REFERENCES

1. UNAIDS. 90-90-90 an ambitious treatment target to help end the AIDS epidemic 2014. Available at: http://www.unaids.org/sites/default/files/media_asset/90-90-90_en.pdf. Accessed September 18, 2018.
2. Joint United Nations Programme on HIV/AIDS. UNAIDS Data 2018. Geneva (Switzerland): 2018. https://www.unaids.org/sites/default/files/media_asset/unaids-data-2018_en.pdf. Accessed May 20, 2019.
3. Commonwealth Secretariat. Guidelines for implementing a multi-sectoral approach to HIV and AIDS in Commonwealth countries. London: Commonwealth Secretariat Health Section; 2003.
4. Cook C, Phelan M, Sander G, et al. The case for a harm reduction decade: progress, potential and paradigm shifts. Harm reduction international 2016. Available at: https://www.hri.global/files/2016/03/10/Report_The_Case_for_a_Harm_Reduction_Decade.pdf. Accessed December 28, 2018.
5. Gray RH, Kigozi G, Serwadda D, et al. Male circumcision for HIV prevention in men in Rakai, Uganda: a randomised trial. Lancet 2007;369(9562):657–66.
6. Cepeda JA, Eritsyan K, Vickerman P, et al. Potential impact of implementing and scaling up harm reduction and antiretroviral therapy on HIV prevalence and

mortality and overdose deaths among people who inject drugs in two Russian cities: a modelling study. Lancet HIV 2018;5(10):e578–87.

7. US Centers for Disease Control and Prevention. Updated guidelines for antiretroviral postexposure prophylaxis after sexual, injection-drug use, or other nonoccupational exposure to HIV — United States, 2016. Morb Mortal Wkly Rep. https://doi.org/10.15585/mmwr.mm6517a5.

8. Kuhar DT, Henderson DK, Struble KA, et al. Updated US Public Health service guidelines for the management of occupational exposures to human immunodeficiency virus and recommendations for postexposure prophylaxis. Infect Control Hosp Epidemiol 2013;34(09):875–92.

9. Henderson DK, Gerberding JL. Prophylactic zidovudine after occupational exposure to the human immunodeficiency virus: an interim analysis. J Infect Dis 1989; 160(2):321–7.

10. Tokars JI, Marcus R, Culver DH, et al. Surveillance of HIV infection and zidovudine use. Ann Intern Med 1993;118(12):913–9.

11. Polder J, Bell D, Barker E, et al. Public health service statement on management of occupational exposure to human immunodeficiency virus, including considerations regarding zidovudine postexposure use. vol. 39. 1990. Available at: http://www.cdc.gov/mmwr/preview/mmwrhtml/00001556.htm. Accessed September 19, 2018.

12. Cardo DM, Culver DH, Ciesielski CA, et al. A case-control study of HIV seroconversion in health care workers after percutaneous exposure. N Engl J Med 1997; 337(21):1485–90.

13. Roland ME, Neilands TB, Krone MR, et al. Seroconversion following nonoccupational postexposure prophylaxis against HIV. Clin Infect Dis 2005;41(10): 1507–13.

14. Cresswell F, Waters L, Briggs E, et al. UK Guideline for the use of HIV Post-Exposure Prophylaxis Following Sexual Exposure, 2015. Int J STD AIDS 2016; 27(9):713–38.

15. World Health Organization. Guidelines on post-exposure prophylaxis for HIV and the use of Co-Trimoxazole prophylaxis for HIV-related infections among adults, adolescents and Children: recommendations for a public health approach 2014. Available at: https://www.who.int/hiv/pub/guidelines/arv2013/arvs2013upplement_dec2014/en/. Accessed December 10, 2018.

16. Tan DHS, Hull MW, Yoong D, et al. Canadian guideline on HIV pre-exposure prophylaxis and nonoccupational postexposure prophylaxis. Can Med Assoc J 2017;189(47):E1448–58.

17. Patel P, Barkowf craig b, Brooks john t, et al. Estimating per-act HIV transmission risk: a systematic review. AIDS 2014;28(10):1509–19.

18. Rodger AJ, Cambiano V, Bruun T, et al. Sexual activity without condoms and risk of HIV transmission in serodifferent couples when the HIV-positive partner is using suppressive antiretroviral therapy. J Am Med Assoc 2016. https://doi.org/10.1001/jama.2016.5148.

19. Rawal S, Bogoch II. Evaluation of non-sexual, non-needlestick, non-occupational HIV post-exposure prophylaxis cases. AIDS 2017;31(10):1500–2.

20. Zash R, Makhema J, Shapiro RL. Neural-tube defects with dolutegravir treatment from the time of conception. N Engl J Med 2018;379(10):979–81.

21. Zash R, Jacobson DL, Diseko M, et al. Comparative safety of dolutegravir-based or efavirenz-based antiretroviral treatment started during pregnancy in Botswana: an observational study. Lancet Glob Health 2018;6(7):e804–10.

22. Mallal S, Phillips E, Carosi G, et al. HLA-B*5701 screening for hypersensitivity to abacavir. N Engl J Med 2008;358:568–79.

23. Ford N, Calmy A, Mofenson L. Safety of efavirenz in the first trimester of pregnancy: an updated systematic review and meta-analysis. AIDS 2011;25(18): 2301–4.

24. World Health Organization. Consolidated guidelines on the use of antiretroviral drugs for treating and preventing HIV infection: recommendations for a public health approach. Geneva (Switzerland): World Health Organization; 2013.

25. Food and Drug Administration. CRIXIVAN® (Indinavir Sulfate) Capsules 2015. Available at: http://www.accessdata.fda.gov/drugsatfda_docs/label/2015/0206 85s077lbl.pdf. Accessed December 13, 2018.

26. Timmermans S, Tempelman C, Godfried MH, et al. Nelfinavir and nevirapine side effects during pregnancy. AIDS 2005;19(8):795–9.

27. Schillie S, Murphy TV, Sawyer M. CDC guidance for evaluating health-care personnel for hepatitis B virus protection and for administering postexposure management. MMWR Recomm Rep 2013;62(RR-10):1–19, rr6210a1 [pii].

28. Freidl GS, Sonder GJ, Bovée LP, et al. Hepatitis A outbreak among men who have sex with men (MSM) predominantly linked with the EuroPride, the Netherlands, July 2016 to February 2017. Euro Surveill 2017. https://doi.org/10.2807/1560-7917.ES.2017.22.8.30468.

29. Friesema IHM, Sonder GJB, Petrignani MWF, et al. Spillover of a hepatitis A outbreak among men who have sex with men (MSM) to the general population, the Netherlands, 2017. Euro Surveill 2018;23(23) [pii:1800265].

30. Stall R, Mills TC, Williamson J, et al. Association of co-occurring psychosocial health problems and increased vulnerability to HIV/AIDS among urban men who have sex with men. Am J Public Health 2003;93(6):939–42.

31. Parsons JT, Millar BM, Moody RL, et al. Syndemic conditions and HIV transmission risk behavior among HIV-negative gay and bisexual men in a U.S. national sample. Health Psychol 2016;36(7):695–703.

32. Morrison SA, Yoong D, Hart TA, et al. High prevalence of syndemic health problems in patients seeking post-exposure prophylaxis for sexual exposures to HIV. PLoS One 2018;13(5):1–16.

33. Bogoch II, Scully EP, Zachary KC, et al. Patient attrition between the emergency department and clinic among individuals presenting for HIV nonoccupational postexposure prophylaxis. Clin Infect Dis 2014;58(11):1618–24.

34. Bogoch II, Siemieniuk RAC, Andrews JR, et al. Changes to initial postexposure prophylaxis regimens between the emergency department and clinic. J Acquir Immune Defic Syndr 2015;69(5):e182–4.

35. Mayer KH, Mimiaga MJ, Gelman M, et al. Raltegravir, tenofovir DF, and emtricitabine for postexposure prophylaxis to prevent the sexual transmission of HIV: safety, tolerability, and adherence. J Acquir Immune Defic Syndr 2012;59(4): 354–9.

36. Mulka L, Annandale D, Richardson C, et al. Raltegravir-based HIV postexposure prophylaxis (PEP) in a real-life clinical setting: fewer drug drug interactions (DDIs) with improved adherence and tolerability. Sex Transm Infect 2016;92(2):107.

37. Thomas R, Galanakis C, Vézina S, et al. Adherence to post-exposure prophylaxis (PEP) and incidence of HIV seroconversion in a major North American cohort. PLoS One 2015;10(11):1 10.

38. Siemieniuk RAC, Sivachandran N, Murphy P, et al. Transitioning to HIV pre-exposure prophylaxis (PrEP) from non-occupational post-exposure prophylaxis

(nPEP) in a comprehensive HIV prevention clinic: a prospective cohort study. AIDS Patient Care STDS 2015;29(8):431–6.

39. CDC. Diagnoses of HIV infection among adults aged 50 Years and older in the United States and dependent areas, 2011–2016, vol. 23, 2018. Available at: http://www.cdc.gov/hiv/library/reports/hiv-surveillance.html. Accessed October 5, 2018.

40. CDC. Estimated HIV incidence and prevalence in the United States, 2010–2015, vol. 23, 2018. Available at: http://www.cdc.gov/hiv/library/reports/hiv-surveillance.html. Accessed October 5, 2018.

41. Public Health Agency of Canada. Summary: estimates of HIV incidence, prevalence and Canada's progress on Meeting the 90-90-90 HIV targets, 2016 2018. Available at: https://www.canada.ca/content/dam/phac-aspc/documents/services/publications/diseases-conditions/summary-estimates-hiv-incidence-prevalence-canadas-progress-90-90-90/pub-eng.pdf. Accessed October 5, 2018.

42. Joint United Nations Programme on HIV/AIDS. UNAIDS Data 2018. Geneva, Switzerland, 2018. Available at: https://www.unaids.org/sites/default/files/media_asset/unaids-data-2018_en.pdf. Accessed May 20, 2019.

43. Mbonu NC, van den Borne B, De Vries NK. Stigma of people with HIV/AIDS in Sub-Saharan Africa: a literature review. J Trop Med 2009;1–14. https://doi.org/10.1155/2009/145891.

44. HIV, TB and human rights in Southern and East Africa: report 2016. Available at: http://www.arasa.info/files/3314/8119/1044/ARASA_2016_Human_Rights_report.pdf. Accessed December 29, 2018.

45. Truvada for PrEP fact Sheet: ensuring safe and proper use. U.S. Food and Drug Administration. Available at: https://www.fda.gov/downloads/Drugs/DrugSafety/.../UCM312290.pdf. Accessed October 10, 2018.

46. New South Wales Ministry of Health. Pre-exposure prophylaxis of HIV with antiretroviral medications - NSW guideline summary. Sydney (Australia); 2016. Available at: https://www1.health.nsw.gov.au/pds/ActivePDSDocuments/GL2016_011.pdf. Accessed October 5, 2018.

47. NSW M of H. Pre-exposure prophylaxis of HIV with antiretroviral medications - NSW guideline summary. Sydney (Australia): NSW Government; 2016. Available at: https://www1.health.nsw.gov.au/pds/ActivePDSDocuments/GL2016_011.pdf. Accessed October 5, 2018.

48. CDC. Preexposure prophylaxis for the prevention of HIV infection in the United States—2017 update: a clinical practice guideline 2018. Available at: https://www.cdc.gov/hiv/pdf/risk/prep/cdc-hiv-prep-guidelines-2017.pdf. Accessed October 10, 2018.

49. Asboe D, Cambiano V, Clutterbuck D, et al. BHIVA/BASHH guidelines on the use of HIV pre-exposure prophylaxis (PrEP) 2018. London: BHIVA; 2018. Available at: http://www.bhiva.org/documents/Publications/PrEP_BHIVA_BASHH_Update-2-FINAL_19-Apr-16.pdf. Accessed October 10, 2018.

50. Grulich AE, Guy R, Amin J, et al. Population-level effectiveness of rapid, targeted, high-coverage roll-out of HIV pre-exposure prophylaxis in men who have sex with men: the EPIC-NSW prospective cohort study. Lancet HIV 2018;3018(18):30215–7.

51. Tsai C, Follis KE, Sabo A, et al. Prevention of SIV infection in macaques by (R)-9-(2-Phosphonylmethoxypropyl)adenine. Science 1995;270(5239):1197–9.

52. Grant RM, Lama JR, Anderson PL, et al. Preexposure chemoprophylaxis for HIV prevention in men who have sex with men. N Engl J Med 2010;363(27):2587–99.

53. Van Damme L, Corneli A, Ahmed K, et al. Preexposure prophylaxis for HIV infection among African Women. N Engl J Med 2012;367(5):411–22.
54. Marrazzo JM, Ramjee G, Richardson BA, et al. Tenofovir-based preexposure prophylaxis for HIV Infection among African Women. N Engl J Med 2015;372(6): 509–18.
55. Baeten JM, Donnell D, Ndase P, et al. Antiretroviral prophylaxis for HIV-1 prevention among heterosexual men and women. N Engl J Med 2013;367(5):399–410.
56. Thigpen MC, Kebaabetswe PM, Paxton LA, et al. Antiretroviral preexposure prophylaxis for heterosexual HIV transmission in Botswana. N Engl J Med 2012; 367(5):423–34.
57. McCormack S, Dunn DT, Desai M, et al. Pre-exposure prophylaxis to prevent the acquisition of HIV-1 infection (PROUD): effectiveness results from the pilot phase of a pragmatic open-label randomised trial. Lancet 2016;387(10013):53–60.
58. Choopanya K, Martin M, Suntharasamai P, et al. Antiretroviral prophylaxis for HIV infection in injecting drug users in Bangkok, Thailand (the Bangkok Tenofovir Study): a randomised, double-blind, placebo-controlled phase 3 trial. Lancet 2013;381(9883):2083–90.
59. Liu AY, Cohen SE, Vittinghoff E, et al. Preexposure prophylaxis for HIV infection integrated with municipal-and community-based sexual health services. JAMA Intern Med 2016;176(1):75–84.
60. Marcus JL, Hurley LB, Hare CB, et al. Preexposure prophylaxis for HIV prevention in a large integrated health care system: adherence , renal safety , and discontinuation. J Acquir Immune Defic Syndr 2016;73(5):540–6.
61. Rajchgot J, Siemieniuk RAC, Sivachandran N, et al. Feasibility of HIV preexposure prophylaxis as part of routine care in Toronto, Canada. J Acquir Immune Defic Syndr 2016;72(3):80–1.
62. Volk JE, Marcus JL, Phengrasamy T, et al. No new HIV infections with increasing use of HIV preexposure prophylaxis in a clinical practice setting. Clin Infect Dis 2015;61(10):1601–3.
63. Schmidt HA, Mciver R, Houghton R, et al. Nurse-led pre-exposure prophylaxis: a non-traditional model to provide HIV prevention in a resource-constrained , pragmatic clinical trial. Sex Health 2018;15(6):595–7.
64. Wilton J, Noor SW, Schnubb A, et al. High HIV risk and syndemic burden regardless of referral source among MSM screening for a PrEP demonstration project in Toronto, Canada. BMC Public Health 2018;18(1):1–11.
65. Wilton J, Mishra S, Tan DHS. Considerations for using the HIRI-MSM screening tool to identify MSM who would benefit most from PrEP. J Acquir Immune Defic Syndr 2017;76(2):e58–61.
66. Charre C, Ramiere C, Roque-Afonso AM, et al. Hepatitis A outbreak in HIV-infected MSM and in PrEP-using MSM despite a high level of immunity, Lyon, France, January to June 2017. Euro Surveill 2017;22(48):1–4.
67. Ismail MF, Wong DK, Bogoch II. The role for hepatitis A vaccination in HIV preexposure prophylaxis. AIDS 2018;32(5):675–6.
68. Hare C, Coll J, Ruane P, et al. The phase 3 discover study: daily F/TAF or F/TDF For HIV preexposure prophylaxis, Abstract 104. In: Conference on Retroviruses and Opportunistic Infections. Seattle, WA; 2019. Available at: http://www.croiconference.org/sessions/phase-3-discover-study-daily-ftaf-or-ftdf-hiv-preexposure-prophylaxis. Accessed March 25, 2019.
69. Molina J-M, Capitant C, Spire B, et al. On-demand preexposure prophylaxis in men at high risk for HIV-1 infection. N Engl J Med 2015;373(23):2237–46.

70. Tumarkin E, Heendeniya A, Murphy P, et al. HIV post-exposure prophylaxis-in-pocket ("PIP") for individuals with low frequency, high risk, HIV exposures. J Acquir Immune Defic Syndr 2018;1. https://doi.org/10.1097/QAI.0000000000001639.

71. Mugo NR, Hong T, Celum C, et al. Pregnancy incidence and outcomes among women receiving preexposure prophylaxis for HIV prevention a randomized clinical trial. J Am Med Assoc 2014;312(4):362–71.

72. Gibb DM, Kizito H, Russell EC, et al. Pregnancy and infant outcomes among HIV-infected women taking long-term ART with and without Tenofovir in the DART trial. PLoS Med 2012;9(5):1–16.

73. Mugwanya KK, Wyatt C, Celum C, et al. Changes in glomerular kidney function among HIV-1- uninfected men and women receiving emtricitabine- tenofovir disoproxil fumarate preexposure prophylaxis a randomized clinical trial. JAMA Intern Med 2015;175(2):246–54.

74. Mugwanya KK, Wyatt C, Celum C, et al. Reversibility of glomerular renal function decline in HIV-uninfected men and women discontinuing emtricitabine-tenofovir disoproxil fumarate pre-exposure prophylaxis. J Acquir Immune Defic Syndr 2016;71(4):374–80.

75. Mulligan K, Glidden DV, Anderson PL, et al. Effects of emtricitabine/tenofovir on bone mineral density in HIV-negative persons in a randomized, double-blind, placebo-controlled trial. Clin Infect Dis 2015;61(4):572–80.

76. Weston E, T Wi JP. Surveillance for antimicrobial drug-resistant Neisseria gonorrhoeae through the enhanced gonococcal antimicrobial surveillance program. Emerg Infect Dis 2017;23:47–52.

77. Traeger MW, Schroeder SE, Wright EJ, et al. Effects of pre-exposure prophylaxis for the prevention of HIV infection on sexual risk behavior in men who have sex with men: a systematic review and meta-analysis. Clin Infect Dis 2018;67(5). https://doi.org/10.1093/cid/ciy182.

78. Knox DC, Anderson PL, Harrigan PR, et al. Multidrug-resistant HIV-1 infection despite preexposure prophylaxis. N Engl J Med 2017;376(5):501–2.

79. Cohen MS, Chen YQ, McCauley M, et al. Prevention of HIV-1 infection with early antiretroviral therapy. N Engl J Med 2011;365(6):493–505.

80. Attia S, Egger M, Müller M, et al. Sexual transmission of HIV according to viral load and antiretroviral therapy: systematic review and meta-analysis. AIDS 2009. https://doi.org/10.1097/QAD.0b013e32832b7dca.

81. Donnell D, Baeten JM, Kiarie J, et al. Heterosexual HIV-1 transmission after initiation of antiretroviral therapy: a prospective cohort analysis. Lancet 2010. https://doi.org/10.1016/S0140-6736(10)60705-2.

82. Fang C, Hsu H, Twu S-H, et al. JID - 2004 - HAART in HIV transmission. J Infect Dis 2004;190:879–85.

83. Lima VD, Lepik KJ, Zhang W, et al. Regional and temporal changes in HIV-related mortality in British Columbia, 1987-2006. Can J Public Health 2010;101(5):415–9. Available at: http://www.ncbi.nlm.nih.gov/pubmed/21214059.

84. Lawn SD, Kranzer K, Wood R. Antiretroviral therapy for control of the HIV-associated tuberculosis epidemic in resource-limited settings. Clin Chest Med 2009. https://doi.org/10.1016/j.ccm.2009.08.010.

85. Rodger AJ, Cambiano V, Bruun T, et al, Risk of HIV transmission through condomless sex in serodifferent gay couples with the HIV-positive partner taking suppressive antiretroviral therapy (PARTNER): final results of a multicentre, prospective, observational study. Lancet 2019. [Epub ahead of print].

86. The Lancet HIV. U=U taking off in 2017. Lancet 2017;4(11):e475.

87. UNAIDS. Undetectable = untransmittable: public health and HIV viral load suppression. Geneva (Switzerland): UNAIDS; 2018. Available at: http://www.unaids.org/sites/default/files/media_asset/undetectable-untransmittable_en.pdf. Accessed December 10, 2018.

88. Bavinton BR, Pinto AN, Phanuphak N, et al. Viral suppression and HIV transmission in serodiscordant male couples: an international, prospective, observational, cohort study. Lancet HIV 2018;5:e438-47.

89. Kojima N, Davey DJ, Jeffrey D. Pre-exposure prophylaxis for HIV infection and new sexually transmitted infections among men who have sex with men. AIDS 2016;30:2251-2.

HIV Initial Assessment and Routine Follow-up

What Tests to Order and Why

Daniel A. Solomon, MD

KEYWORDS

- HIV • Laboratory • Testing • Assessment • Follow-up • Diagnosis • Evaluation
- Management

KEY POINTS

- Laboratory testing is an important component of initial evaluation and routine follow-up care of patients with HIV.
- Initial evaluation is focused on confirming diagnosis, characterizing degree of immune suppression, and preparing for treatment initiation.
- Screening for coinfections and latent infections has an important impact on management, counseling, and education.
- Frequency of routine monitoring is reduced once patients are stable on therapy.
- Laboratory testing for patients with well-controlled HIV should be focused on health promotion and preventative care.

INTRODUCTION

With marked advances in human immunodeficiency virus (HIV) therapy over the past 30 years, HIV has transformed from a terminal diagnosis to a chronic disease.[1] Life expectancy of patients with HIV who are treated with antiretroviral therapy (ART) now approaches that of the general population.[2,3] The clinical care of patients with HIV is centered around disease control, medication adherence, and preventative care, akin to other chronic diseases. Laboratory testing is an important component of initial evaluation and routine follow-up care, but the number of tests can seem overwhelming to clinicians and patients alike. Framing the objectives of HIV care around the model of chronic disease management and health promotion may allow clinicians to organize the necessary laboratory tests, and contextualize the testing for patients.

Disclosure Statement: The author has no financial disclosures.
Division of Infectious Disease, Brigham and Women's Hospital, 75 Francis Street, PBB 4A, Boston, MA 02115, USA
E-mail address: dasolomon@bwh.harvard.edu

Infect Dis Clin N Am 33 (2019) 647–662
https://doi.org/10.1016/j.idc.2019.05.001
0891-5520/19/© 2019 Elsevier Inc. All rights reserved.

There are six goals of testing in the management of HIV: (1) confirm the diagnosis, (2) assess the degree of immunosuppression, (3) prepare for treatment initiation, (4) evaluate for coinfections and prior exposures, (5) monitor response to therapy and for medication side effects, and (6) provide appropriate preventative care. This article defines which tests are necessary (and unnecessary) to accomplish each of the goals, and explains how each test is useful. As a quick reference guide, a summary of all the tests, and when each test is indicated, is included in **Table 1**. Tests that are not routinely recommended are included in **Table 2**.

GOAL 1: CONFIRM THE DIAGNOSIS
Human Immunodeficiency Virus RNA

The most important test to confirm the diagnosis of HIV is the plasma quantitative HIV RNA (viral load). If the HIV RNA is detectable, the diagnosis is confirmed.

HIV RNA is also helpful to assess infectious risk because patients with a high viral load have higher rates of HIV transmission, an important point of education for patients.[4]

Repeat Human Immunodeficiency Virus Screening Test

Patients who have a positive screening test and a detectable HIV RNA do not need a repeat screening test for confirmation. However, if the confirmatory differentiation assay is negative and/or the HIV RNA is undetectable, the patient may have a false-positive screening test. False-positive screening tests are common, especially in a low-prevalence population, whereas false-positive differentiation assays are rare.[5] The most common cause of a false-positive screening test is the presence of a cross-reactive antibody, often in the setting of an intercurrent infection. Some patients have persistent false-positive tests on repeat screening, but many have a negative screening test on repeat evaluation. For patients with discordant results suggesting a false-positive screen, a repeat screening test may be performed after 3 months to help guide the interpretation of HIV surveillance testing in the future.[6]

GOAL 2: ASSESS DEGREE OF IMMUNOSUPPRESSION
CD4 Cell Count

The CD4 cell count with percentage is the most helpful test to characterize the degree of immunosuppression in patients with active HIV. Patients with CD4 cell counts less than 200 cells/μL are at increased risk for opportunistic infections, with the greatest risk less than 50 cells/μL. Although all patients with HIV should be treated with ART, the absolute CD4 count can help guide urgency for treatment initiation.[7]

The degree of immunosuppression helps clinicians guide prophylactic antibiotics. For patients with CD4 cell counts less than 200 cells/μL, primary prophylaxis against *Pneumocystis jirovecii* should be initiated and continued until CD4 cell count is greater than 200 cells/μL.

The CD4 cell count also helps to guide timing for vaccine administration. There are two considerations for appropriate timing of vaccines: safety and efficacy. Live vaccines including measles, mumps, and rubella, yellow fever vaccine, and Zostavax, should not be administered to patients with CD4 cell count less than 200 cells/μL because of the risk of disease acquisition.[8] For vaccines that are T-lymphocyte dependent, antibody development relies on the patient's CD4 cell count and function. Although inactivated vaccines, such as the conjugate pneumonia vaccine, hepatitis A vaccine, and hepatitis B vaccine, are considered safe in individuals with low CD4 cell count, antibody response is more robust when CD4 cell count is greater than

Table 1
Routine tests, and when they are recommended

Laboratory Test	At Entry to Care	Follow-up, CD4 <200 cells/μL or AIDS	Follow-up, Stable on ART, CD4 >200 cells/μL	Virologic Failure	Regimen Change
			Time Point		
HIV RNA	Yes	Every 1–3 mo until virologically suppressed	Every 6 mo	Every 4–6 wk until virologically suppressed	4–6 wk after change
CD4 count	Yes	Every 1–3 mo	Yearly until CD4 >300 cells/μL, then no longer indicated	Repeat at time of virologic failure; trend if <200 cells/μL or persistent viremia	Not indicated if remains virologically suppressed
Standard genotype	Yes	No	No	Yes	Not indicated if remains virologically suppressed
HLA B*5701	Yes, if ABC included in regimen; consider in all patients	No	No	No	Yes, if ABC included in new regimen and not performed at entry to care
G6PD	Yes	No	No	No	No
CBC, BMP, LFTs	Yes	Every 1–3 mo	Every 6 mo	Yes	4–6 wk after change

(continued on next page)

Table 1 (continued)

		Time Point			
Laboratory Test	At Entry to Care	Follow-up, CD4 <200 cells/µL or AIDS	Follow-up, Stable on ART, CD4 >200 cells/µL	Virologic Failure	Regimen Change
Urinalysis	Yes	Every 1–3 mo if TDF or TAF included in ART	Every 6 mo if TDF or TAF included in ART	Yes	At time of change and repeat 4–6 wk after change if TDF or TAF included in ART
Urine hCG	Yes, women of childbearing age	As indicated by pregnancy risk	As indicated by pregnancy risk	As indicated by pregnancy risk	As indicated by pregnancy risk
TST or IGRA	Yes	No	Repeat once if initial test performed at CD4 <200 cells/µL	No	No
Hepatitis B serology (anti-HBs, anti-HBc, HB SAg)	Yes	No	No	No	No
Hepatitis A serology (HAV IgG)	Yes	No	No	No	No
Hepatitis C serology (HCV Ab)	Yes	No	Every 6–12 mo for MSM at risk for STI, people who inject drugs	No	No
GC, chlamydia (all appropriate sites)	Yes	Every 3 mo to yearly; frequency depends on risk	Every 3 mo to yearly; frequency depends on risk	No	No

Syphilis (treponemal Ab or RPR)	Yes	Every 3 mo to yearly; frequency depends on risk	Every 3 mo to yearly; frequency depends on risk	No
Toxoplasma IgG CMV IgG, varicella IgG	Yes	No	No	No
HgbA$_{1c}$, lipid panel	Yes	Yearly	Yearly	No
Cervical cytology, HPV (women)	Yes	Yearly	Every 1–3 y	No
Anal cytology (MSM, women who practice anal sex)	Yes	Yearly	Every 1–3 y	No
DEXA	No	No	Age 50 for patients on TDF or TAF	No

Abbreviations: ABC, abacavir; BMP, basic metabolic panel; CBC, complete blood count; GC, gonorrhea; CMV, cytomegalovirus; G6PD, glucose-6-phosphate dehydrogenase; HAV, hepatitis A virus; hCG, human chorionic gonadotropin; HCV, hepatitis C virus; HgbA$_{1c}$, hemoglobin A$_{1c}$; HPV, human papilloma virus; IGRA, interferon-γ release assay; LFT, liver function test; MSM, men who have sex with men; RPR, rapid plasma reagin; STI, sexually transmitted infection; TAF, tenofovir alafenamide; TDF, tenofovir disoproxil fumarate; TST, tuberculin skin test.

Table 2
Tests that are not routinely recommended for all patients

Test	When Should These Tests Be Ordered?
Repeat HIV screening test	Only if confirmatory HIV RNA is undetectable
Integrase genotype	At entry to care for patients who acquired HIV from someone on INSTI or with known INSTI resistance Virologic failure while on INSTI
CCR5/CXCR4 tropism assay	If entry inhibitor is being considered for salvage therapy
Chest radiograph	Positive screening test for latent tuberculosis (TST or IGRA) Guided by symptoms
Serum cryptococcal antigen	Symptomatic patients with CD4 count <100 cells/μL
Lumbar puncture	Positive syphilis test in a patient with neurologic or ocular symptoms As guided by neurologic symptoms and degree of immunosuppression

Abbreviations: IGRA, interferon-γ release assay; INSTI, integrase inhibitor; TST, tuberculin skin test.

200 cells/μL.[9] Many clinicians choose to defer immunizations until patients are on ART and have had significant immune reconstitution to optimize immunologic response to vaccines. Finally, the CD4 cell count can help estimate the duration of infection. After a transient drop at the time of acute infection, the CD4 cell count typically returns near to baseline and declines steadily at a mean rate between 20 and 50 cells/μL per year in patients not on ART.[10] Although the rate of decline varies by patient, a low CD4 count typically correlates with a longer duration of infection.

GOAL 3: PREPARE FOR TREATMENT

It is well understood that HIV-infected individuals on ART cannot transmit the virus if they are virologically suppressed, and patients on ART have better health outcomes regardless of the degree of immunosuppression.[11,12] In the modern era of simple, well-tolerated, and highly effective ART regimens, all patients with HIV should be initiated on treatment at the time of diagnosis with few caveats. The following laboratory tests are helpful to guide appropriate choice of initial ART and plan for alternative future regimens in case of side effects.

Human Immunodeficiency Virus Resistance Testing

Standard HIV genotype is recommended at the time of diagnosis for all patients to assess for transmitted drug resistance. Resistance tests are most reliable when performed soon after HIV acquisition. In chronic HIV infection, over time resistant mutant strains may revert to wild-type virus. The resistant virus persists in the host HIV reservoir and can have an impact on response to therapy, but it may be present at levels too low for detection by standard genotype assays.[13]

It should be noted that the standard genotype does not assess for resistance to integrase inhibitors (INSTIs). Transmitted resistance to INSTIs is rare, so obtaining an integrase genotype at the time of diagnosis is not currently recommended, although this may change with increased use of INSTIs in clinical practice.[14] Baseline integrase genotype should be considered in a patient who may have acquired HIV from an individual who is currently on treatment with INSTIs or has a known history of INSTI resistance.

With INSTI-based regimens as preferred first-line therapy, results of standard genotype at the time of diagnosis typically do not influence first-line ART. The results are more relevant for second-line ART selection for people who experience an adverse event on INSTIs or require an ART switch for an alternative reason. A recent analysis shows that in the current era of INSTI-based ART, the standard genotype is not cost-effective.[15] Guidelines continue to support obtaining a genotype at baseline, but this is an area of active controversy.

HIV genotype should also be obtained for patients who are experiencing virologic failure (as defined by HIV RNA >200 copies/μL) on their current regimen to help guide changes in ART. If patients are failing therapy that includes an INSTI, an integrase genotype must be performed in addition to standard genotype.

HLA B*5701

The presence of this HLA haplotype is associated with a high risk for hypersensitivity to abacavir, a potentially life-threatening adverse reaction. As a result, abacavir is contraindicated in individuals who are HLA B*5701 positive. Some clinicians obtain baseline HLA B*5701 testing even for patients who will not be started on abacavir in their initial regimen to plan for alternative regimens in the future should patients experience adverse effects on their first-line therapy; others defer this testing until abacavir treatment is being considered.[16,17]

Glucose-6-Phosphate Dehydrogenase Deficiency

Screening for glucose-6-phosphate dehydrogenase deficiency is recommended before starting patients on an oxidant drug, such as dapsone, primaquine, or sulfonamides. Black men and women and men from the Mediterranean, India, and Southeast Asia have a higher prevalence of glucose-6-phosphate dehydrogenase deficiency, so a reasonable approach is targeted testing in these populations either at entry to care or before starting one of these medications.[18]

CCR5/CXCR4 Tropism Assay

Tropism assay should be performed for patients who are being considered for treatment with maraviroc.[19] This CCR5 antagonist is rarely used today, except in the rare patient with multiclass resistance, or in patients who have an adverse reaction to multiple alternative classes of medications. Because this class of medications is infrequently needed, a tropism assay is not recommended for patients at entry to care.

"Safety" Laboratory Tests

The following laboratory tests should be obtained help to characterize the health status of the patient, establish baseline values that can be monitored on therapy, and determine any complications related to HIV infection.

- Complete blood count at the time of diagnosis may show leukopenia, anemia, and thrombocytopenia, all of which are common in patients with HIV infection.
- Basic metabolic panel and urinalysis should be obtained for initial assessment of renal function. Presence of chronic kidney disease or proteinuria may alter the choice of ART, and renal function must be monitored while on therapy especially for patients on regimens that include tenofovir disoproxil fumarate (TDF) or tenofovir alafenamide (TAF).

- Liver function tests should be evaluated to establish a baseline before starting treatment. Elevation in baseline transaminases should raise consideration for viral hepatitis coinfection. Drug-induced liver injury is an uncommon but well characterized side effect of several antiretrovirals, so transaminases should be monitored intermittently when patients are on ART.
- Urinary human chorionic gonadotropin (hCG) should be performed in all women of childbearing age. Nonpregnant women should have a detailed discussion regarding birth control options, and should have yearly pregnancy test or more frequently depending on sexual behavior/risk. Pregnant women or women desiring pregnancy should have an informed discussion with a clinician about the risks of HIV for the patient and the fetus, and pregnancy may alter the choice of ART.

GOAL 4: EVALUATE FOR COINFECTIONS, AND PRIOR EXPOSURES

Patients with HIV are at higher risk for additional infections for multiple reasons. First, many infections are transmitted via the same route as HIV, so behavior that exposed the patient to HIV also introduces risk for other sexually transmitted or blood-borne diseases. Second, patients with HIV may be at increased risk for additional infections because of host immunosuppression, which is influenced by the absolute CD4 cell count and uncontrolled viremia. It is important to assess for concomitant infections at the time of HIV diagnosis, and screen for prior exposures to characterize the patient's risk for future primary infections and the risk of reactivation of latent infections.

Sexually Transmitted Infections

Gonorrhea and chlamydia
Nucleic acid amplification tests have the highest sensitivity for diagnosis of gonorrhea and chlamydia. For diagnosis of genital infections, urine tests are available for women and men. However, vaginal and cervical swabs have a higher sensitivity than urine tests in women and are the preferred screening modality.[20] Self-collected vaginal swabs have excellent sensitivity and specificity, so this should be an option depending on patient preference.[21] Screening for extragenital infections is particularly important in patients who practice receptive anal and/or oral intercourse. Although clinicians often consider extragenital infections in men who have sex with men (MSM), pharyngeal and rectal infections in women who practice oral or anal intercourse are underrecognized and often go undiagnosed.[22-24]

Syphilis
There is a high rate of syphilis in HIV-infected individuals, especially among MSM.[25] This is because of the similar mode of transmission of both infections, and enhanced transmission of one infection in the setting of the other.[26] The presentation of syphilis in patients with HIV individuals is similar as in HIV-uninfected individuals, although atypical and aggressive presentations of syphilis are more common in patients who have HIV.[27] Testing is performed with a traditional two-step algorithm (nontreponemal test, such as rapid plasma reagin (RPR), followed by confirmatory treponemal test) or a reverse algorithm (treponemal enzyme immunoassay followed by confirmatory RPR and an additional antitreponemal test). A lumbar puncture should be considered in patients who have a positive test along with neurologic or ocular symptoms to evaluate for neurosyphilis, but does not need to be performed for asymptomatic individuals.

Hepatitis C
The rate of sexual transmission of hepatitis C virus (HCV) in the general population is low, but significantly higher in HIV-infected individuals, especially MSM.[28,29] HCV

antibody should be included as part of sexually transmitted disease screening in this population. Because prior infection does not confer immunity, HCV viral load should be considered in patients with a history of treated or cleared infection with ongoing sexual risk factors.

Frequency of testing
The interval for testing for all sexually transmitted infections depends on the patient's sexual risk factors. Sexually active patients should be screened at least once yearly, but for patients with high-risk sexual behavior, screening every 3 to 6 months may be indicated. This includes patients with multiple anonymous sexual partners, commercial sex workers, or patients whose primary partner has multiple additional sex partners.

Viral Hepatitis

Hepatitis B
Evaluation for hepatitis B virus (HBV) is important for two reasons. First, HIV/HBV co-infection is associated with rapid progression of liver fibrosis.[30,31] Second, the presence of HBV coinfection may have an impact on choice of initial ART regimen. Tenofovir is highly effective against HBV, even in the setting of multidrug-resistant HBV infection, so most patients should be treated with a tenofovir-containing regimen.[32] Patients should be screened for evidence of chronic hepatitis B infection and/or prior immunity with hepatitis B surface antibody, hepatitis B surface antigen, and hepatitis B core antibody. Individuals who are nonimmune should be vaccinated. All patients with chronic HBV (hepatitis B surface antigen positive) should be treated with tenofovir-containing HIV regimens; TDF and TAF are both active against HBV, with the latter having better renal and bone safety.

Hepatitis C
Similar to HIV/HBV coinfection, HIV accelerates the course of HCV-related chronic liver disease.[33] HIV/HCV-coinfected patients suffer more liver-related morbidity and mortality, nonhepatic organ dysfunction, and overall mortality than HCV-monoinfected patients.[34,35] Direct-acting antivirals for HCV are highly effective with similar rates of HCV eradication in people with and without HIV.[36] Patients should be screened with an HCV antibody, and clinicians should be aware of potential drug interactions between ART for HIV and direct-acting antivirals for HCV.

Hepatitis A
Patients should be screened for immunity to hepatitis A virus (HAV) with a hepatitis A IgG antibody test. HAV vaccination is recommended for susceptible HIV-infected individuals (HAV IgG negative) with an additional risk factor, such as chronic liver disease, injection drug use, MSM, homelessness, or travel to a hepatitis A endemic area. Given the recent hepatitis A outbreaks along with the availability and safety of the vaccine, it is reasonable to vaccinate all susceptible individuals.[37,38]

Tuberculosis

Tuberculosis (TB) is a leading cause of morbidity and mortality in HIV-infected individuals globally, although it is uncommon in the United States and Canada.[39] Patients with HIV are at higher risk for reactivation of latent TB (LTBI).[40] All patients with HIV should be evaluated for LTBI with either a tuberculin skin test (TST) or interferon-γ release assay (IGRA). A history of bacillus Calmette-Guérin vaccination can cause a positive TST, so IGRAs are favored in patients who have received the vaccine. The sensitivity of the TST and IGRA are decreased in the setting of low CD4 cell count, so for patients who are immunocompromised at the time of diagnosis, repeat screening should be performed once the CD4 cell count is greater than 200/μL. Repeat screening should be performed yearly thereafter only in patients who have ongoing exposure to TB-infected individuals, such as health care workers.

If a screening test is positive, patients should be queried about history of TB exposure and evaluated for active disease with a clinical history, physical examination, and chest radiograph. Treatment of LTBI is indicated in all HIV-infected individuals.

Toxoplasma

Prior exposure to toxoplasmosis should be evaluated with toxoplasma IgG. Seropositive patients are at risk of reactivation disease if severely immunosuppressed (CD4 cell counts <100), and need primary prophylaxis until they respond to ART. Patients who are seronegative should be counseled regarding risk factors for acquisition, including exposure to cat feces, gardening, and eating undercooked meat.[41] People with HIV need not part with their cats or have their cats tested for toxoplasmosis.

Cytomegalovirus

In the Western world, the rate of cytomegalovirus (CMV) positivity is high among people with HIV, but patients with a negative CMV IgG are at risk for primary infection, which is particularly severe in immunocompromised individuals.[42] Patients who are seronegative should receive CMV-negative or leukocyte-reduced blood products if they need a blood transfusion. Patients should also be counseled that CMV is sexually transmitted, so barrier protection for sex with new partners is advised until immune reconstitution has occurred.[43]

Varicella

Most individuals in the United States are seropositive for varicella (varicella IgG positive), either from primary infection or through vaccination. Although universal vaccination was recommended in the United States in 1995, it has not been adopted worldwide, so patients born outside the United States may not have received the vaccine. Primary infection is less common in the postvaccine era, so individuals who were not vaccinated during childhood or received only one dose of the vaccine may remain susceptible to infection.[44]

Varicella vaccine is a live vaccine and should be avoided in patients who are immunocompromised. HIV-infected individuals without evidence of immunity may be vaccinated if CD4 count is greater than 200 cells/μL. Susceptible individuals with CD4 count less than 200 cells/μL should be considered for treatment with varicella immunoglobulin (VariZIG) after a suspected exposure to an individual with primary varicella, or to an individual with reactivation (herpes zoster) with open lesions.[45]

Cryptococcal Antigen

Evaluation for disseminated cryptococcal infection with cryptococcal antigen from the serum and cerebrospinal fluid should be considered in symptomatic patients with CD4 count less than 100 cells/μL.[46] In highly endemic areas, such as sub-Saharan Africa, some recommend screening even asymptomatic individuals with a serum cryptococcal antigen. However, in developing countries, routine serum cryptococcal antigen in asymptomatic individuals or patients with CD4 count greater than 100 cells/μL is not recommended.

Imaging

There are no routine radiology studies needed for asymptomatic individuals, and imaging should only be ordered for patients with additional indications. Chest radiograph should be performed for patients who are diagnosed with LTBI. For patients with CD4 count less than 200 cells/μL, clinicians should have a low threshold to pursue appropriate targeted imaging for symptomatic individuals.

GOAL 5: MONITORING RESPONSE TO TREATMENT AND EVALUATING FOR SIDE EFFECTS

Testing for treatment monitoring is divided into laboratory testing for efficacy and safety.

Efficacy Laboratory Tests

Human immunodeficiency virus RNA

Pretreatment viral load is considered the patient's "baseline." Follow-up quantitative HIV RNA tests performed after initiation of therapy are compared with the baseline viral load to assess treatment efficacy and is a helpful marker of patient adherence. Viral load declines rapidly after initiation of ART, especially with INSTI-based therapy.[47] Clinicians should repeat a viral load 4 to 6 weeks after initiation of therapy and then every 1 to 3 months until viral suppression is achieved. Once patients are stable on therapy, the viral load should be monitored every 6 months, or more frequently after any change in regimen.

CD4 cell count

Recovery of CD4 cell count after treatment initiation is less predictable than the decline in HIV viral load. There are many factors that contribute to the pace of immune recovery including age, duration of infection, baseline CD4 count, and baseline HIV viral load.[48,49] The rate of recovery is typically greatest at the onset of therapy, and continues at mean rate of 50 to 100 cells/μL until steady state is achieved.[50] Some studies show that CD4 recovery may continue greater than 10 years later.[51] Clinicians should be aware that CD4 count naturally fluctuates and is affected by some medications and intercurrent illnesses. For patients with a CD4 cell count less than 200 cells/μL, serial testing every 1 to 3 months is recommended to track immune reconstitution and to guide the need for ongoing prophylactic medications. Once patients have achieved a stable CD4 cell count greater than 300 cells/μL, routine monitoring is no longer recommended because the results do not change clinical management.[8] Some patients continue to request the test, but they should be informed that variation in the CD4 cell count does not warrant changes in ART provided viral suppression is maintained.

Safety Laboratory Tests

All patients should be monitored with complete blood count, basic metabolic panel, and liver function tests while on therapy to track abnormalities attributed to HIV infection and assess for medication side effects. Urinalysis should also be obtained for patients on tenofovir-based therapy. Safety laboratory studies should be monitored 4 to 6 weeks after treatment initiation or change in ART. For patients who are stable on therapy, safety laboratory studies can be obtained every 6 months.

GOAL 6: PREVENTATIVE CARE AND HEALTH PROMOTION

Improvement in life expectancy for patients with HIV is largely caused by the effectiveness of modern ART, but can also be attributed to engagement in routine health care and enhanced preventative measures. All patients with HIV should have the following preventative tests.

- Hemoglobin A_{1c}: There is an increased prevalence of diabetes in patients with HIV.[52] Hemoglobin A_{1c} should be obtained at entry to care and repeated yearly thereafter in patients considered to be at high risk for diabetes.
- Lipid panel: As infectious complications of HIV have become less common with current ART, cardiovascular disease has become a leading driver of morbidity and mortality. Patients with HIV are at increased risk of cardiovascular disease because of increased inflammation and immune activation. Although the risk is highest in patients with circulating virus, cardiovascular risk is increased even in patients who are on suppressive ART.[53] Patients should have a lipid panel at the time of diagnosis and yearly thereafter with aggressive lipid management to decrease cardiovascular risk.
- Bone density (DEXA) scan: HIV and its treatment reduce bone density. As a result, all patients should undergo evaluation of bone density at age 50.[54] Tenofovir-containing regimens in particular may lower bone density; the risk is lower with TAF compared with TDF, but active surveillance for osteoporosis is still recommended.[55]
- Tobacco screening: Epidemiologic studies show an increased risk of lung cancer in patients with HIV.[56] All patients with HIV should be screened for tobacco use, and provided appropriate resources to assist in smoking cessation.
- Cervical cancer screening: Abnormal cervical cytology secondary to human papilloma virus (HPV) infection is 10 to 11 times higher in HIV-infected women as compared with the general population with increased risk correlating with lower CD4 count.[57,58] Women should have cervical pap smears every 1 to 3 years, with more intensive follow-up if abnormal results are identified.
- Anal cancer screening: HIV-infected individuals who practice receptive anal intercourse are at increased risk for HPV-related anal dysplasia.[59] Anal pap smear with reflex to HPV cotesting is recommended in this population. This is most relevant for MSM, but an underrecognized risk group is HIV-infected women who practice anal sex. A careful and sensitive sexual history can help identify women who are candidates for cervical and anal cancer screening. The appropriate interval for screening is not known but most clinicians perform anal pap smears every 1 to 3 years.
- Age-appropriate cancer screening: There is no change in recommended surveillance for colorectal cancer, prostate cancer, breast cancer, or lung cancer for patients with HIV infection.

SUMMARY

Laboratory testing is an essential component of care to guide treatment of HIV and monitor patients on therapy. An organized approach to laboratory ordering can help clinicians to understand the utility of each test, ensure a comprehensive evaluation, and decrease the use of unnecessary tests. A scaffold that reinforces the model of chronic disease management is a tool to educate patients about the natural history of disease, engage patients as active participants in their care, and empower patients with HIV to live healthy lives.

REFERENCES

1. Deeks SG, Lewin SR, Havlir DV. The end of AIDS: HIV infection as a chronic disease. Lancet 2013;382(9903):1525.

2. Nakagawa F, May M, Phillips A. Life expectancy living with HIV: recent estimates and future implications. Curr Opin Infect Dis 2013;26(1):17–25.
3. Samji H, Cescon A, Hogg RS, et al. Closing the gap: increases in life expectancy among treated HIV-positive individuals in the United States and Canada. PLoS One 2013;8(12):e81355.
4. Quinn TC, Wawer MJ, Sewankambo N, et al. Viral load and heterosexual transmission of human immunodeficiency virus type 1. Rakai Project Study Group. N Engl J Med 2000;342(13):921–9.
5. Kim S, Lee J-H, Choi JY, et al. False-positive rate of a "fourth-generation" HIV antigen/antibody combination assay in an area of low HIV prevalence. Clin Vaccine Immunol 2010;17(10):1642–4.
6. Centers for Disease Control and Prevention (U.S.), Bernard MB, Association of Public Health Laboratories, et al. Laboratory testing for the diagnosis of HIV infection: updated recommendations. Atlanta (GA): Centers for Disease Control and Prevention; 2014. https://doi.org/10.15620/cdc.23447. Accessed November 26, 2018.
7. Panel on Antiretroviral Guidelines for Adults and Adolescents. Guidelines for the use of antiretroviral agents in adults and adolescents living with HIV. Department of Health and Human Services. Available at: http://www.aidsinfo.nih.gov/ContentFiles/AdultandAdolescentGL.pdf. Accessed November 26, 2018.
8. Panel on Opportunistic Infections in HIV-Infected Adults and Adolescents. Guidelines for the prevention and treatment of opportunistic infections in HIV-infected adults and adolescents: recommendations from the Centers for Disease Control and Prevention, the National Institutes of Health, and the HIV Medicine Association of the Infectious Diseases Society of America. Available at: http://aidsinfo.nih.gov/contentfiles/lvguidelines/adult_oi.pdf. Accessed December 22, 2018.
9. Kroon FP, van Dissel JT, de Jong JC, et al. Antibody response to influenza, tetanus and pneumococcal vaccines in HIV-seropositive individuals in relation to the number of CD4+ lymphocytes. AIDS 1994;8(4):469–76. Available at: https://www.ncbi.nlm.nih.gov/pubmed/7912086.
10. Patrikar S, Basannar DR, Bhatti VK, et al. Rate of decline in CD4 count in HIV patients not on antiretroviral therapy. Armed Forces Med J India 2014;70(2):134.
11. Rodger AJ, Cambiano V, Bruun T, et al. Sexual activity without condoms and risk of HIV transmission in serodifferent couples when the HIV-positive partner is using suppressive antiretroviral therapy. JAMA 2016;316(2):171–81.
12. INSIGHT START Study Group, Lundgren JD, Babiker AG, Gordin F, et al. Initiation of antiretroviral therapy in early asymptomatic HIV infection. N Engl J Med 2015;373(9):795–807.
13. Castro H, Pillay D, Cane P, et al. Persistence of HIV-1 transmitted drug resistance mutations. J Infect Dis 2013;208(9):1459–63.
14. Kim Y, Chin BS, Kim G, et al. Integrase strand transfer inhibitor resistance mutations in antiretroviral treatment-naïve patients in Korea: a prospective, observational study. J Korean Med Sci 2018;33(25). https://doi.org/10.3346/jkms.2018.33.e173.
15. Hyle E, Scott J, Sax P et al. Baseline resistance testing in the current treatment era – no longer cost-effective? Abstract presented at: International AIDS Conference. Amsterdam, the Netherlands, July 23-27, 2018.
16. Ma JD, Lee KC, Kuo GM. HLA-B*5701 testing to predict abacavir hypersensitivity. PLoS Curr 2010;2:RRN1203.
17. Mallal S, Phillips E, Carosi G, et al. HLA-B*5701 screening for hypersensitivity to abacavir. N Engl J Med 2008;358(6):568–79.

18. Tungsiripat M, Drechsler H, Sarlone C, et al. Prevalence and significance of G6PD deficiency in patients of an urban HIV clinic. J Int Assoc Physicians AIDS Care 2008;7(2):88–90.

19. Soriano V, Geretti AM, Perno C-F, et al. Optimal use of maraviroc in clinical practice. AIDS 2008;22(17):2231–40.

20. Centers for Disease Control and Prevention. Recommendations for the laboratory-based detection of Chlamydia trachomatis and Neisseria gonorrhoeae–2014. MMWR Recomm Rep 2014;63(RR-02):1–19. Available at: https://www.ncbi.nlm.nih.gov/pubmed/24622331.

21. Lunny C, Taylor D, Hoang L, et al. Self-collected versus clinician-collected sampling for chlamydia and gonorrhea screening: a systemic review and meta-analysis. PLoS One 2015;10(7):e0132776.

22. Danby CS, Cosentino LA, Rabe LK, et al. Patterns of extragenital chlamydia and gonorrhea in women and men who have sex with men reporting a history of receptive anal intercourse. Sex Transm Dis 2016;43(2):105–9.

23. Bazan JA, Carr Reese P, Esber A, et al. High prevalence of rectal gonorrhea and Chlamydia infection in women attending a sexually transmitted disease clinic. J Womens Health 2015;24(3):182–9.

24. Llata E, Braxton J, Asbel L, et al. Rectal Chlamydia trachomatis and Neisseria gonorrhoeae infections among women reporting anal intercourse. Obstet Gynecol 2018;132(3):692–7.

25. Sexually transmitted disease surveillance 2017. Available at: https://www.cdc.gov/std/stats17/2017-STD-Surveillance-Report_CDC-clearance-9.10.18.pdf. Accessed November 26, 2018.

26. Solomon MM, Mayer KH, Glidden DV, et al. Syphilis predicts HIV incidence among men and transgender women who have sex with men in a preexposure prophylaxis trial. Clin Infect Dis 2014;59(7):1020–6.

27. Zetola NM, Klausner JD. Syphilis and HIV infection: an update. Clin Infect Dis 2007;44(9):1222–8.

28. Bradshaw D, Matthews G, Danta M. Sexually transmitted hepatitis C infection: the new epidemic in MSM? Curr Opin Infect Dis 2013;26(1):66–72.

29. van de Laar TJW, Matthews GV, Prins M, et al. Acute hepatitis C in HIV-infected men who have sex with men: an emerging sexually transmitted infection. AIDS 2010;24(12):1799–812.

30. Hawkins C, Christian B, Fabian E, et al. Brief report: HIV/HBV coinfection is a significant risk factor for liver fibrosis in Tanzanian HIV-infected adults. J Acquir Immune Defic Syndr 2017;76(3):298–302.

31. Thio CL, Seaberg EC, Skolasky R Jr, et al. HIV-1, hepatitis B virus, and risk of liver-related mortality in the Multicenter Cohort Study (MACS). Lancet 2002;360(9349):1921–6. Available at: https://www.ncbi.nlm.nih.gov/pubmed/12493258.

32. Lee HW, Park JY, Lee JW, et al. Long-term efficacy of tenofovir disoproxil fumarate monotherapy for multidrug-resistant chronic HBV infection. Clin Gastroenterol Hepatol 2018. https://doi.org/10.1016/j.cgh.2018.10.037.

33. Hernandez MD, Sherman KE. HIV/hepatitis C coinfection natural history and disease progression. Curr Opin HIV AIDS 2011;6(6):478–82.

34. Lo Re V 3rd, Kallan MJ, Tate JP, et al. Hepatic decompensation in antiretroviral-treated patients co-infected with HIV and hepatitis C virus compared with hepatitis C virus-monoinfected patients: a cohort study. Ann Intern Med 2014;160(6):369–79.

35. Chen T-Y, Ding EL, Seage GR Iii, et al. Meta-analysis: increased mortality associated with hepatitis C in HIV-infected persons is unrelated to HIV disease progression. Clin Infect Dis 2009;49(10):1605–15.
36. Bhattacharya D, Belperio PS, Shahoumian TA, et al. Effectiveness of all-oral antiviral regimens in 996 human immunodeficiency virus/hepatitis C virus genotype 1-coinfected patients treated in routine practice. Clin Infect Dis 2017;64(12): 1711–20.
37. Freidl GS, Sonder GJ, Bovée LP, et al. Hepatitis A outbreak among men who have sex with men (MSM) predominantly linked with the EuroPride, the Netherlands, July 2016 to February 2017. Euro Surveill 2017;22(8). https://doi.org/10.2807/ 1560-7917.ES.2017.22.8.30468.
38. Iverson SA, Narang J, Garcia MJ, et al. Hepatitis A outbreak among persons experiencing homelessness—Maricopa County, Arizona, 2017. Open Forum Infect Dis 2017;4(Suppl 1):S245.
39. WHO | Global tuberculosis report 2018. 2018. Available at: https://www.who.int/ tb/publications/global_report/en/. Accessed December 10, 2018.
40. Shea KM, Steve Kammerer J, Winston CA, et al. Estimated rate of reactivation of latent tuberculosis infection in the United States, overall and by population subgroup. Am J Epidemiol 2014;179(2):216.
41. Basavaraju A. Toxoplasmosis in HIV infection: an overview. Trop Parasitol 2016; 6(2):129–35.
42. Adland E, Klenerman P, Goulder P, et al. Ongoing burden of disease and mortality from HIV/CMV coinfection in Africa in the antiretroviral therapy era. Front Microbiol 2015;6:1016.
43. Gianella S, Scheffler K, Mehta SR, et al. Seminal shedding of CMV and HIV transmission among men who have sex with men. Int J Environ Res Public Health 2015;12(7):7585–92.
44. Papaloukas O, Giannouli G, Papaevangelou V. Successes and challenges in varicella vaccine. Ther Adv Vaccines 2014;2(2):39–55.
45. FDA approval of an extended period for administering VariZIG for postexposure prophylaxis of varicella. Available at: https://www.cdc.gov/mmwr/preview/ mmwrhtml/mm6112a4.htm. Accessed December 10, 2018.
46. Warkentien T, Crum-Cianflone NF. An update on *Cryptococcus* among HIV-infected patients. Int J STD AIDS 2010;21(10):679–84.
47. Karen Jacobson OO. Integrase inhibitor-based regimens result in more rapid virologic suppression rates among treatment-naïve human immunodeficiency virus–infected patients compared to non-nucleoside and protease inhibitor–based regimens in a real-world clinical setting: a retrospective cohort study. Medicine 2018;97(43). https://doi.org/10.1097/MD.0000000000013016.
48. Stirrup OT, Copas AJ, Phillips AN, et al. Predictors of CD4 cell recovery following initiation of antiretroviral therapy among HIV-1 positive patients with well-estimated dates of seroconversion. HIV Med 2018;19(3):184–94.
49. Lawn SD, Myer L, Bekker L-G, et al. CD4 cell count recovery among HIV-infected patients with very advanced immunodeficiency commencing antiretroviral treatment in sub-Saharan Africa. BMC Infect Dis 2006;6:59.
50. Kaufmann GR, Perrin L, Pantaleo G, et al. CD4 T-lymphocyte recovery in individuals with advanced HIV-1 infection receiving potent antiretroviral therapy for 4 years: the Swiss HIV Cohort Study. Arch Intern Med 2003;163(18):2187–95.
51. Bishop JD, DeShields S, Cunningham T, et al. CD4 count recovery after initiation of antiretroviral therapy in patients infected with human immunodeficiency virus. Am J Med Sci 2016;352(3):239–44.

52. Samaras K. Prevalence and pathogenesis of diabetes mellitus in HIV-1 infection treated with combined antiretroviral therapy. J Acquir Immune Defic Syndr 2009; 50(5):499–505.
53. Triant VA. Cardiovascular disease and HIV infection. Curr HIV/AIDS Rep 2013; 10(3):199.
54. Philip M, Grant AGC. Tenofovir and bone health. Curr Opin HIV AIDS 2016; 11(3):326.
55. Mills A, Arribas JR, Andrade-Villanueva J, et al. Switching from tenofovir diso-proxil fumarate to tenofovir alafenamide in antiretroviral regimens for virologically suppressed adults with HIV-1 infection: a randomised, active-controlled, multi-centre, open-label, phase 3, non-inferiority study. Lancet Infect Dis 2016;16(1): 43–52.
56. Reddy KP, Kong CY, Hyle EP, et al. Lung cancer mortality associated with smok-ing and smoking cessation among people living with HIV in the United States. JAMA Intern Med 2017;177(11):1613.
57. Paramsothy P, Duerr A, Heilig CM, et al. Abnormal vaginal cytology in HIV-infected and at-risk women after hysterectomy. J Acquir Immune Defic Syndr 2004;35(5):484–91. Available at: https://www.ncbi.nlm.nih.gov/pubmed/15021313.
58. Harris TG, Burk RD, Palefsky JM, et al. Incidence of cervical squamous intraepi-thelial lesions associated with HIV serostatus, CD4 cell counts, and human papil-lomavirus test results. JAMA 2005;293(12):1471–6.
59. Leeds IL, Fang SH. Anal cancer and intraepithelial neoplasia screening: a review. World J Gastrointest Surg 2016;8(1):41–51.

Why Everyone (Almost) with HIV Needs to Be on Treatment
A Review of the Critical Data

Claire E. Farel, MD, MPH*, Ann M. Dennis, MD, MS

KEYWORDS

- HIV • AIDS • Antiretroviral therapy • Rapid start • Treatment as prevention
- Guidelines • CD4

KEY POINTS

- Antiretroviral therapy (ART) is recommended for all individuals with human immunodeficiency virus (HIV), regardless of CD4 count, to reduce the morbidity and mortality associated with HIV infection and to prevent transmission of HIV.
- The evidence for immediate and universal ART is strong, clearly showing individual and population-level benefits, and is supported by all major guidelines groups.
- ART should be initiated as soon as possible after HIV diagnosis, including at the time of diagnosis if feasible and acceptable to the patient.
- ART should be continued without interruption to maintain virologic suppression.
- Delayed ART may be warranted in the setting of active tuberculosis or cryptococcal meningitis; the benefits of treatment of HIV controllers is also unknown.

INTRODUCTION: MOVING BEYOND CD4 COUNT THRESHOLDS

The introduction of potent combination antiretroviral therapy (ART) in the mid-1990s changed the landscape of human immunodeficiency virus (HIV), bringing marked improvements in morbidity and mortality.[1,2] The designation of these regimens as highly active antiretroviral therapy [HAART], represented a shift in how these medications were perceived. ART had evolved from pills that may slow the devastating progress of HIV to regimens that could more reliably and sustainably suppress viral replication and restore a person to health. The development of plasma HIV viral load assays allowed clinicians and people with HIV (PWH) to monitor this progress. In the present

Disclosure: Neither author has any disclosures.
Division of Infectious Diseases, University of North Carolina at Chapel Hill, 130 Mason Farm Road, CB# 7030, Chapel Hill, NC 27599, USA
* Corresponding author.
E-mail address: cfarel@med.unc.edu

day, more than 20 years after the introduction of effective ART, the term ART is routinely used and reflects the current state of the science: all ART is highly active, potent, durable, and generally well tolerated (**Fig. 1**A).

Despite these advances, over the 20 years following the introduction of effective therapy, guidelines remained conflicted on when to initiate ART. Early regimens, following the introduction of protease inhibitors and combination ART, were expensive and carried the risk of adverse effects and resistance caused by incomplete viral suppression. From 1998 until 2000, the US Department of Health and Human Services guidelines recommended that all PWH be offered treatment, but these recommendations were amended, reflecting uncertainty about the optimal use of these powerful and often toxic medications. CD4 thresholds became the focus of efforts to maximize the benefits of ART while minimizing associated risks. Guidelines agreed that PWH with a CD4 threshold less than 200 cells/mm^3 should receive ART. This threshold was then increased to 350 cells/mm^3 from 2006 to 2009, then to 500 cells/mm^3 from 2009 to 2013.

Since 2014, a consensus of landmark studies has justified starting ART regardless of CD4 count and, in many cases, before getting the results of this test. The evidence for immediate and universal ART is strong, clearly showing individual and population-level benefits and is supported by all major guidelines groups (**Table 1**). Altogether, improvements in ART and recognition of its clinical and epidemiologic benefits justify near-universal ART (**Fig. 1**), preferably as soon after the diagnosis of HIV as possible.

This article reviews the evidence supporting near-universal ART regardless of CD4 count and the shift in practice to ART initiation immediately following HIV diagnosis. It provides case-based discussions to explore the evidence behind the current recommendation for ART for all PWH and discusses specific situations showing the rare scenarios in which ART initiation may be delayed.

NEW HUMAN IMMUNODEFICIENCY VIRUS DIAGNOSIS

Case 1: a 21-year-old male college student was diagnosed with HIV when he developed a rash and presented to student health. He was diagnosed concomitantly with secondary syphilis (rapid plasma reagin 1:256) and treated at the local county health department. His most recent negative HIV test was 6 months before HIV diagnosis. Apart from the rash, now resolved, he is asymptomatic. His CD4 is 579 cells/mm^3 (29%), HIV viral load 180,000 copies/μL. He is still on his parents' insurance and worried about medication cost and accidental disclosure. His partner, who accompanies him, is confirmed to be HIV negative.

Clinical Benefits

Initiation of ART as soon as possible after confirmation of HIV diagnosis is beneficial for almost all PWH, with the exception of those with cryptococcal meningitis or tuberculosis (see case 5). Some of the most convincing evidence for this recommendation comes from 2 large clinical trials (Strategic Timing of Antiretroviral Therapy [START] and TEMPRANO), which clearly showed a reduced risk of both AIDS and non-AIDS clinical events among participants who initiated ART at CD4 greater than 500 cells/mm^3 or higher (see **Fig. 1**B).[7,8] **Table 2** summarizes these and other key trials and cohort studies that have shaped current practice.

In considering this patient and his concerns regarding initiating ART, note that, in addition to preventing the progression of HIV, ART reduces HIV-associated immune activation and inflammation, helping to reduce risk of vascular and end-organ damage and malignancy.[8] For a young, asymptomatic patient this may be a less compelling

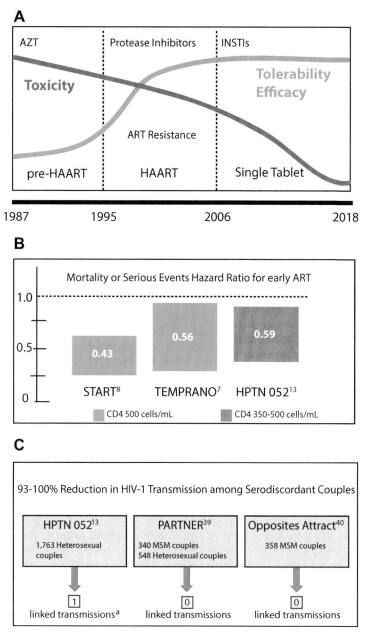

Fig. 1. Summary of major advances and clinical trials supporting universal ART for HIV infection regardless of CD4 count. (*A*) Improvements in ART. The advent of HAART in 1995 led to significant improvements in ART efficacy but initially carried substantial side effects limiting tolerability of regimens. Single-tablet regimens and integrase strand inhibitors changed the landscape of ART after 2006. Modern ART regimens are more potent, durable, and efficacious, with substantially improved tolerability. (*B*) Clinical benefits. Summary of the 3 randomized clinical trials showing significant reductions in mortality or serious adverse events when ART is initiated at higher CD4 cell counts. (*C*) Decreased transmission. Three trials showed substantial reduction in HIV transmission among serodiscordant couples, including men who have sex with men. [a] In HPTN 052, no phylogenetically linked infections were observed when HIV-1 infection was stably suppressed in the HIV-positive partner.[36] INSTI, integrase strand transfer inhibitor.

Table 1
Guideline recommendations: when to start antiretroviral therapy

Current Guidelines	Recommendation
International Antiviral Society -USA Panel 2018[3]	ART is recommended for virtually all individuals infected with HIV, as soon as possible after diagnosis
World Health Organization 2017[4]	Rapid ART initiation should be offered to all people with HIV following a confirmed HIV diagnosis and clinical assessment
US Department of Health and Human Services 2018[5]	ART is recommended for all individuals with HIV, regardless of CD4 count, to reduce the morbidity and mortality associated with HIV infection
European AIDS Clinical Society 2018[6]	ART is recommended in all adults with chronic HIV infection, irrespective of CD4 counts. Rapid start at time of HIV diagnosis is feasible, acceptable, and should be considered when possible

consideration, but ART initiation greatly decreases his risk of further complications and associated hospitalizations.[14] ART initiation is likely to increase his life expectancy; in a recent study, disparity between life expectancy for persons with HIV and without HIV in the United States was reduced from 13.1 to 7.9 years by ART initiation at CD4 greater than or equal to 500 cells/mm^3.[15] Another important benefit of ART for this patient is prevention of transmission of HIV to his current partner or others if he remains virologically suppressed on ART.[13,16] Individual patient readiness to initiate ART is of utmost importance, but every effort should be made to start ART as soon as is feasible. When possible, leveraging support resources within the clinic and community is critical in ensuring ongoing engagement in HIV care. This case also shows the importance of screening for sexually transmitted infections, including viral hepatitides, at the time of HIV testing and at appropriate intervals thereafter.

Medication Cost and Access

This patient's concern about medication cost and insurance implications is common. ART is expensive, with manufacturer wholesale pricing for a typical branded combination regimen averaging more than $3000/mo[5] Most private and federal plans offer full or partial coverage of many acceptable regimens and patient copays may vary depending on plans. Many PWH qualify for resources such as pharmaceutical company copay assistance programs or Ryan White programs such as the AIDS Drug Assistance Program. Team-based support, including nurses, social workers, case managers, and pharmacists, for PWH initiating ART is invaluable in navigating the specific challenges associated with ART initiation and adherence. For this patient, options may include accessing a manufacturer assistance program, seeking independent insurance, or considering participation in a research study if available.

Improvements in Antiretroviral Therapy Tolerability and Efficacy

For most PWH newly initiating ART, a typical regimen consists of a combination of agents from at least 2 classes, usually nucleoside or nucleotide reverse transcriptase inhibitors and integrase strand transfer inhibitors.[3] The pill burden for a new regimen is 1 to 2 pills taken daily, compared with the numerous pills, prominent side effects, and frequent dosing that were hallmarks of earlier generations of ART. Side effects of modern ART, most commonly headache and nausea, generally diminish after the first few weeks of therapy. The integrase strand transfer inhibitor dolutegravir may cause mild neuropsychiatric side effects, including insomnia, but is well tolerated in most patients and rarely requires discontinuation because of side effects. The authors advise

Table 2
Key practice-changing studies influencing recommendations for near-universal antiretroviral therapy

Year Findings Made Public	Study	Key Findings
2006	SMART[9]	Deferred ART initiation until CD4<250 cells/mm^3 was associated with higher morbidity and mortality compared with initiation of ART at CD4 >350 cells/mm^3. Continuous ART prevented both AIDS and non-AIDS events; episodic use of ART increased risk of opportunistic infection or death and did not prevent adverse effects associated with ART
2009	ART CC[10]	Deferred ART initiation until CD4<350 cells/mm^3 was associated with higher mortality than initiation at higher CD4. Earlier ART initiation conferred increased life expectancy
2009	NA-ACCORD[11]	ART initiation in CD4 350–500 cells/mm^3 range decreased mortality vs deferred initiation; mortality reduced further with ART initiation at CD4 >500 cells/mm^3 vs deferred
2010	CIPRA HT 001[12]	ART initiation at CD4>350 cells/mm^3 decreased rates of death and incident tuberculosis compared with deferred initiation at CD4<200 cells/mm^3 among participants in Haiti
2011	HPTN 052[13]	Treatment as prevention: HIV transmission was essentially eliminated in serodiscordant couples when the HIV-positive partner was on ART; morbidity and mortality benefits were seen for partners on ART
2015	TEMPRANO[7]	Early ART (CD4>800 cells/mm^3) and isoniazid preventive therapy independently reduced the risk of severe morbidity among participants in Côte d'Ivoire
2015	START[8]	Immediate ART reduces risk of AIDS and non-AIDS events regardless of CD4 count. Notably, study halted by independent Data and Safety Monitoring Board to recommend that participants in arm deferring ART until CD4 count reached 350 cells/mm^3 should receive ART

involving the patient in decision making in selecting the optimal ART regimen and establishing close follow-up to monitor for any side effects, concerns, or barriers to accessing ART. PWH should be educated regarding the risks of self-discontinuing or modifying ART, including rebound of hepatitis B (if applicable) and concern for development of resistance with inconsistent administration.

DIAGNOSIS DURING ACUTE HUMAN IMMUNODEFICIENCY VIRUS INFECTION: THE CASE FOR URGENT ANTIRETROVIRAL THERAPY INITIATION

Case 2: a 44-year-old previously healthy man presented for evaluation and management of newly diagnosed HIV. He was seen at an emergency department in a nearby town after the acute onset of severe headache, fever of 38.9°C (102°F), arthralgias, loose stools, tremor, malaise, and diaphoresis. He was given supportive care with intravenous fluids and discharged home. His symptoms persisted and he developed a painful pharyngitis. Three days after onset of these symptoms he presented to an urgent care clinic and was prescribed amoxicillin and a brief prednisone taper after rapid testing for HIV, *Streptococcus*, influenza, and mononucleosis were negative. Nine days after his initial symptom onset he was seen by his primary care physician, who noted diffuse lymphadenopathy, lymphopenia (absolute lymphocyte count <1000 cells/mm^3), thrombocytopenia (70,000 platelets/mm^3), and an increased aspartate aminotransferase (AST) of 78 IU/L. Screening HIV antigen/antibody (Ag/Ab) testing was positive, but Multispot was negative. A confirmatory HIV viral load was 750,000 copies/μL, consistent with acute HIV.

Acute or early HIV infection (AHI) is generally defined as the weeks to months following HIV infection before development of antibodies to HIV.[17] Most AHI is symptomatic, although symptoms may be nonspecific and persons with AHI may not seek medical care for their symptoms, or their disclosed history may not prompt HIV testing by medical providers. The increased use of fourth-generation HIV Ag/Ab testing allows a greater proportion of new HIV diagnoses to be identified during the acute period. The importance of HIV diagnosis during AHI is underscored by the increased transmission potential caused by the typically high viral load burden.[17] A study in North Carolina identified AHI using pooled nucleic acid amplification for antibody-negative samples and individual HIV RNA for antibody-indeterminate samples found that 3.4% of individuals diagnosed with HIV during the study time period (2003–2012) had AHI.[18]

Benefit of Antiretroviral Therapy During Acute Human Immunodeficiency Virus Infection: Curbing Human Immunodeficiency Virus Progression and Inflammation

Symptomatic presentation with AHI has been associated with high levels of HIV viremia and more rapid progression of disease, highlighting the importance of immediate ART initiation during this period (**Box 1**).[19] The robust viral replication that occurs in AHI triggers widespread immune cell activation, increases the viral reservoir, and has longer-term implications for disease progression.[20,21] Early ART decreases CD4 and CD8+ T-cell activation and results in smaller HIV proviral DNA and RNA reservoir size.[20,21] CD4 counts typically decline markedly in the setting of AHI and early ART may increase the trajectory and extent of CD4 count recovery, particularly if initiated as close to seroconversion as is possible.[17,22] However, studies to date indicate that ART does attenuate but not fully resolve chronic inflammation.[23] Very early immune damage by HIV is durable and potential irreversible in inflammation biomarker studies (RV254/SEARCH010) and early initiation does not resolve the chronic inflammation associated with all-cause morbidity and mortality risk in treated HIV infection.[23] Nonetheless, early ART initiation attenuates inflammation more than when ART is initiated in chronic HIV infection. However, more research is needed to determine whether reduction in viral reservoir correlates with improvement in end-organ function or other clinical benefits.[24]

Box 1
Initiation of antiretroviral therapy during acute human immunodeficiency virus infection

- May allow greater recovery of CD4+ T-lymphocyte count and function
- Reduction in the latent viral reservoir
- Attenuates but does not fully resolve the chronic inflammation associated with all-cause morbidity and mortality risk in treated HIV infection
- Prevents HIV transmission

Reduction of Latent Viral Reservoir

Early ART limits the size of HIV reservoirs compared with later treatment and may be the necessary foundation for reservoir containment.[21] The size of the viral reservoir during chronic HIV infection is established in early AHI with a set-point viral load reached within the first 2 months.[21] Infection persists in long-lived memory CD4+ T cells in peripheral blood and mononuclear cells in tissues. Initiation of ART during AHI reduces proviral DNA early in infection and with marked reduction in HIV DNA set-point; further, HIV DNA is persistently reduced with continuation of long-term ART.[25] The semen reservoir is established later and more gradually than the blood reservoir; however, the semen viral reservoir is reduced during early ART treatment, thereby reducing the high transmission risk during AHI.[26] The clinical impact of viral load reduction through ART and behavior change has been shown among 88 MSM with AHI in Thailand, where transmission over the first year following infection was estimated to be reduced by 89%.[27]

RAPID ANTIRETROVIRAL THERAPY INITIATION AT HUMAN IMMUNODEFICIENCY VIRUS DIAGNOSIS

Rapid ART is defined as initiation within 14 days of confirmed HIV diagnosis and is a component of a growing movement to facilitate streamlined entry into HIV care with same-day ART initiation.[28–30] There is mounting evidence indicating the benefits of early ART initiation, including initiation of ART on the same day the diagnosis of HIV is confirmed (**Box 2**). Although multiple barriers to initiating rapid ART exist (**Box 3**), persons with no contraindication to early ART should be offered rapid ART initiation. World Health Organization guidelines now recommend ART initiation as soon as possible after an HIV diagnosis is confirmed.[31]

A meta-analysis of 22 studies, including 2 randomized controlled trials (in Haiti and South Africa), 2 cluster randomized trials (in Uganda and Lesotho), and 11 observational studies (in 8 countries including the United States), showed that accelerated ART, including ART started on the day of diagnosis, can lead to improved clinical outcomes.[30] In Haiti, same-day HIV testing and ART initiation were assessed in a randomized controlled trial for PWH with CD4 less than 500 cells/mm^3 and compared with standard ART initiation (approximately 3 weeks after testing).[28] The study found improvements in retention in care with virologic suppression at 12 months (53% vs 44% in the standard group had RNA<50 copies/μL at 12 months).

Two clinic-based studies in the United States show feasibility and reductions in time to virologic suppression.[32,33] In San Francisco, a clinic-based cohort prioritized same-day ART for PWH diagnosed during acute/recent infection or for those with CD4 less than 200 cells/mm^3.[32] The study was successful in starting ART within 24 hours for more than 90% of eligible PWH and found reductions in time to virologic suppression compared with nonintervention PWH. The feasibility and effectiveness of rapid ART

Box 2
Rapid antiretroviral therapy initiation

- Reduces time to viral suppression and confers associated immunologic benefits
- May improve retention in HIV care
- Requires coordinated multidisciplinary services and a commitment to streamline access to ART

Box 3
Challenges to implementing rapid antiretroviral therapy

- PWH may not be ready to initiate ART on the day of diagnosis.
  - Risks and benefits of immediate ART should be offered; rapid ART initiation should be presented as standard of care to maximize therapeutic benefit.
- Securing access to same-day ART supply and a reliable mechanism for ongoing ART supply is challenging.
  - There are numerous bureaucratic barriers to immediate access to ART regardless of payor source; burdensome eligibility requirements for patient assistance programs create further delay.
  - Coordinating rapid ART start is resource intensive and may not be feasible without multidisciplinary collaboration by care teams.
- Health care providers are faced with competing demands during the initial visit.
  - HIV counseling, addressing comorbid psychiatric and medical conditions, addressing substance abuse, food and housing insecurity, and helping PWH navigate insurance and pharmaceutical assistance programs can shift focus from ART initiation.
  - Clear delineation of roles within a multidisciplinary care team may help providers focus on medical issues and ART start.
- Health care providers may be reluctant to start ART without complete laboratory data.
  - Several first-line regimens are appropriate for initiation in the absence of baseline genotypic data. Similarly, prior regimens and laboratory data may be used to guide choice of ART in patients reentering care. The Rapid Entry and ART in Clinic for HIV (REACH) program in Atlanta successfully implemented an ART rapid start program and used provider education to streamline this process.[33]
- Rapid ART start confers additional risk for adverse effects of therapy, particularly among patients with advanced HIV.
  - PWH considered for rapid start of ART should be screened for signs and symptoms of opportunistic infections, particularly cryptococcal meningitis or tuberculosis, to avoid immune reconstitution inflammatory syndrome.
- Early ART initiation raises concern for development of drug resistance.
  - The HIV-CAUSAL collaboration, a large multisite cohort, found a low risk of acquired drug resistance with longer durations of ART, supporting the safety of early initiation of ART.[35]

---

start was also shown in a clinical cohort of mostly uninsured and underinsured PWH in Atlanta.[33] This study found reductions in time to viral suppression and time to first provider visit.[33] Other studies also found shorter time to viral suppression among an observational cohort in San Diego with initiation of ART within 30 days of diagnosis; immediate ART was offered at first intake visit.[34]

PUBLIC HEALTH BENEFITS OF IMMEDIATE ANTIRETROVIRAL THERAPY: TREATMENT AS PREVENTION

Numerous studies have shown that ART markedly reduces risk of HIV transmission from PWH to their partners, eliminating risk of sexual transmission in the setting of durable viral suppression (see **Fig. 1**C).[13,36–39] Widespread recognition of this concept, known as treatment as prevention (TasP), occurred in 2011 with the early release of data from HPTN 052, a large study of serodiscordant, mostly heterosexual couples in 9 countries.[13] The HIV-positive partners in the study were asymptomatic, with CD4 count of 350 to 550 cells/mm^3, and randomized to start ART at time of enrollment versus delaying ART. Early ART reduced rates of sexual transmission of HIV to the uninfected partner by 96%.[13] No phylogenetically linked incident infections were observed when the HIV-positive partners were virologically suppressed (1 transmission event occurred before virologic suppression of the infected partner).[13] The Partners of People on ART-A New Evaluation of the Risks (PARNTER), PARTNER2, and Opposites Attract studies reported strong evidence that TasP is effective among men who have sex with men, with zero linked HIV transmission events among couples in any of these studies.[40–42] Together, these data have formed the basis for the compelling Undetectable = Untransmittable (U=U) campaign, which has gained worldwide support since 2016 and is an important tool in counseling PWH and their partners and reducing stigma associated with HIV.[43]

Despite this galvanizing progress, challenges to implementing universal TasP remain, particularly in areas with highly prevalent and incident HIV. A population-based cohort in a high-HIV-prevalence (30%) district of KwaZulu-Natal, South Africa, showed substantial reductions in household HIV incidence among PWH with immediate eligibility to receive ART (CD4<350 cells/mm^3).[44] However, in the ANRS (French National Agency for Research on AIDS) 12249 TasP trial, performed in the same district, there was no significant difference in cumulative incidence by arms, a finding attributed to low linkage to HIV care and subsequent limited increase in ART coverage.[45] Further analysis of population dynamics in this study revealed that the high incidence of HIV essentially outpaced the benefit of suppressive ART in this population.[46] Although TasP is an immensely promising tool, these results highlight the need for robust linkage and retention efforts for all PWH.

ANTIRETROVIRAL THERAPY AND SPECIAL POPULATIONS
Pregnancy

Case 3: a 24-year-old woman presents after a new diagnosis of HIV in the context of a prenatal visit. Her partner is HIV positive and she is not sure whether he is on ART. Her last HIV test was 2 years before the current visit. This pregnancy is her first. Ultrasonography reveals a fetus at 12 weeks' gestational age. Laboratory results show CD4 446 cells/mm^3 (36%), and HIV RNA 140,000 copies/μL. She is committed to following medical advice to maximize the chances for a healthy baby but is also concerned about toxicity of ART for the fetus.

Reduction of Perinatal Human Immunodeficiency Virus Transmission

Initiation of ART in pregnant women carries particular urgency both to ensure the health of the mother and to prevent perinatal transmission of HIV. Worldwide, enormous strides have been made in reducing mother-to-child transmission of HIV, largely attributable to effective combination ART and maternal virologic suppression.[47] Although viral suppression at the time of delivery is an important focus of monitoring during pregnancy, several studies have also shown that earlier ART initiation, optimally before conception, further reduces risk of transmission.[48,49]

Antiretroviral Therapy and the Developing Fetus

This patient's concern regarding the toxicity of ART for a developing fetus is common and an important consideration. There are a variety of preferred (well-validated) and acceptable (less well-studied, particularly with regard to pharmacokinetics) ART regimens for pregnant women with HIV, and almost any ART regimen is preferred to no ART.[50] Uncontrolled maternal HIV presents the greatest risk to the fetus and is associated with adverse fetal outcomes and transmission risk. However, concerns for ART association with preterm birth and low birth weight merit ongoing monitoring and discussion with the patient.[51] In addition, new data suggesting a possible increased risk of neural tube defects among women in Botswana who took dolutegravir around the time of conception have raised concerns about the use of this medication in the first trimester.[52] HIV-positive women of childbearing age who take dolutegravir and are not on effective contraception should be counseled regarding these findings and switched to alternative ART if appropriate.

Engagement in Care and the Fourth Trimester

Special efforts should be made to ensure engagement in HIV care for pregnant women, using medical case management resources and coordinating HIV and prenatal care visits when possible. A time of particular risk for HIV-positive pregnant women is the so-called fourth trimester postpartum period when engagement in care may flag because of postpartum depression, focus on the infant, and reduced intensity of efforts by medical providers.[53] A recent study in the United States examined retention in HIV care postpartum and found that receiving less than 12 weeks of antenatal ART was negatively associated with HIV care retention at 24 months postpartum, underscoring the importance of efforts to maximize engagement in care throughout the peripartum period.[54] Maintaining adherence to ART is important for all women, but of particular concern in this scenario are women who may experience repeat pregnancies during this time period.

Human Immunodeficiency Virus Controllers

Case 4: a 62-year-old woman presented to establish care after moving from another part of the country. She was referred for her current visit after a hospitalization for abdominal aortic aneurysm repair, at which time she reported a history of HIV. Her past medical history also includes hypertension, mild renal insufficiency, and a history of treated latent tuberculosis infection. She was diagnosed with HIV in 1994 and has never been on ART. She had been told that she has a low viral load and high CD4 count and did not require ART, and has not received care for her HIV in several years. Review of available records reveals that 4 years after HIV diagnosis her CD4 count was 590 cells/mm^3 (45%) and her HIV viral load was less than 400 copies/μL, the lower limit of detection of the assay. Additional CD4 counts over an 8-year period ranged from 500 to 900 cells/mm^3, with HIV viral load measurements less than the level of detection of the assay and most recently less than 50 copies/μL. She is reluctant to initiate ART based on her discussions with her prior HIV medical providers.

A small proportion (<1%) of people with HIV have low or undetectable levels of viral replication and maintain high CD4 counts. This group is referred to as HIV controllers, with those who never have detectable HIV viremia further categorized as elite controllers. Among elite controllers, some HIV replication occurs (although less than the typical limits of detection) and this population shows sequelae of inflammation and immune activation more commonly associated with HIV in their noncontroller counterparts.[55] An examination of coronary atherosclerosis among a group of elite controllers not on ART compared with PWH on ART and HIV-negative controls revealed that rates of coronary artery disease among the elite controllers were comparable with those of the noncontrollers on ART, and some inflammatory markers were higher.[56]

Further, an analysis of non–AIDS-related events and all-cause hospitalizations among elite controllers and other HIV-positive persons on ART showed a 3-fold higher rate of cardiovascular hospitalizations among elite controllers compared with their treated counterparts.[57] Additional studies have shown that ART is of benefit in reducing markers of inflammation and immune activation among elite controllers, likely because of further reduction in viral replication.[58,59] It is concerning that these studies have also shown less CD4 recovery than expected in elite controllers with ART initiation, reflecting possible harm in deferring ART.[60,61]

For this patient, a careful discussion of these data is warranted. Conceptually, initiating a medication without measurable benefit on standard laboratory monitoring (eg, HIV RNA) may be a difficult case to make, particularly given the counseling she received in the past. Given her evolving clinical status with regard to her vascular disease (including her chronic renal insufficiency), the authors recommend focusing on ART as a component of health optimization and a logical measure in an effort to avoid further vascular inflammation. For PWH with less dramatic and demonstrable vascular disease or other comorbidities, the opportunity to prevent so-called silent vascular damage, malignancy, and other sequelae of inflammation and immune activation should be discussed. If ART is not initiated, regular engagement in HIV care is recommended to monitor for viremia and to assess readiness to initiate ART.

WHEN SHOULD ANTIRETROVIRAL THERAPY BE DELAYED?

Case 5: a 40-year-old man was brought to the emergency department by his family because of confusion. He reported mild headaches and weight loss over the prior 2 weeks, and had an abrupt onset of severe headache and confusion 1 day before presentation. In the emergency department, he became agitated and was unable to speak. A computed tomography scan of the head showed no mass lesions or other gross abnormalities. Lumbar puncture was performed with opening pressure increased at 30 cm H_2O. Cerebrospinal fluid (CSF) examination showed 25 nucleated cells with 88% lymphocytes, protein 151 mg/dL, and glucose of 36 mg/dL. Cryptococcal antigen level in CSF was increased to 1:10,000. A Gram stain of the CSF revealed 2+ yeast, and culture grew *Cryptococcus neoformans*. HIV Ag/Ab testing was reactive. CD4 count was 27 cells/mm^3 (5%) and HIV RNA was 645,300 copies/μL.

In patients with AIDS and most opportunistic infections (OIs), major guidelines have recommended initiation or reinitiation of ART within the first 2 weeks after diagnosis of OI.[3,62] In the setting of AIDS-related malignancy, immediate ART initiation is supported.[63] However, 2 specific clinical entities warrant consideration of a delay in ART initiation after initiation of OI therapy because of concern for paradoxic clinical worsening secondary to immune reconstitution inflammatory syndrome (IRIS): cryptococcal meningoencephalitis and active tuberculosis (particularly tuberculosis involving the central nervous system) (**Box 4**).

Cryptococcal Meningoencephalitis

Cryptococcal meningoencephalitis is a hallmark of advanced AIDS and is often fatal within weeks of presentations such as this patient's. It is more common at CD4 counts less than 100 cells/mm^3 and most common at CD4 counts less than 50 cells/mm^3, representing severely delayed diagnosis or difficulty accessing HIV care and ART. Although assessment for increased intracranial pressure (ICP) and initiation of induction therapy is a priority, planning should begin immediately for linkage to HIV care and

---

Box 4
When to delay antiretroviral therapy

- Cryptococcal meningoencephalitis
- Tuberculosis
- Certain HIV controllers

access to ART once the patient is clinically ready, as well as medical case management if available. Once treatment is underway, virologic suppression is critical to allow a chance for recovery and to avoid relapse.

The concern for starting ART sooner than 2 weeks after completion of induction therapy for this patient is the risk of ICP secondary to IRIS while significant fungal burden remains. Debate persists regarding the safest time to initiate ART in presentations like this patient's, particularly with low CSF lymphocyte count and increased ICP.[3,62,64,65] In high-resourced settings, when close monitoring is possible and the clinical setting allows easy access to monitoring of ICP, a more nuanced decision regarding timing of ART is possible, with acceptable intervals ranging from 2 weeks after completion of antifungal induction therapy until completion of the induction/consolidation phase (10 weeks). This approach requires treatment or prevention of concomitant OIs and hinges on a commitment to initiate ART at the earliest safe interval.

Trials evaluating early ART (within 2 weeks of diagnosis) in sub-Saharan Africa found significantly higher mortality with early ART, particularly within 2 to 5 weeks after diagnosis.[66] High rates of unmasking subclinical cryptococcal meningitis after ART initiation also remain a concern in these settings.[67] A review of pooled data suggests higher mortality risk associated with ART initiation within 4 weeks of diagnosis of cryptococcal meningoencephalitis in low-income and middle-income countries, although it is unclear whether this higher risk can be attributed to IRIS.[68]

Tuberculosis

For PWH with pulmonary tuberculosis and CD4 counts less than 50 cells/mm^3, results of a randomized clinical trial support starting ART within 2 weeks after initiation of antituberculosis therapy.[69] Although IRIS was more common with earlier versus later ART, PWH with low CD4 counts who started early ART had significantly lower rates of new AIDS-defining illnesses and death. This effect was not seen in PWH who started early ART with CD4 counts greater than or equal to 50 cells/mm^3, for whom ART within 8 weeks of initiating treatment of tuberculosis is recommended. For PWH and tuberculosis involving the central nervous system, a delay in ART initiation is recommended for at least 8 weeks following start of antituberculosis treatment.[3,69,70]

Certain human immunodeficiency virus controllers

Case 4 is an example of an HIV controller who was found to have intermittent low-level viremia and concomitant vascular disease who initiated ART. In the absence of detectable viremia or relevant comorbidities, the benefit of ART is less clear. PWH who are HIV controllers and have maintained an undetectable HIV viral load for years may be observed off ART. Routine viral load monitoring is warranted.[5]

SUMMARY

The concordance of major guidelines groups regarding the benefit of ART at all stages of HIV infection and the advent of effective, well-tolerated, and durable ART have made the decision to initiate therapy easier for many providers and PWH. However, the importance of comprehensive support measures to ensure access to the projected long-term benefits of ART for all PWH, particularly low-income persons and the working poor, cannot be understated and is consistently under threat of funding shortfalls. Despite viral suppression, disparities in health outcomes for many men and women with HIV underscore the need for uninterrupted, frictionless access to health care. Further evaluation is needed to determine the most cost-effective and well-tolerated regimens, including generics, in a time of increased scrutiny of health care costs. Most importantly, HIV stigma continues to be the most persistent barrier to universal ART, the most common indirect cause of death from AIDS, and the obstacle to the deserved benefits of longevity and improved quality of life for all persons with HIV.

REFERENCES

1. Hammer SM, Squires KE, Hughes MD, et al. A controlled trial of two nucleoside analogues plus indinavir in persons with human immunodeficiency virus infection and CD4 cell counts of 200 per cubic millimeter or less. AIDS Clinical Trials Group 320 Study Team. N Engl J Med 1997;337(11):725–33.
2. Gulick RM, Mellors JW, Havlir D, et al. Treatment with indinavir, zidovudine, and lamivudine in adults with human immunodeficiency virus infection and prior antiretroviral therapy. N Engl J Med 1997;337(11):734–9.
3. Saag MS, Benson CA, Gandhi RT, et al. antiretroviral drugs for treatment and prevention of HIV infection in adults: 2018 recommendations of the International Antiviral Society-USA Panel. JAMA 2018;320(4):379–96.
4. Guidelines for managing advanced HIV disease and rapid initiation of antiretroviral therapy, July 2017. World Health Organization; 2017. Available at: https://apps. who.int/iris/bitstream/handle/10665/255884/9789241550062-eng.pdf;jsessionid= 47F9653C0B6124B33903B924C64FC409?sequence=1.
5. Department of Health and Human Services. Panel on antiretroviral guidelines for adults and adolescents. Guidelines for the use of antiretroviral agents in adults and adolescents living with HIV 2018. Available at: http://aidsinfo.nih.gov/ contentfiles/lvguidelines/AdultandAdolescentGL.pdf. Accessed December 15, 2018.
6. Battegay M, Ryom L. European AIDS Clinical Society EACS guidelines version 9.1 2018. Available at: http://www.eacsociety.org/files/2018_guidelines-9.1-english.pdf. Accessed December 23, 2018.
7. TEMPRANO ANRS 12136 Study Group, Danel C, Moh R, Gabillard D, et al. A trial of early antiretrovirals and isoniazid preventive therapy in Africa. N Engl J Med 2015;373(9):808–22.
8. INSIGHT START Study Group, Lundgren JD, Babiker AG, Gordin F, et al. Initiation of antiretroviral therapy in early asymptomatic HIV infection. N Engl J Med 2015; 373(9):795–807.
9. Strategies for Management of Antiretroviral Therapy (SMART) Study Group, El-Sadr WM, Lundgren JD, Neaton JD, et al. CD4+ count-guided interruption of antiretroviral treatment. N Engl J Med 2006;355(22):2283–96.
10. When To Start Consortium, Sterne JAC, May M, Costagliola D, et al. Timing of initiation of antiretroviral therapy in AIDS-free HIV-1-infected patients: a collaborative analysis of 18 HIV cohort studies. Lancet 2009;373(9672):1352–63.
11. Kitahata MM, Gange SJ, Abraham AG, et al. Effect of early versus deferred antiretroviral therapy for HIV on survival. N Engl J Med 2009;360(18):1815–26.
12. Severe P, Juste MAJ, Ambroise A, et al. Early versus standard antiretroviral therapy for HIV-infected adults in Haiti. N Engl J Med 2010;363(3):257–65.
13. Cohen MS, Chen YQ, McCauley M, et al. Prevention of HIV-1 infection with early antiretroviral therapy. N Engl J Med 2011;365(6):493–505.
14. Crum-Cianflone NF, Grandits G, Echols S, et al. Trends and causes of hospitalizations among HIV-infected persons during the late HAART era: what is the impact of CD4 counts and HAART use? J Acquir Immune Defic Syndr 2010; 54(3):248–57.

15. Marcus JL, Chao CR, Leyden WA, et al. narrowing the gap in life expectancy between HIV-infected and HIV-uninfected individuals with access to care. J Acquir Immune Defic Syndr 2016;73(1):39–46.

16. LeMessurier J, Traversy G, Varsaneux O, et al. Risk of sexual transmission of human immunodeficiency virus with antiretroviral therapy, suppressed viral load and condom use: a systematic review. CMAJ 2018;190(46):E1350–60.

17. Cohen MS, Shaw GM, McMichael AJ, et al. Acute HIV-1 infection. N Engl J Med 2011;364(20):1943–54.

18. Kuruc JD, Cope AB, Sampson LA, et al. Ten years of screening and testing for acute HIV infection in North Carolina. J Acquir Immune Defic Syndr 2016;71(1): 111–9.

19. Daar ES, Pilcher CD, Hecht FM. Clinical presentation and diagnosis of primary HIV-1 infection. Curr Opin HIV AIDS 2008;3(1):10–5.

20. Jain V, Hartogensis W, Bacchetti P, et al. Antiretroviral therapy initiated within 6 months of HIV infection is associated with lower T-cell activation and smaller HIV reservoir size. J Infect Dis 2013;208(8):1202–11.

21. Ananworanich J, Dubé K, Chomont N. How does the timing of antiretroviral therapy initiation in acute infection affect HIV reservoirs? Curr Opin HIV AIDS 2015; 10(1):18–28.

22. Le T, Wright EJ, Smith DM, et al. Enhanced CD4+ T-cell recovery with earlier HIV-1 antiretroviral therapy. N Engl J Med 2013;368(3):218–30.

23. Sereti I, Krebs SJ, Phanuphak N, et al. Persistent, albeit reduced, chronic inflammation in persons starting antiretroviral therapy in acute HIV infection. Clin Infect Dis 2017;64(2):124–31.

24. Henrich TJ, Gandhi RT. Early treatment and HIV-1 reservoirs: a stitch in time? J Infect Dis 2013;208(8):1189–93.

25. Ananworanich J, Chomont N, Eller LA, et al. HIV DNA set point is rapidly established in acute HIV infection and dramatically reduced by early ART. EBioMedicine 2016;11:68–72.

26. Chéret A, Durier C, Mélard A, et al. Impact of early cART on HIV blood and semen compartments at the time of primary infection. PLoS One 2017;12(7):e0180191.

27. Kroon EDMB, Phanuphak N, Shattock AJ, et al. Acute HIV infection detection and immediate treatment estimated to reduce transmission by 89% among men who have sex with men in Bangkok. J Int AIDS Soc 2017;20(1):21708.

28. Koenig SP, Dorvil N, Dévieux JG, et al. Same-day HIV testing with initiation of antiretroviral therapy versus standard care for persons living with HIV: a randomized unblinded trial. PLoS Med 2017;14(7):e1002357.

29. Geng EH, Havlir DV. The science of rapid start-From the when to the how of antiretroviral initiation. PLoS Med 2017;14(7):e1002358.

30. Ford N, Migone C, Calmy A, et al. Benefits and risks of rapid initiation of antiretroviral therapy. AIDS 2018;32(1):17–23.

31. World Health Organization. Guidelines for managing advanced HIV disease and rapid initiation of antiretroviral therapy, July 2017 2017. Available at: http://apps. who.int/iris/bitstream/handle/10665/255884/9789241550062-eng.pdf. Accessed December 15, 2018.

32. Pilcher CD, Ospina-Norvell C, Dasgupta A, et al. The effect of same-day observed initiation of antiretroviral therapy on HIV viral load and treatment outcomes in a US Public Health setting. J Acquir Immune Defic Syndr 2017;74(1): 44–51.

33. Colasanti J, Sumitani J, Mehta CC, et al. Implementation of a rapid entry program decreases time to viral suppression among vulnerable persons living with HIV in the Southern United States. Open Forum Infect Dis 2018;5(6):ofy104.
34. Hoenigl M, Chaillon A, Moore DJ, et al. Rapid HIV viral load suppression in those initiating antiretroviral therapy at first Visit after HIV diagnosis. Sci Rep 2016;6: 32947.
35. Lodi S, Günthard HF, Dunn D, et al. Effect of immediate initiation of antiretroviral treatment on the risk of acquired HIV drug resistance. AIDS 2018;32(3):327–35.
36. Attia S, Egger M, Müller M, et al. Sexual transmission of HIV according to viral load and antiretroviral therapy: systematic review and meta-analysis. AIDS 2009;23(11):1397–404.
37. Cohen MS, Chen YQ, McCauley M, et al. Antiretroviral therapy for the prevention of HIV-1 transmission. N Engl J Med 2016;375(9):830–9.
38. McNairy ML, El-Sadr WM. Antiretroviral therapy for the prevention of HIV transmission: what will it take? Clin Infect Dis 2014;58(7):1003–11.
39. Cohen MS. Treatment for HIV prevention, one couple at a time. Lancet HIV 2018; 5(8):e408–9.
40. Rodger AJ, Cambiano V, Bruun T, et al. sexual activity without condoms and risk of HIV transmission in serodifferent couples when the HIV-positive partner is using suppressive antiretroviral therapy. JAMA 2016;316(2):171–81.
41. Bavinton BR, Jin F, Prestage G, et al. The opposites attract Study of viral load, HIV treatment and HIV transmission in serodiscordant homosexual male couples: design and methods. BMC Public Health 2014;14:917.
42. Rodger A. Risk of HIV transmission through condomless sex in MSM couples with suppressive ART: the PARTNER2 Study extended results in gay men. AIDS 2018. 23-27 July 2018, Amsterdam. Late breaker oral abstract WEAX0104LB. Available at: https://programme.aids2018.org/PAGMaterial/PPT/6213_8403/WEAX0104LB_ RODGER_PARTNER2_AIDS2018%20.pdf. Accessed December 15, 2018.
43. The Lancet Hiv. U=U taking off in 2017. Lancet HIV 2017;4(11):e475.
44. Oldenburg CE, Bor J, Harling G, et al. Impact of early antiretroviral therapy eligibility on HIV acquisition: household-level evidence from rural South Africa. AIDS 2018;32(5):635–43.
45. Iwuji CC, Orne-Gliemann J, Larmarange J, et al. Universal test and treat and the HIV epidemic in rural South Africa: a phase 4, open-label, community cluster randomised trial. Lancet HIV 2018;5(3):e116–25.
46. Larmarange J, Diallo MH, McGrath N, et al. The impact of population dynamics on the population HIV care cascade: results from the ANRS 12249 treatment as prevention trial in rural KwaZulu-Natal (South Africa). J Int AIDS Soc 2018; 21(Suppl 4):e25128.
47. Cooper ER, Charurat M, Mofenson L, et al. Combination antiretroviral strategies for the treatment of pregnant HIV-1-infected women and prevention of perinatal HIV-1 transmission. J Acquir Immune Defic Syndr 2002;29(5):484–94.
48. Townsend CL, Byrne L, Cortina-Borja M, et al. Earlier initiation of ART and further decline in mother-to-child HIV transmission rates, 2000-2011. AIDS 2014;28(7): 1049–57.
49. Mandelbrot L, Tubiana R, Le Chenadec J, et al. No perinatal HIV-1 transmission from women with effective antiretroviral therapy starting before conception. Clin Infect Dis 2015;61(11):1715–25.
50. Panel on Treatment of HIV-Infected Pregnant Women and Prevention of Perinatal Transmission. Recommendations for use of antiretroviral drugs in pregnant HIV-1-infected women for maternal health and interventions to reduce perinatal HIV

transmission in the United States. AIDSinfo. Available at: https://aidsinfo.nih.gov/guidelines/html/3/perinatal-guidelines/0/. Accessed December 14, 2018.

51. Chen JY, Ribaudo HJ, Souda S, et al. Highly active antiretroviral therapy and adverse birth outcomes among HIV-infected women in Botswana. J Infect Dis 2012;206(11):1695–705.

52. Zash R, Makhema J, Shapiro RL. Neural-tube defects with dolutegravir treatment from the time of conception. N Engl J Med 2018;379(10):979–81.

53. Tully KP, Stuebe AM, Verbiest SB. The fourth trimester: a critical transition period with unmet maternal health needs. Am J Obstet Gynecol 2017; 217(1):37–41.

54. Chen JS, Pence BW, Rahangdale L, et al. Postpartum HIV care continuum outcomes in the Southeastern USA. AIDS 2018. https://doi.org/10.1097/QAD.0000000000002094.

55. Crowell TA, Hatano H. Clinical outcomes and antiretroviral therapy in "elite" controllers: a review of the literature. J Virus Erad 2015;1(2):72–7.

56. Pereyra F, Lo J, Triant VA, et al. Increased coronary atherosclerosis and immune activation in HIV-1 elite controllers. AIDS 2012;26(18):2409–12.

57. Crowell TA, Gebo KA, Blankson JN, et al. Hospitalization rates and reasons among HIV elite controllers and persons with medically controlled HIV infection. J Infect Dis 2015;211(11):1692–702.

58. Boufassa F, Lechenadec J, Meyer L, et al. Blunted response to combination antiretroviral therapy in HIV elite controllers: an international HIV controller collaboration. PLoS One 2014;9(1):e85516.

59. Hatano H, Yukl SA, Ferre AL, et al. Prospective antiretroviral treatment of asymptomatic, HIV-1 infected controllers. PLoS Pathog 2013;9(10):e1003691.

60. Okulicz JF, Marconi VC, Landrum ML, et al. Clinical outcomes of elite controllers, viremic controllers, and long-term nonprogressors in the US Department of Defense HIV natural history study. J Infect Dis 2009;200(11):1714–23.

61. Hunt PW, Brenchley J, Sinclair E, et al. Relationship between T cell activation and CD4+ T cell count in HIV-seropositive individuals with undetectable plasma HIV RNA levels in the absence of therapy. J Infect Dis 2008;197(1):126–33.

62. Panel on opportunistic infections in HIV-infected adults and adolescents. Guidelines for the prevention and treatment of opportunistic infections in HIV-infected adults and adolescents: recommendations from the Centers for Disease Control and Prevention, the National Institutes of Health, and the HIV Medicine Association of the Infectious Diseases Society of America. AIDSinfo. Available at: https://aidsinfo.nih.gov/guidelines/html/4/adult-and-adolescent-opportunistic-infection/318/introduction. Accessed December 15, 2018.

63. Gopal S, Patel MR, Yanik EL, et al. Association of early HIV viremia with mortality after HIV-associated lymphoma. AIDS 2013;27(15):2365–73.

64. Ingle SM, Miro JM, Furrer H, et al. Impact of ART on mortality in cryptococcal meningitis patients: high-income settings. Presented at: 22nd Conference on Retroviruses and Opportunistic Infections. Seattle, WA, February 23–26, 2015. Available at: http://www.croiconference.org/sessions/impact-art-mortality-cryptococcal-meningitis-patients-high-income-settings.

65. Perfect JR, Dismukes WE, Dromer F, et al. Clinical practice guidelines for the management of cryptococcal disease: 2010 update by the infectious diseases society of america. Clin Infect Dis 2010;50(3):291–322.

66. Boulware DR, Meya DB, Muzoora C, et al. Timing of antiretroviral therapy after diagnosis of cryptococcal meningitis. N Engl J Med 2014;370(26): 2487–98.

67. Rhein J, Hullsiek KH, Evans EE, et al. detrimental outcomes of unmasking cryp-tococcal meningitis with recent ART initiation. Open Forum Infect Dis 2018;5(8): ofy122.
68. Eshun-Wilson I, Okwen MP, Richardson M, et al. Early versus delayed antiretroviral treatment in HIV-positive people with cryptococcal meningitis. Cochrane Database Syst Rev 2018;(7):CD009012.
69. Havlir DV, Kendall MA, Ive P, et al. Timing of antiretroviral therapy for HIV-1 infection and tuberculosis. N Engl J Med 2011;365(16):1482–91.
70. Blanc F-X, Sok T, Laureillard D, et al. Earlier versus later start of antiretroviral therapy in HIV-infected adults with tuberculosis. N Engl J Med 2011;365(16): 1471–81.

Initial Antiretroviral Therapy in an Integrase Inhibitor Era: Can We Do Better?

Sean G. Kelly, MD[a],*, Mary Clare Masters, MD[b],
Babafemi O. Taiwo, MBBS[b]

KEYWORDS

- Integrase stand transfer inhibitors • Dolutegravir • Bictegravir • Dual therapy
- Rapid start

KEY POINTS

- Regimens containing a second-generation integrase inhibitor constitute most widely-recommended initial therapies.
- Emerging dual therapy regimens may further enhance cost effectiveness and tolerability.
- Alternative medication delivery through rapid start may further improve clinical outcomes.

INTRODUCTION

Since the world first encountered the AIDS epidemic almost four decades ago,[1] the culprit retrovirus has been identified,[2] its interplay with human immunity increasingly unraveled,[3] and steady progress made in antiretroviral therapy (ART).[4] The human immunodeficiency virus (HIV) field has now embraced integrase strand transfer inhibitor (INSTI)-based three-drug regimens for first-line (initial) ART, because of their virologic and tolerability properties. Herein, we review initial ART in an INSTI era, and the emerging concepts of two-drug therapy and rapid ART initiation.

OVERVIEW OF INITIAL ANTIRETROVIRAL THERAPY IN 2019

INSTI-containing three-drug regimens are now recommended for initial ART by the US Department of Health and Human Services (DHHS), the International Antiviral Society

Disclosure Statement: B.O. Taiwo has served as a consultant for ViiV, GSK, Gilead, Merck, and Janssen; and received research funding through Northwestern University from ViiV. S.G. Kelly and M.C. Masters have no potential conflicts of interest.
^a Division of Infectious Diseases, Vanderbilt University Medical Center, A2200 MCN, 1161 21st Avenue South, Nashville, TN 37232, USA; ^b Division of Infectious Diseases, Northwestern University Feinberg School of Medicine, 645 North Michigan Avenue, Suite 900, Chicago, IL 60611, USA
* Corresponding author.
E-mail address: sean.g.kelly@vumc.org

Infect Dis Clin N Am 33 (2019) 681–692
https://doi.org/10.1016/j.idc.2019.05.003
id.theclinics.com
0891-5520/19/© 2019 Elsevier Inc. All rights reserved.

(IAS)-USA, the World Health Organization, and the European AIDS Clinical Society.[5–8] The full set of guidelines from each of these expert groups, however, diverge (**Table 1**); IAS-USA is the most focused because it recommends second-generation INSTI (dolutegravir [DTG] and bictegravir [BIC])-based regimens above all others. Regimens containing the first-generation INSTIs (raltegravir [RAL] and elvitegravir [EVG]), protease inhibitors (PIs), and nonnucleoside reverse transcription inhibitors (NNRTIs) are assigned varying levels of support among the different guidelines.

The current dominance of INSTIs in recommended initial three-drug regimens is a testament to the strengths of this class of antiretroviral drugs.[9] Compared with PIs, no pharmacologic boosting (via inhibition of cytochrome P-450 3A4) is required for INSTIs, with the exception of EVG. As such, their potential for drug-drug interactions is lower. Furthermore, PIs have been linked with metabolic adverse effects (AEs), including treatment-limiting hyperbilirubinemia with boosted atazanavir[10] and concerns about possible cardiovascular risk with cumulative exposure to boosted darunavir (DRV).[11] NNRTI-containing regimens also have certain disadvantages relative to INSTI-containing regimens. Rilpivirine must be taken with food, it has multiple medication interactions, a low barrier against resistance, and compromised efficacy in the setting of high HIV viremia (HIV-1 RNA >100,000 copies/mL) or severe immunosuppression (CD4 count <200 cells/μL).[12] Efavirenz (EFV) dominated the global landscape for several years, but has declined in popularity because of a high incidence of neuropsychiatric AEs[13]; requirement of dosing on an empty stomach[12]; low resistance barrier; and the potential for generation of the K103N mutation,[14] an EFV-resistant variant that can also be transmitted. Doravirine is a recently-approved NNRTI with no food requirement, activity against some EFV-resistant variants, and better tolerability than EFV and boosted DRV.[15,16] Although doravirine has not been directly compared with an INSTI, resistance has been documented during virologic failure of initial doravirine-containing ART,[16] unlike the second-generation INSTI-based three-drug regimens. Overall, the characteristics of doravirine are insufficient to challenge the dominance of INSTIs in initial ART.

INTEGRASE INHIBITOR–BASED THREE-DRUG REGIMENS

Across studies, INSTI-based three-drug regimens have exhibited high efficacy and tolerability in initial ART.[9] RAL was shown to be noninferior to EFV and with fewer neuropsychiatric AEs.[17] EVG demonstrated similar efficacy compared with EFV[18] and boosted-PI based regimens,[19] along with better clinical and/or laboratory tolerability. However, INSTI-specific resistance mutations have been reported during failure of RAL- or EVG-based regimens.[20,21]

The second-generation INSTIs are potent, well-tolerated, and have raised the barrier to resistance.[22,23] In the SINGLE study, DTG demonstrated superiority to EFV, primarily because of lower discontinuation rates from AEs, such as rash and neuropsychiatric events.[24] In SPRING-2, DTG was shown to be noninferior to RAL,[25] whereas in the FLAMINGO trial, DTG was superior to boosted DRV.[26] Another large randomized trial (ARIA) demonstrated superiority of DTG over boosted atazanavir in treatment-naive women.[27] BIC is the most recent INSTI, and has shown noninferior virologic efficacy compared with DTG in multiple trials.[28–30] Virologic failure was exceedingly rare among individuals who adhered to and tolerated these regimens. There have been no reports of resistance emergence in clinical trials of DTG- or BIC-based triple therapy in treatment-naive persons with HIV (PWH)

Several INSTIs are available in fixed dose combination (FDC) tablets, which are often preferred by patients and may aid in adherence.[31] EVG was the first INSTI-containing FDC as EVG/cobicistat/emtricitabine (FTC)/tenofovir disoproxil fumarate

Table 1
Recommended initial ART regimens as of October 2018

	DHHS	IAS	WHO	EACS
Initial regimens	DTG/ABC/3TC[a] DTG + tenofovir[b]/FTC EVG/c/tenofovir[b]/FTC RAL + tenofovir[b]/FTC	BIC/TAF/FTC DTG/ABC/3TC DTG + TAF/FTC	DTG + 2 NRTIs EFV + 2 NRTIs	DTG/ABC/3TC[a] DTG + tenofovir[b]/FTC EVG/c/tenofovir[b]/FTC RAL + tenofovir[b]/FTC RPV/tenofovir/FTC[b,c] (DRV/c or DRV/r) + tenofovir[b]/FTC
Alternative regimens if first-line therapy unavailable or contraindicated	(DRV/c or DRV/r) + tenofovir[b]/FTC (ATV/c or ATV/r) + tenofovir[b]/FTC (DRV/c or DRV/r) + ABC/3TC[a] (ATV/c or ATV/r) + ABC/3TC[a] EFV + tenofovir[b]/FTC RPV/tenofovir/FTC[b,c] RAL + ABC/3TC[a,d] DRV/r + RAL (BID)[c,e] LPV/r + 3TC (BID)[e]	DRV/c + TAF (or TDF)/FTC DRV/r + TAF (or TDF)/FTC EFV/TDF/FTC EVG/c/TAF (or TDF)/FTC RAL + TAF (or TDF)/FTC RPV/TAF (or TDF)/FTC[c]	ATV/r + 2 NRTIs LPV/r + 2 NRTIs DTG + 2 NRTIs DRV/r + DTG + 1–2 NRTIs	RAL + ABC/3TC[a,d] EFV + ABC/3TC[a,d] EFV/TDF/FTC (ATV/c or ATV/r) + tenofovir[b]/FTC (DRV/c or DRV/r) + ABC/3TC[a] (ATV/c or ATV/r) + ABC/3TC[a,d] (DRV/r or DRV/c) + RAL (BID)[c]

Abbreviations: 3TC, lamivudine; ABC, abacavir; ATV, atazanavir; BIC, bictegravir; BID, twice daily; c, cobicistat; DRV, darunavir; DTG, dolutegravir; EACS, European AIDS Clinical Society; EFV, efavirenz; EVG, elvitegravir; FTC, emtricitabine; LPV, lopinavir; NRTI, nucleos(t)ide reverse transcriptase inhibitor; r, ritonavir; RAL, raltegravir; RPV, rilpivirine; TAF, tenofovir alafenamide; TDF, tenofovir disoproxil fumarate; WHO, World Health Organization.

[a] If HLA-B*5701-negative.
[b] Either TAF or TDF.
[c] If pretreatment HIV RNA level is <100,000 copies/mL and CD4 cell count is >200 cells/mm^3.
[d] If HIV RNA <100,000 copies/mL.
[e] Recommended only if ABC, TDF, or TAF cannot be used.

(TDF). Nonetheless, a propensity for drug-drug interactions (because of cobicistat) and a lower barrier to resistance relative to DTG and BIC are potential shortcomings of this regimen. DTG and BIC are available as the FDC tablets DTG/abacavir (ABC)/lamivudine (3TC) and BIC/FTC/tenofovir alafenamide (TAF), respectively, and they do not require a pharmacologic booster.[23,30] PWH with end-stage renal disease receiving hemodialysis require careful ART consideration and dosing adjustments, because such FDC tablets are not recommended in such patients.

The need for HLA-B 5701 allele testing before ABC initiation and reported associations between recent ABC use and increased risk of cardiovascular events are barriers to DTG/ABC/3TC use in some scenarios.[32] In addition, DTG/ABC/3TC was associated with more gastrointestinal side effects than BIC/FTC/TAF in a head-to-head comparison, likely because of the effects of ABC.[30,33] There were also more neuropsychiatric symptoms with DTG/ABC/3TC, but no significant differences in treatment discontinuation rates.[29,33] Significant increases in total and low-density lipoprotein cholesterol were seen in the BIC/FTC/TAF arm at 96 weeks, but lipid-lowering medication use was low in each arm.[30] Of note, some cohort studies reported rates of neuropsychiatric adverse events with DTG that exceed those reported in randomized clinical trials,[34] but this is not a consistent observation among other large cohorts.[35]

Understanding of the tolerability profile of INSTIs continues to evolve. Recently, unintentional weight gain has been associated with INSTI use in initial ART.[36–38] In the North American AIDS Cohort Collaboration on Research and Design (NA-ACCORD), weight gain with INSTIs was significantly greater than was seen with NNRTI-based (but not PI-based) initial regimens, and there was an indication that the propensity for weight gain may differ between INSTIs.[39] Studies are ongoing to better understand the underlying mechanisms, to ascertain populations that may be at higher risk of moderate to severe weight gain,[40] and to determine the attributable risk for the different INSTIs and the metabolic/cardiovascular consequences, if any.

Some precautions and contraindications apply to INSTIs. For example, concurrent dosing with medications containing multivalent metal cations (eg, iron or calcium) may impair INSTI absorption.[41] Furthermore, PWH receiving treatment of tuberculosis with rifampin experience enhanced DTG metabolism through cytochrome P-450 3A4 induction,[42] but increasing the dosing of DTG to twice daily during concomitant rifampin use has been shown to overcome this effect and maintain antiviral efficacy.[43] RAL may also be used if the dose is increased to 800 mg twice daily.[44] Use of BIC, however, is precluded by concurrent rifampin use, even with twice-daily dosing.[45] Careful consideration is also needed in women who are pregnant or of child-bearing potential. Although RAL remains among first-line ART regimens for pregnant women with HIV,[12] serum EVG concentrations decline throughout pregnancy with standard dosing, which may result in virologic failure and mother-to-child transmission,[46] thus its use is not recommended as initial ART in pregnancy by DHHS or IAS-USA.[6,12] Preliminary data have also indicated an association between early DTG exposure and neural tube defects.[47] Pending additional investigation, guidelines now recommend avoiding DTG in the early stages of pregnancy and in women of child-bearing potential unless they are on effective contraception.[6,7,12] Little is known about BIC in pregnancy and it is not currently recommended.

As INSTIs take center stage in three-drug ART, so too does TAF as a replacement for TDF. TAF has more favorable renal and bone profiles, and is approved for use in individuals with glomerular filtration rate as low as 30 mL/min.[48,49] TAF can also replace TDF in those with chronic hepatitis B virus (HBV) coinfection.[50,51] Nonetheless, TDF/FTC remains among recommended initial NRTIs in the major guidelines except IAS-USA.[6] TDF/FTC has been approved as a generic formulation, but this is not yet commercially available in the United States. Similarly, a generic TDF/3TC formulation was recently approved but is also not yet commercially available.

DUAL THERAPY

Initial ART with a second-generation INSTI plus two NRTIs has brought us closer than ever before to the ceiling of virologic efficacy and convenience, but can we do better? A frequently targeted area for improvement is the number of medications in ART regimens. The imperative for this is to lower the AEs (short- and long-term) and possibly cost of therapy without compromising efficacy or future treatment options. Although some guidelines already include boosted DRV + RAL twice daily and boosted lopinavir (LPV) + 3TC,[6,12] these regimens fail to meet the high bar set by contemporary INSTI-based three-drug ART, and are only listed as options when tenofovir or ABC cannot be used. Boosted DRV + RAL is further restricted to patients with viral load <100,000 copies/mL and CD4 greater than 200 cells/μL.[12] The risk of AEs including metabolic derangement, propensity for drug interactions (given the need for pharmacologic boosting), and inconvenient dosing are additional reasons why there has been limited uptake of PI-containing two-drug regimens in initial ART to date.

The prospect for broader adoption of dual therapy for initial ART has been enhanced by the advent of DTG + 3TC. This dual regimen benefits from the robust potency, resistance barrier, and tolerability of DTG coupled with 3TC, the only antiretroviral agent that has been in the DHHS guidelines since they were first published.[52] Tolerability and long-term safety of DTG + 3TC are improved by excluding ABC and TDF, whereas the benefits of excluding TAF are less clear. It is, however, plausible that limiting NRTI exposure in general (eg, DTG + 3TC) may reduce the risk of mitochondrial toxicity. Recently, long-term use of TDF and, to a lesser extent, ABC, was associated with shortened telomere length, which may hasten immunosenescence.[53] Although this finding remains under investigation and no clinical associations have been made, there is a need to investigate the telomere effects of TAF, which results in higher intracellular drug exposure than TDF. 3TC, in contrast, has a remarkable record of safety, the evidence for which was recently summarized by Quercia and colleagues[54]: (1) no effect *in vitro* on cell growth, lactate production, intracellular lipids, mitochondrial DNA (mtDNA), or mtDNA-encoded respiratory chain subunit II of cytochrome c oxidase after a long-term treatment[55]; (2) weaker inhibition of the mtDNA polymerase gamma by the 3TC(−) enantiomer[56]; and (3) 87% reduced risk of hyperlactatemia/lactic acidosis compared with regimens containing other NRTIs (including TDF, ABC, zidovudine, stavudine, and didanosine).[57] Furthermore, dual therapy with DTG + 3TC could also be a more cost-effective option if widely used. A modeling study found that if DTG + generic 3TC was used as initial therapy or for induction-maintenance by 50% of persons initiating ART in the United States and 25% of those currently virally suppressed switched to DTG+ 3TC, cost savings over 5 years could exceed $3 billion.[58]

Clinical trial data in support of DTG + 3TC as initial ART have begun to accumulate. The strategy of using 3TC as part of a two-drug regimen started when Cahn and colleagues[59] reported that boosted LPV + 3TC was noninferior to standard three-drug therapy in treatment-naive PWH, regardless of baseline viral load. To sidestep the shortcomings of boosted LPV, the same group conducted the PADDLE study of DTG + 3TC and showed 90% virologic efficacy through Week 96 in 20 patients with baseline viral load less than 100,000 copies/mL and CD4 count greater than 200 cells/μL.[60] Subsequently, AIDS Clinical Trials Group (ACTG) A5353 confirmed the high efficacy of DTG + 3TC in treatment-naive participants and extended the evidence to those with baseline viral load greater than 100,000 copies/mL.[61] Notably, one participant with virologic failure in A5353 developed resistance mutations to 3TC and DTG, prompting concerns about the resistance barrier of this dual regimen. Two ongoing fully powered studies (GEMINI 1 and GEMINI 2) are now providing definitive data about DTG + 3TC. Noninferiority of DTG + 3TC to DTG + TDF/FTC has been demonstrated through Week 48, and follow-up will continue through Week 144.[62] Importantly, no resistance has been reported to date in any of the individuals who have experienced virologic failure on DTG + 3TC in the GEMINI studies. As expected, changes in renal and bone biomarkers favored the TDF-free DTG + 3TC regimen. An FDC formulation of DTG + 3TC was approved in 2019.

Boosted DRV + 3TC is also being investigated for initial therapy. Although this regimen was noninferior to boosted DRV + TDF/TFC at 48 weeks in the ANDES trial,[63] there is reduced enthusiasm for boosted PIs in initial ART, except in specific situations. Looking into the future, the combination of doravirine and the investigational MK 8591 (a novel nucleoside reverse transcriptase translocation inhibitor) stands out as a possible two-drug candidate for treatment. Pharmacologic compatibility of this regimen was demonstrated recently,[64] and the combination is already being investigated in the induction-maintenance DRIVE2SIMPLIFY study (ClinicalTrials. gov; NCT03272347).

Although dual therapy offers some potential advantages in initial ART, there are limitations that will constrain its use. For example, the GEMINI studies excluded participants with screening viral load greater than 500,000 copies/mL, hence little is known in that subgroup, which might be of particular relevance for patients with either acute HIV or very advanced HIV disease. Furthermore, DTG + 3TC and other tenofovir-free dual regimens are contraindicated in HIV/HBV coinfection, and the strategy has not been investigated in tuberculosis coinfection or pregnancy. Data are also lacking in PWH with advanced renal disease or on hemodialysis. Notably, the current 3TC renal dosing recommendations are based on small pharmacokinetic studies that demonstrated large serum concentration increases with renal impairment. Subjects in these studies, however, tolerated 300-mg single doses or continuous 150-mg daily doses without AEs.[65,66] Because DTG does not require renal dosing adjustment, it is reasonable to consider investigating DTG + 3TC in dialysis patients.

RAPID ANTIRETROVIRAL THERAPY START

Guidelines globally now recommend ART initiation regardless of immune status.[5–8] However, treatment initiation is often delayed while waiting for results of recommended pretherapy tests, which may include CD4 count, viral load, HIV resistance genotype, hepatitis B serologies, complete metabolic panel, and HLA B5701 genotype.[5,7,8] There is now momentum toward rapid ART initiation, provided it is not contraindicated by untreated opportunistic infections.[6] Although the definition of rapid ART has varied from ART initiation on the day of HIV diagnosis to within a few days or even 2 weeks of diagnosis, new infrastructure is commonly needed to support its implementation. Pilot programs in the United States have demonstrated significant reduction in time between HIV diagnosis and ART initiation, shorter time to viral suppression, and higher rates of durable viral suppression with early ART start,[67–69] consistent with similarly promising results from randomized trials in Haiti and sub-Saharan Africa.[70–73] By accelerating the time to suppression of plasma HIV-1, rapid ART initiation can also help optimize the benefits of undetectable = untransmissible at the population level. Rapid ART start (particularly same-day initiation) has limitations, however. It may not be for the ideal treatment strategy for every patient, and concerns about its feasibility or financial sustainability in some settings, and the potential for racial and other disparities in its implementation have surfaced.[67,69]

Clearly, initiation of ART before the availability of results of baseline tests has become easier with availability of three-drug regimens that include second-generation INSTIs and TAF/FTC (ie, DTG + TAF/FTC and BIC/TAF/FTC). These regimens are safe, effective even in individuals with the most commonly transmitted resistance mutations (eg, K103N, M184V, and thymidine-analogue mutations),[74] and active against HBV. Correspondingly, the recently available FDC tablet containing boosted DRV + TAF/FTC may also be suitable for rapid ART initiation. However, two-drug regimens, including DTG + 3TC, are not recommended currently for rapid ART initiation because of concerns about potential monotherapy[75] (eg, in patients with transmitted drug resistance) and limited data on efficacy at viral loads greater than 500,000 copies/mL. Carefully designed studies with safeguards for participant safety may help understand whether there is a role for selected two-drug regimens in rapid ART initiation.

SUMMARY

INSTIs are transforming the paradigm of HIV treatment and have the potential to revolutionize HIV care delivery worldwide. DTG- or BIC-containing three-drug regimens are well-tolerated, and highly effective with a high resistance barrier, hence their dominance in initial ART. Dual therapy, such as with DTG + 3TC, is an emerging treatment option for initial ART that may promote long-term success in some patients by lowering cost and reducing AEs. Although it is generally safe to initiate DTG, BIC, or boosted DRV + TAF/FTC before the availability of baseline laboratory testing results, two-drug combinations, including DTG+3TC, are not recommended currently for rapid ART initiation.

REFERENCES

1. Gottlieb MS, Schroff R, Schanker HM, et al. *Pneumocystis carinii* pneumonia and mucosal candidiasis in previously healthy homosexual men: evidence of a new acquired cellular immunodeficiency. N Engl J Med 1981;305(24):1425–31.
2. Barre-Sinoussi F, Chermann JC, Rey F, et al. Isolation of a T-lymphotropic retrovirus from a patient at risk for acquired immune deficiency syndrome (AIDS). Science 1983;220(4599):868–71.
3. Dalgleish AG, Beverley PC, Clapham PR, et al. The CD4 (T4) antigen is an essential component of the receptor for the AIDS retrovirus. Nature 1984;312(5996): 763–7.
4. Fischl MA, Richman DD, Grieco MH, et al. The efficacy of azidothymidine (AZT) in the treatment of patients with AIDS and AIDS-related complex. A double-blind, placebo-controlled trial. N Engl J Med 1987;317(4):185–91.
5. Guidelines for the use of antiretroviral agents in adults and adolescents living with HIV. Available at: https://aidsinfo.nih.gov/guidelines/html/1/adult-and-adolescent-arv/0. Accessed September 13, 2018.
6. Saag MS, Benson CA, Gandhi RT, et al. Antiretroviral drugs for treatment and prevention of HIV infection in adults: 2018 recommendations of the International Antiviral Society–USA panel. JAMA 2018;320(4):379–96.
7. Updated recommendations on first-line and second-line antiretroviral regimens and post-exposure prophylaxis and recommendations on early infant diagnosis of HIV: interim guidance. 2018. Available at: http://apps.who.int/iris/bitstream/handle/

10665/273632/WHO-CDS-HIV-18.18-eng.pdf?ua=1. Accessed September 13, 2018.

8. EACS; European AIDS Clinical Society Guidelines. 2017. Available at: http://www.eacsociety.org/files/guidelines_9.0-english.pdf. Accessed September 13, 2018.

9. Messiaen P, Wensing AM, Fun A, et al. Clinical use of HIV integrase inhibitors: a systematic review and meta-analysis. PLoS One 2013;8(1):e52562.

10. Lennox JL, Landovitz RJ, Ribaudo HJ, et al. Efficacy and tolerability of 3 nonnucleoside reverse transcriptase inhibitor-sparing antiretroviral regimens for treatment-naive volunteers infected with HIV-1: a randomized, controlled equivalence trial. Ann Intern Med 2014;161(7):461–71.

11. Ryom L, Lundgren JD, El-Sadr W, et al. Cardiovascular disease and use of contemporary protease inhibitors: the D:A:D international prospective multicohort study. Lancet HIV 2018;5(6):e291–300.

12. (OARAC) DPoAGfAaAAWGotOoARAC. Guidelines for the use of antiretroviral agents in HIV-1-infected adults and adolescents. 2017. Available at: https://aidsinfo.nih.gov/guidelines. Accessed June 22, 2018.

13. Ford N, Shubber Z, Pozniak A, et al. Comparative safety and neuropsychiatric adverse events associated with efavirenz use in first-line antiretroviral therapy: a systematic review and meta-analysis of randomized trials. J Acquir Immune Defic Syndr 2015;69(4):422–9.

14. Levintow SN, Okeke NL, Hue S, et al. Prevalence and transmission dynamics of HIV-1 transmitted drug resistance in a southeastern cohort. Open Forum Infect Dis 2018;5(8):ofy178.

15. Orkin C, Squires KE, Molina JM, et al. Doravirine/lamivudine/tenofovir disoproxil fumarate is non-inferior to efavirenz/emtricitabine/tenofovir disoproxil fumarate in treatment-naive adults with human immunodeficiency virus-1 infection: week 48 results of the DRIVE-AHEAD trial. Clin Infect Dis 2018;68(4):535–44.

16. Molina JM, Squires K, Sax PE, et al. Doravirine versus ritonavir-boosted darunavir in antiretroviral-naive adults with HIV-1 (DRIVE-FORWARD): 48-week results of a randomised, double-blind, phase 3, non-inferiority trial. Lancet HIV 2018;5(5):e211–20.

17. Markowitz M, Nguyen BY, Gotuzzo E, et al. Sustained antiretroviral effect of raltegravir after 96 weeks of combination therapy in treatment-naive patients with HIV-1 infection. J Acquir Immune Defic Syndr 2009;52(3):350–6.

18. Sax PE, DeJesus E, Mills A, et al. Co-formulated elvitegravir, cobicistat, emtricitabine, and tenofovir versus co-formulated efavirenz, emtricitabine, and tenofovir for initial treatment of HIV-1 infection: a randomised, double-blind, phase 3 trial, analysis of results after 48 weeks. Lancet 2012;379(9835):2439–48.

19. DeJesus E, Rockstroh JK, Henry K, et al. Co-formulated elvitegravir, cobicistat, emtricitabine, and tenofovir disoproxil fumarate versus ritonavir-boosted atazanavir plus co-formulated emtricitabine and tenofovir disoproxil fumarate for initial treatment of HIV-1 infection: a randomised, double-blind, phase 3, non-inferiority trial. Lancet 2012;379(9835):2429–38.

20. Malet I, Fourati S, Morand-Joubert L, et al. Risk factors for raltegravir resistance development in clinical practice. J Antimicrob Chemother 2012;67(10):2494–500.

21. Kulkarni R, Abram ME, McColl DJ, et al. Week 144 resistance analysis of elvitegravir/cobicistat/emtricitabine/tenofovir DF versus atazanavir+ritonavir+emtricitabine/tenofovir DF in antiretroviral-naive patients. HIV Clin Trials 2014;15(5):218–30.

22. Oliveira M, Ibanescu RI, Anstett K, et al. Selective resistance profiles emerging in patient-derived clinical isolates with cabotegravir, bictegravir, dolutegravir, and elvitegravir. Retrovirology 2018;15(1):56.

23. Tsiang M, Jones GS, Goldsmith J, et al. Antiviral activity of bictegravir (GS-9883), a novel potent HIV-1 integrase strand transfer inhibitor with an improved resistance profile. Antimicrob Agents Chemother 2016;60(12):7086–97.

24. Walmsley SL, Antela A, Clumeck N, et al. Dolutegravir plus abacavir-lamivudine for the treatment of HIV-1 infection. N Engl J Med 2013;369(19):1807–18.

25. Raffi F, Rachlis A, Stellbrink HJ, et al. Once-daily dolutegravir versus raltegravir in antiretroviral-naive adults with HIV-1 infection: 48 week results from the randomised, double-blind, non-inferiority SPRING-2 study. Lancet 2013;381(9868): 735–43.

26. Molina JM, Clotet B, van Lunzen J, et al. Once-daily dolutegravir versus darunavir plus ritonavir for treatment-naive adults with HIV-1 infection (FLAMINGO): 96 week results from a randomised, open-label, phase 3b study. Lancet HIV 2015;2(4):e127–36.

27. Orrell C, Hagins DP, Belonosova E, et al. Fixed-dose combination dolutegravir, abacavir, and lamivudine versus ritonavir-boosted atazanavir plus tenofovir disoproxil fumarate and emtricitabine in previously untreated women with HIV-1 infection (ARIA): week 48 results from a randomised, open-label, non-inferiority, phase 3b study. Lancet HIV 2017;4(12):e536–46.

28. Sax PE, Pozniak A, Montes ML, et al. Coformulated bictegravir, emtricitabine, and tenofovir alafenamide versus dolutegravir with emtricitabine and tenofovir alafenamide, for initial treatment of HIV-1 infection (GS-US-380-1490): a randomised, double-blind, multicentre, phase 3, non-inferiority trial. Lancet 2017;390(10107): 2073–82.

29. Gallant J, Lazzarin A, Mills A, et al. Bictegravir, emtricitabine, and tenofovir alafenamide versus dolutegravir, abacavir, and lamivudine for initial treatment of HIV-1 infection (GS-US-380-1489): a double-blind, multicentre, phase 3, randomised controlled non-inferiority trial. Lancet 2017;390(10107):2063–72.

30. Wohl DA, Yazdanpanah Y, Baumgarten A, et al. A phase 3, randomized, controlled clinical trial of bictegravir in a fixed-dose combination, B/F/TAF, vs ABC/DTG/3TC in treatment-naïve adults at Week 96. Paper presented at: IDWeek. San Francisco, CA, October 3–7, 2018.

31. Ramjan R, Calmy A, Vitoria M, et al. Systematic review and meta-analysis: patient and programme impact of fixed-dose combination antiretroviral therapy. Trop Med Int Health 2014;19(5):501–13.

32. Elion RA, Althoff KN, Zhang J, et al. Recent abacavir use increases risk of type 1 and type 2 myocardial infarctions among adults with HIV. J Acquir Immune Defic Syndr 2018;78(1):62–72.

33. Wohl D, Clarke A, Maggiolo F, et al. Patient-reported symptoms over 48 weeks among participants in randomized, double-blind, phase III non-inferiority trials of adults with HIV on co-formulated bictegravir, emtricitabine, and tenofovir alafenamide versus co-formulated abacavir, dolutegravir, and lamivudine. Patient 2018;11(5):561–73.

34. Hoffmann C, Welz T, Sabranski M, et al. Higher rates of neuropsychiatric adverse events leading to dolutegravir discontinuation in women and older patients. HIV Med 2017;18(1):56–63.

35. Batista CJB, Meireles MV, Fonseca FF, et al. Safety profile of dolutegravir: real-life data of large scale implementation in Brazil. Paper presented at: Conference on Retroviruses and Opportunistic Infections. Boston, MA, March 4–7, 2018.

36. Norwood J, Turner M, Bofill C, et al. Brief report: weight gain in persons with HIV switched from efavirenz-based to integrase strand transfer inhibitor-based regimens. J Acquir Immune Defic Syndr 2017;76(5):527–31.

37. Menard A, Meddeb L, Tissot-Dupont H, et al. Dolutegravir and weight gain: an unexpected bothering side effect? AIDS 2017;31(10):1499–500.

38. Bakal DR, Coelho LE, Luz PM, et al. Obesity following ART initiation is common and influenced by both traditional and HIV-/ART-specific risk factors. J Antimicrob Chemother 2018;73(8):2177–85.

39. Lake JE, Jenkins CA, Rebeiro PF, et al. ART initiation with integrase inhibitors is associated with greater weight gain than with PI- or NNRTI-based ART in the US and Canada Paper presented at: 20th International Workshop on Comorbidities and Adverse Drug Reactions in HIV. New York, NY, October 13–14, 2018.

40. Bedimo R, Adams-Huet B, Xilong L, et al. Integrase inhibitors-based HAART is associated with greater BMI Gains in blacks and Hispanics. Paper presented at: IDWeek. San Francisco, CA, October 3–7, 2018.

41. Griessinger JA, Hauptstein S, Laffleur F, et al. Evaluation of the impact of multivalent metal ions on the permeation behavior of dolutegravir sodium. Drug Dev Ind Pharm 2016;42(7):1118–26.

42. Dooley KE, Sayre P, Borland J, et al. Safety, tolerability, and pharmacokinetics of the HIV integrase inhibitor dolutegravir given twice daily with rifampin or once daily with rifabutin: results of a phase 1 study among healthy subjects. J Acquir Immune Defic Syndr 2013;62(1):21–7.

43. Dooley K, Kaplan R, Mwelase N, et al. Safety and efficacy of dolutegravir-based ART in TB/HIV coinfected adults at week 24. Paper presented at: Conference on Retroviruses and Opportunistic Infections. Boston, MA, March 4–7, 2018.

44. Taburet AM, Sauvageon H, Grinsztejn B, et al. Pharmacokinetics of raltegravir in HIV-infected patients on rifampicin-based antitubercular therapy. Clin Infect Dis 2015;61(8):1328–35.

45. Custodio JM, West SK, Collins S, et al. Pharmacokinetics of bictegravir administered twice daily in combination with rifampin. Paper presented at: Conference on Retroviruses and Opportunistic Infections. Boston, MA, March 4–7, 2018.

46. Momper JD, Best BM, Wang J, et al. Elvitegravir/cobicistat pharmacokinetics in pregnant and postpartum women with HIV. AIDS 2018;32(17):2507–16.

47. Zash R, Makhema J, Shapiro RL. Neural-tube defects with dolutegravir treatment from the time of conception. N Engl J Med 2018;379(10):979–81.

48. Hagins D, Orkin C, Daar ES, et al. Switching to coformulated rilpivirine (RPV), emtricitabine (FTC) and tenofovir alafenamide from either RPV, FTC and tenofovir disoproxil fumarate (TDF) or efavirenz, FTC and TDF: 96-week results from two randomized clinical trials. HIV Med 2018;19(10):724–33.

49. DeJesus E, Haas B, Segal-Maurer S, et al. Superior efficacy and improved renal and bone safety after switching from a tenofovir disoproxil fumarate- to a tenofovir alafenamide-based regimen through 96 weeks of treatment. AIDS Res Hum Retroviruses 2018;34(4):337–42.

50. Buti M, Gane E, Seto WK, et al. Tenofovir alafenamide versus tenofovir disoproxil fumarate for the treatment of patients with HBeAg-negative chronic hepatitis B virus infection: a randomised, double-blind, phase 3, non-inferiority trial. Lancet Gastroenterol Hepatol 2016;1(3):196–206.

51. Chan HL, Fung S, Seto WK, et al. Tenofovir alafenamide versus tenofovir disoproxil fumarate for the treatment of HBeAg-positive chronic hepatitis B virus

infection: a randomised, double-blind, phase 3, non-inferiority trial. Lancet Gastroenterol Hepatol 2016;1(3):185–95.

52. Prevention CfDCa. Report of the NIH panel to define principles of therapy of HIV infection and guidelines for the use of antiretroviral agents in HIV-infected adults and adolescents. 1998. Available at: https://aidsinfo.nih.gov/contentfiles/adultandadolescentgl04241998014.pdf. Accessed October 18, 2018.

53. Montejano R, Stella-Ascariz N, Monge S, et al. Impact of nucleos(t)ide reverse transcriptase inhibitors on blood telomere length changes in a prospective cohort of aviremic HIV-1 infected adults. J Infect Dis 2018;218(10):1531–40.

54. Quercia R, Perno CF, Koteff J, et al. Twenty-five years of lamivudine: current and future use for the treatment of HIV-1 infection. J Acquir Immune Defic Syndr 2018; 78(2):125–35.

55. Venhoff N, Setzer B, Melkaoui K, et al. Mitochondrial toxicity of tenofovir, emtricitabine and abacavir alone and in combination with additional nucleoside reverse transcriptase inhibitors. Antivir Ther 2007;12(7):1075–85.

56. Martin JL, Brown CE, Matthews-Davis N, et al. Effects of antiviral nucleoside analogs on human DNA polymerases and mitochondrial DNA synthesis. Antimicrob Agents Chemother 1994;38(12):2743–9.

57. Risk factors for lactic acidosis and severe hyperlactataemia in HIV-1-infected adults exposed to antiretroviral therapy. AIDS 2007;21(18):2455–64.

58. Girouard MP, Sax PE, Parker RA, et al. The cost-effectiveness and budget impact of 2-drug dolutegravir-lamivudine regimens for the treatment of HIV infection in the United States. Clin Infect Dis 2016;62(6):784–91.

59. Cahn P, Andrade-Villanueva J, Arribas JR, et al. Dual therapy with lopinavir and ritonavir plus lamivudine versus triple therapy with lopinavir and ritonavir plus two nucleoside reverse transcriptase inhibitors in antiretroviral-therapy-naive adults with HIV-1 infection: 48 week results of the randomised, open label, noninferiority GARDEL trial. Lancet Infect Dis 2014;14(7):572–80.

60. Figueroa MI, Rolon MJ, Patterson P, et al. Dolutegravir-lamivudine as initial therapy in HIV-infected, ARV naive patients: 96 week results of the PADDLE trial. Paper presented at: IAS 2017: Conference on HIV Pathogenesis Treatment and Prevention. Paris, France, July 23–26, 2017.

61. Taiwo BO, Zheng L, Stefanescu A, et al. ACTG A5353: a pilot study of dolutegravir plus lamivudine for initial treatment of human immunodeficiency virus-1 (HIV-1)-infected participants with HIV-1 RNA <500000 copies/mL. Clin Infect Dis 2018; 66(11):1689–97.

62. Cahn P, Sierra Madero P, Arribas J, et al. Non-inferior efficacy of dolutegravir (DTG) plus lamivudine (3TC) vs DTG plus tenofovir/emtricitabine (TDF/FTC) fixed-dose combination in antiretroviral treatment–naive adults with HIV-1 infection—Week 48 results from the GEMINI Studies. Paper presented at: 22nd International AIDS Conference. Amsterdam, the Netherlands, July 23–27, 2018.

63. Figueroa MI, Sued OG, Gun AM, et al. DRV/r/3TC FDC for HIV-1 treatment naive patients: week 48 results of the ANDES study. Paper presented at: 25th Conference on Retroviruses and Opportunistic Infections (CROI). Boston, MA, March 4–7, 2018.

64. Matthews R, Rudd D, Fillgrove K, et al. No difference in MK-8591 and doravirine pharmacokinetics after co-administration. Paper presented at: IDWeek. San Francisco, CA, October 3–7, 2018.

65. Bohjanen PR, Johnson MD, Szczech LA, et al. Steady-state pharmacokinetics of lamivudine in human immunodeficiency virus-infected patients with end-stage

renal disease receiving chronic dialysis. Antimicrob Agents Chemother 2002; 46(8):2387–92.

66. Heald AE, Hsyu PH, Yuen GJ, et al. Pharmacokinetics of lamivudine in human immunodeficiency virus-infected patients with renal dysfunction. Antimicrob Agents Chemother 1996;40(6):1514–9.

67. Colasanti J, Sumitani J, Mehta CC, et al. Implementation of a rapid entry program decreases time to viral suppression among vulnerable persons living with HIV in the Southern United States. Open Forum Infect Dis 2018;5(6):ofy104.

68. Pilcher CD, Ospina-Norvell C, Dasgupta A, et al. The effect of same-day observed initiation of antiretroviral therapy on HIV viral load and treatment outcomes in a US public health setting. J Acquir Immune Defic Syndr 2017;74(1): 44–51.

69. Bacon O, Chin JC, Hsu L, et al. The rapid ART program initiative for HIV diagnosis (RAPID) in San Francisco. Paper presented at: Conference on Retroviruses and Opportunistic Infections. Boston, MA, March 4–7, 2018.

70. Labhardt ND, Ringera I, Lejone TI, et al. Effect of offering same-day art vs usual health facility referral during home-based HIV testing on linkage to care and viral suppression among adults with HIV in Lesotho: the CASCADE randomized clinical trial. JAMA 2018;319(11):1103–12.

71. Rosen S, Maskew M, Fox MP, et al. Initiating antiretroviral therapy for HIV at a patient's first clinic visit: the RAPIT randomized controlled trial. PLoS Med 2016; 13(5):e1002015.

72. Amanyire G, Semitala FC, Namusobya J, et al. Effects of a multicomponent intervention to streamline initiation of antiretroviral therapy in Africa: a stepped-wedge cluster-randomised trial. Lancet HIV 2016;3(11):e539–48.

73. Koenig SP, Dorvil N, Devieux JG, et al. Same-day HIV testing with initiation of antiretroviral therapy versus standard care for persons living with HIV: a randomized unblinded trial. PLoS Med 2017;14(7):e1002357.

74. Margot NA, Wong P, Kulkarni R, et al. Commonly transmitted HIV-1 drug resistance mutations in reverse-transcriptase and protease in antiretroviral treatment-naive patients and response to regimens containing tenofovir disoproxil fumarate or tenofovir alafenamide. J Infect Dis 2017;215(6):920–7.

75. Wijting I, Rokx C, Boucher C, et al. Dolutegravir as maintenance monotherapy for HIV (DOMONO): a phase 2, randomised non-inferiority trial. Lancet HIV 2017; 4(12):e547–54.

Switching Antiretroviral Therapy in the Setting of Virologic Suppression
A Why and How-To Guide

Brian R. Wood, MD*

KEYWORDS

- HIV • Antiretroviral agents • Drug substitution • Viral load

KEY POINTS

- There may be benefits to switching antiretroviral therapy (ART) for an individual with a suppressed viral load, such as reduced short- or long-term toxicity, lower pill burden, avoidance of drug-drug interactions, and others.
- Before any ART regimen switch, several factors must be considered, including past ART experience and history of virologic failures or resistance, which is especially important if switching from a regimen of high barrier to resistance to one of lower barrier or switching to a regimen with fewer active agents.
- Growing data support switching to 2-drug maintenance ART for carefully selected individuals, although the optimal candidates and long-term advantages when compared with tenofovir alafenamide fumarate–based 3-drug ART regimens have not been established.

INTRODUCTION

With advances in human immunodeficiency virus (HIV) treatment, a person diagnosed with HIV who adheres to antiretroviral therapy (ART) is expected to live a near-normal lifespan and thus may take ART for 30 to 40 years or more.[1] In addition, as persons with HIV age, medical comorbidities accumulate (called "multimorbidity") and polypharmacy worsens.[2–4] For these reasons, clinical HIV practice often concentrates on optimizing ART to reduce risks of long-term toxicity. Although a proportion of people with HIV have not yet achieved viral suppression, most of those who are engaged in care have achieved this important benchmark, and thus a frequent focus of clinical visits is potential ART switches to "update" or simplify the regimen to improve quality of life.

Disclosure Statement: None.

Division of Allergy and Infectious Diseases, University of Washington, Mountain West AIDS Education and Training Center, Seattle, WA, USA

* Harborview Medical Center, 325 9th Avenue, Mailstop 359932, Seattle, WA 98104.

E-mail address: bwood2@uw.edu

Infect Dis Clin N Am 33 (2019) 693–705
https://doi.org/10.1016/j.idc.2019.04.003
0891-5520/19/© 2019 Elsevier Inc. All rights reserved.

id.theclinics.com

There may be benefits and risks to switching an ART regimen in the setting of virologic suppression. The purpose of this review is to discuss why such a switch may be considered or in certain cases recommended, how to assess the urgency of an ART regimen switch for an individual with a suppressed viral load, and key variables to consider before switching to ensure the regimen change is safe and will maintain virologic suppression. Some controversial areas and potential future developments in the area of switching ART are also discussed.

For the purpose of this review, virologic suppression will be defined as an HIV RNA level that is routinely not detected or detected below the limit of quantification of the assay (eg, detected below 40 or 50 copies/mL). Although some data suggest that an HIV RNA level detected less than the limit of quantification of the assay confers higher risk of virologic failure as compared with a nondetected HIV RNA level, in clinical practice virologic failure in this setting is rare, and most experts and guidelines do not recommend altering ART or laboratory monitoring protocols for individuals with HIV RNA levels in this range.[5–7]

BENEFITS AND RISKS OF AN ANTIRETROVIRAL THERAPY SWITCH IN THE SETTING OF ROUTINELY SUPPRESSED VIRAL LOADS

Potential benefits of an ART switch in the setting of consistently suppressed HIV RNA levels include reduced short- or long-term toxicity, lower pill burden, and avoidance of interactions with other medications. These benefits tend to be greatest for people taking older antiretroviral (ARV) agents due to greater toxicity. If a patient reports side effects to an ARV or the ARV is inducing obvious laboratory abnormalities, the decision to switch to a newer agent may be easy; however, a frequent question that arises in HIV clinical practice is whether an individual who has stably suppressed viral loads and seems to be tolerating an older ARV needs to switch to a newer agent. This choice requires shared decision-making with the patient; considerations around these switches will be discussed in more detail.

Some individuals may benefit from an ART change due to new or worsening medical comorbidities (such as renal insufficiency, cardiovascular disease, liver dysfunction, or coinfections such as tuberculosis or viral hepatitis). Less commonly, an individual may benefit from an ART switch due to difficulties adhering to food requirements, changes to insurance coverage, or inability to tolerate large tablets or to take oral pills due to surgery or other medical illness.

For women, transgender, or gender nonbinary individuals with HIV who desire conception or become pregnant, a change to ART may be indicated. Although this review does not summarize data for safety or risks of specific ARVs during conception or pregnancy, this is an important point of discussion for individuals with HIV who are of child-bearing potential. Clinicians should assess the current ART regimen and its safety for conception or pregnancy, any current Food and Drug Administration (FDA) warnings about the ARV components and pregnancy, and the pros versus cons of switching to an alternative option. If a person becomes pregnant while taking ART, it is essential to review what is known about the safety of the ARVs; in general, it is preferred to continue a regimen during pregnancy if the individual is tolerating it and has suppressed viral loads, but if there are specific safety concerns around the ARV components or concerns that drug levels may decrease to unacceptable ranges during pregnancy then a switch may be necessary. National treatment guidelines discuss specific ARV considerations in more detail.[7,8]

There are many reasons why an ART regimen switch may be indicated and may be beneficial for an individual with HIV; however, any change to suppressive ART bears risk. Unanticipated side effects may occur. Plus, every switch carries risk of delays or mix-ups due to pharmacy or insurance coverage issues. Therefore, all ART switches should include a discussion of these dangers and a contingency plan if unforeseen side effects or problems arise (eg, a phone call to the patient and/or pharmacy a few days after a new regimen is prescribed helps to identify and address difficulties and eliminate days of missed medication and should be a routine practice).

WEIGHING THE URGENCY OF AN ANTIRETROVIRAL THERAPY SWITCH

Some ART switches should take higher priority than others, and certain factors may increase the urgency of a switch (**Table 1**). For instance, an individual taking an older regimen that is known to have higher risk of long-term toxicity should be considered high priority for a switch, especially if side effects are apparent. For example, the author generally considers individuals taking older nucleoside reverse transcriptase inhibitors (NRTIs) (zidovudine, stavudine, didanosine) and older protease inhibitors

Table 1
Assessing the priority of switching an antiretroviral regimen based on the components

	Examples of Factors that Increase Urgency
High priority to switch	
Older NRTIs (zidovudine, stavudine, didanosine)	Lipodystrophy, dyslipidemia, neuropathy, pancreatitis, lactic acidosis
Older PIs (nelfinavir, indinavir, saquinavir, fosamprenavir, lopinavir)	Lipodystrophy, dyslipidemia, GI intolerance
Enfuvirtide	Injection site reactions
Moderate priority to switch	
Tenofovir disoproxil fumarate (TDF)	Chronic kidney disease or other risk factors for renal insufficiency; osteopenia or osteoporosis or multiple risk factors for osteoporosis
Cobicistat, ritonavir	Drug-drug interactions; GI intolerance
Atazanavir	Renal or gallstones; jaundice; dyslipidemia; renal insufficiency; GI intolerance; drug-drug interactions
Darunavir	Dyslipidemia; GI intolerance; drug-drug interactions
Efavirenz	Mental health symptoms; CNS intolerance; dyslipidemia; hypovitaminosis D
Lower priority to switch	
Nevirapine	Dyslipidemia
Abacavir	Ischemic cardiovascular event or multiple risk factors for ischemic cardiovascular disease; GI intolerance; advanced liver disease
Generally do not switch	
Dolutegravir	Headache, insomnia, other neuropsychiatric intolerance

Risks and benefits of a switch should be discussed with the patient, and factors that may increase the urgency of a switch should be evaluated. This table does not account for conception or pregnancy, which should be considered.

Abbreviations: CNS, central nervous system; GI, gastrointestinal; NRTI, nucleoside reverse transcriptase inhibitor; PI, protease inhibitor.

(PIs) (lopinavir, fosamprenavir, indinavir, nelfinavir, saquinavir) to be high priority for a switch due to elevated rates of adverse effects with these medications. Important considerations for how to switch boosted PIs safely and ensure the new regimen will maintain virologic suppression are discussed in the next section, but generally a switch of these older agents to newer, better tolerated (and often simpler) options is recommended.

Switching other agents may not be as urgent unless certain factors are present. For instance, medications such as cobicistat-boosted elvitegravir, efavirenz, nevirapine, atazanavir, and darunavir are no longer recommended ARVs for treatment-naïve individuals per national treatment guidelines in the United States.[6,7] If a person taking one of these medications has routinely suppressed viral loads and feels well, switching to a newer agent is not necessary. However, in this setting the author always assesses for side effects, drug-drug interactions, and other indications to switch and has a conversation with the patient about the pros and cons of a potential "update" to the regimen.

As an example, cobicistat-boosted elvitegravir, which is a part of combination tablets with emtricitabine/tenofovir alafenamide fumarate (TAF) or emtricitabine/tenofovir disoproxil fumarate (TDF), is more likely to cause gastrointestinal (GI) intolerance and drug-drug interactions as compared with nonboosted integrase strand transfer inhibitors (INSTIs) such as dolutegravir, bictegravir, or raltegravir. Furthermore, virologic failure on elvitegravir is more likely to select for drug resistance than failure on dolutegravir or bictegravir. Therefore, an assessment for GI symptoms, drug-drug interactions, and adherence is especially important for anyone taking elvitegravir/cobicistat. Similarly, efavirenz can cause several side effects, including mental health symptoms such as suicidality and central nervous system (CNS) side effects such as dizziness, vivid dreams, and morning grogginess; plus, efavirenz may increase lipids (especially triglycerides) and lower vitamin D levels and has a low barrier to resistance.[9–11] In addition, the efavirenz combination tablet is combined with emtricitabine and TDF (as opposed to TAF). Consequently, for an individual taking efavirenz, the author always inquires about mental health and CNS side effects, considers lipid and vitamin D levels as well as renal function, and has a conversation about potential benefits of a switch. If a person feels well on an efavirenz-anchored regimen and has regularly suppressed viral loads there is no requirement to switch, although some individuals report feeling better on newer ART and experience improvements in cognition even if they did not believe they were experiencing significant side effects.[12] Occasionally though, patients switch off efavirenz then report feeling worse on the new regimen, leading to a request to switch back, highlighting that the tolerability of new regimens is difficult to predict and clinicians must be ready for unexpected outcomes after any switch.

Similarly, darunavir (boosted by ritonavir or cobicistat) and atazanavir (boosted or unboosted) are ARVs that are no longer on guideline-based lists of first-line regimens for most people with HIV.[6,7] Like efavirenz, these are ARVs that the author always considers updating, depending on several clinical factors. These agents may have more GI intolerability and drug-drug interactions as compared with nonboosted INSTIs and also may be worse for lipids than newer drugs. Atazanavir has a unique side effect profile that includes kidney stones and gallstones, indirect hyperbilirubinemia (which is medically benign but can lead to jaundice), and possibly higher risk of renal insufficiency as compared with newer ARVs.[13,14] On the other hand, the indirect hyperbilirubinemia from atazanavir may be cardioprotective.[15–17] Boosted darunavir, although better in terms of metabolic side effects than older PIs, affects lipids more than newer options and has more tolerability issues than nonboosted INSTIs and the latest nonnucleoside reverse transcriptase inhibitors (NNRTIs).[18–22] Therefore, there may be benefits to updating medications such as boosted darunavir or atazanavir. However, a critical factor to consider before implementing such a switch is that PIs have a high barrier to resistance as compared with some other ARVs (eg, raltegravir, elvitegravir, and NNRTIs). Thus, switching from a PI to a drug of lower barrier to resistance may lead to loss of virologic control in certain individuals and should only be done after a careful review of past ART regimens, virologic failures, and resistance test results (discussed further in the next section).

Another common clinical question is which persons with HIV should switch from TDF to TAF, because TAF likely induces lower risk of renal proximal tubulopathy and less adverse effects on bone mineral density due to lower circulating levels of active metabolites.[23,24] In general, the author has a low threshold to change TDF to TAF, but certain individuals are prioritized for this switch. For example, the author considers individuals with other risk factors for renal insufficiency, such as diabetes mellitus, to be higher priority for this switch. Likewise, certain individuals may have higher risk of TDF-induced renal dysfunction, including those who are older than 50 years of age, taking other nephrotoxic medications, or taking TDF combined with a boosted PI; the author prioritizes such individuals for an update from TDF to TAF.[25,26] He also encourages individuals at high risk for osteoporosis due to low body weight, tobacco dependence, corticosteroid use, family history, or other factors to make this switch. Although TDF leads to lower serum lipid levels as compared with TAF, the clinical significance remains unclear; in general, the author does not consider this to be a reason to avoid the switch from TDF to TAF. For individuals who do not have significant risk factors for renal disease or osteoporosis (eg, young, otherwise healthy persons), the author typically discusses what is known about the switch from TDF to TAF, potential advantages such as reduced long-term risk of renal and bone toxicity and smaller-sized combination tablets, and considers whether their insurance covers the TAF-containing formulation. If the patient is amenable to the switch and the TAF-containing regimen is covered, then the author typically makes this update; if not, then he continues TDF with monitoring of renal function and bone mineral density per guidelines. It should be noted that the effects of TAF in the setting of active TDF-induced renal proximal tubulopathy have not been thoroughly studied (only sparse case reports exist) and the author generally avoids TAF in this situation if safe alternatives are accessible.[27]

CONSIDERATIONS AROUND SWITCHING AND TIPS FOR SWITCHING SAFELY

The goal of any ART regimen switch is to maintain virologic suppression while minimizing the risk of toxicity and improving quality of life. Several factors must be considered before any ART change is made (**Table 2**). Most importantly, a patient's past ARV history should be reviewed with a focus on past drug intolerances, virologic failures, and resistance test results. It is imperative to consider all past resistance test results (as opposed to only the most recent result) and to remember that resistance assays performed off ART (more than 4–6 weeks after ART stoppage) have limited sensitivity.

The reason that it is so important to consider past virologic failures and past resistance results is to ensure adequate activity of the new ART regimen in order to maintain virologic suppression. This is especially important if the preswitch regimen contains agents with high barrier to resistance and if the new regimen does not (meaning the switch leads to a relative reduction in the barrier to resistance). This concept is illustrated by a clinical trial called SWITCHMRK.[28] In this study, individuals with suppressed HIV RNA levels while taking lopinavir/ritonavir (a boosted PI with high barrier

Table 2	
Antiretroviral agents with high- or low-resistance barrier	
Relatively High Barrier to Resistance	**Relatively Low Barrier to Resistance**
Boosted PIs (boosted darunavir, atazanavir, lopinavir, etc.)	NNRTIs (doravirine, rilpivirine, efavirenz, nevirapine)
Dolutegravir, bictegravir	Other INSTIs (raltegravir, elvitegravir)
	NRTIs (TAF, TDF, abacavir, lamivudine, emtricitabine)
	Other agents (maraviroc, enfuvirtide)

When considering a regimen switch, a switch from an agent with high resistance barrier to another agent of high barrier generally has low risk of failing. Similarly, a switch from an agent of low barrier to another agent of low barrier or to an agent of high barrier is considered low risk. However, switching from a high-barrier agent to one of low barrier may be risky if the patient has a history of virologic failure and known or possible NRTI or other resistance mutations and should be done with the consultation of an experienced specialist.

to resistance) plus 2 NRTIs were enrolled and randomized to either continue their current regimen or to switch to raltegravir (an INSTI with lower resistance barrier) plus 2 NRTIs. The group who switched to the raltegravir-containing regimen had statistically lower rates of virologic suppression at 24 weeks, leading to early termination of the trial. However, analyses demonstrated that the subgroup of participants with no past virologic failures or NRTI resistance mutations maintained noninferior rates of virologic suppression after the switch to raltegravir. One can conclude that because the switch in this trial involved transition from a regimen of high barrier to resistance to one of low barrier to resistance, the NRTI mutations, which compromised the NRTI backbone, were overcome by the boosted PI but not by raltegravir, leading to higher risk of virologic rebound after the switch.

Consequently, if a patient is taking a regimen with high barrier to resistance (boosted PI, dolutegravir, or bictegravir) and they have documented NRTI resistance mutations or past virologic failures that raise concern for NRTI resistance, one should generally switch only to another high barrier to resistance option (see **Table 2**). On the other hand, if a patient is taking a regimen with a high barrier to resistance but clearly has no past virologic failures and no resistance to any components of the new regimen, including no NRTI resistance mutations, they can generally switch to any new option, including one of lower barrier to resistance (raltegravir, elvitegravir, or NNRTIs).

In addition to considering the relative barrier to resistance of the preswitch and post-switch regimen and the history of virologic failures or resistance, it is important to consider other factors before any regimen switch: drug-drug interactions (including over-the-counter medications), food requirements, desire for conception or use of contraception for persons of child-bearing potential, pill burden, and insurance coverage. There may be additional considerations when switching to certain agents, such as HLA-B*5701 status for abacavir and CD4 count for rilpivirine (which is generally avoided if the current CD4 count is less than 200 cells/mm^3). Certain comorbidities may also affect the selection of new agents in a regimen; for example, for someone with HIV-hepatitis B coinfection, it is crucial to ensure that the new ART regimen is adequate to treat hepatitis B (generally this means inclusion of TDF or TAF). Similarly, if an individual has chronic renal insufficiency, the creatinine clearance should be calculated to determine if new agents, such as TAF, may be safe.

Although sometimes patients request an ART regimen change, there are instances in which a practitioner may recommend a switch (due to drug-drug interactions, comorbidities, or other indications). In this setting, a patient may be reluctant to modify their regimen, especially if they have been taking it for a long time and feel well. The author finds it helpful to consider whether the patient can safely return to their preswitch regimen if they do not tolerate the new combination and to counsel the patient about options if side effects occur after the switch. If a person switches their regimen for the purpose of simplification, to reduce the risk of long-term toxicity, or for minor side effects, it is generally acceptable to return to the preswitch regimen if needed. However, if they switch due to significant toxicity, comorbidities, or drug-drug interactions, this may not be the case; a conversation about what to do if they experience side effects and whether they can return to their preswitch regimen or not can help both to reassure the patient about the switch and to prepare for possible postswitch complications.

The HIV RNA level should be rechecked approximately 4 weeks after any ART regimen change.[7] Generally a complete metabolic panel is checked as well, keeping in mind that several ARV agents (bictegravir, dolutegravir, cobicistat, and rilpivirine) raise serum creatinine after initiation through blockage of renal tubular secretion. **Box 1** provides a checklist of factors to review before any ART regimen switch.

Box 1
Checklist for switching ART in the setting of virologic suppression. Assess each factor before making an ART regimen change

✔ Review past antiretroviral regimens, intolerances, adherence barriers, virologic failures, and all resistance test results

✔ Check drug-drug interactions (including over-the-counter medications) and food requirements with new regimen

✔ Consider conception or pregnancy desire for persons of child-bearing potential

✔ Assess comorbidities or co-occurring conditions such as renal insufficiency, mental health issues, viral hepatitis co-infection,[a] HLA-B*5701 status (if switching to abacavir)

✔ Verify insurance coverage

✔ Make plan for telephone check-in and lab follow-up and contingency plan for if the new regimen is not tolerated

   [a] If hepatitis B coinfection, ensure new regimen will be adequate for hepatitis B treatment (generally a regimen that includes TDF or TAF). If untreated chronic hepatitis C coinfection, consider drug-drug interactions between the antiretroviral therapy regimen and hepatitis C direct-acting antivirals

---

SWITCHING ANTIRETROVIRAL THERAPY IN THE ABSENCE OF A CLEAR CLINICAL HISTORY

A common clinical conundrum is whether to switch an ART regimen when an individual's ART history is unknown and past resistance results unavailable, especially if they are taking what seems to be a salvage regimen (suggesting past virologic failures and/or resistance). In this setting, the author generally tries to elicit as much history from the patient as possible regarding past regimens, shows them photos of ARV pills to see which medications they recognize, and tries to piece together their treatment history as much as possible. However, in the absence of records confirming past viral loads and resistance results, it can be difficult to feel confident about the history. If the individual has only taken 1 or 2 regimens (and the switch was not for virologic failure), feels certain they have never been called back to clinic for resistance testing, and seems to have excellent adherence (such as by pharmacy refill history), then it is generally safe to switch to any new regimen, assuming there are no other contraindications.

If, however, they are taking what seems to be a salvage regimen, are unsure of their history, remember being called in for resistance testing, report periods in which they struggled with adherence, or took mono- or dual-NRTI therapy in the early years of ART, one should worry about underlying resistance mutations and either maintain a regimen with equivalent number of active agents and comparable resistance barrier or seek more information. For example, a person taking emtricitabine/TDF plus daruna-vir plus ritonavir plus raltegravir could empirically switch to darunavir/cobicistat/emtri-citabine/TAF plus dolutegravir, which would be simpler and would not reduce the number of active agents or the barrier to resistance. However, if this individual wanted 1 pill per day, one should not switch to a single-pill option without additional informa-tion; in this situation, DNA genotype resistance testing should be considered.

A DNA or "archive" genotype is a test that assesses for resistance-associated mu-tations in integrated proviral DNA (as opposed to circulating HIV RNA). The advantage is this assay can be performed at any HIV RNA level, including undetectable. The disad-vantage is the sensitivity and specificity of the test are imperfect and lower than a com-posite of past RNA genotypes; moreover, the clinical significance of mutations in integrated proviral DNA has not been confirmed.[29,30] Therefore, DNA resistance results must be considered in the context of what is known of the patient's ART history to ensure they make clinical sense; results can help inform regimen switches but are not definitive and may miss key mutations. Acknowledging these caveats, if simplifying a complex regimen for a patient who has extensive treatment history and no access to past resistance assay results, the test can add clinical information to help guide switch decisions. It is a test the author orders only in rare circumstances.

SWITCHING TO LESS THAN THREE ANTIRETROVIRAL AGENTS

Typically, an ART regimen includes 3 active drugs. Some individuals maintain a sup-pressed viral load on 2-drug ART, especially if one of the drugs is potent with a high barrier to resistance (such as dolutegravir or a boosted PI). In recent years, data sup-porting transition to 2-drug "maintenance ART" (switch from a standard 3-drug regimen to a 2-drug regimen after viral suppression has been achieved) have expanded.[31] One 2-drug combination tablet has been approved for this in the United States: dolutegravir/rilpivirine.[32] Other combinations such as dolutegravir with lamivu-dine or boosted darunavir plus lamivudine seem promising.[33,34]

Maintenance therapy with dolutegravir plus rilpivirine was studied in 2 large, open-label, multinational, phase 3 studies.[32] Enrollees were required to have a suppressed viral load for at least 6 months on standard 3-drug ART. They were randomized to continue their baseline regimen or switch to dolutegravir with rilpivirine. Exclusion criteria included past virologic failure, major ARV resistance mutations from any class, or hepatitis B coinfection. After 48 weeks, the proportion of participants with HIV RNA less than 50 copies/mL in the 2-drug maintenance ART arm was noninferior to the pro-portion of those who continued 3-drug ART (95% in each group), and this led to the FDA approval of the combination dolutegravir/rilpivirine tablet for maintenance ART for individuals with a suppressed viral load for at least 6 months on a standard 3-drug regimen, no history of treatment failure, and no known resistance mutations to dolutegravir or rilpivirine.[35]

Interest in 2-drug maintenance ART stems from the potential to reduce long-term toxicity by minimizing ARV exposure and from potential to reduce cost if part of the 2-drug regimen is generic (such as lamivudine).[36] The best candidates for switching to 2-drug maintenance therapy have not been clearly defined. Furthermore, 2-drug maintenance options have primarily been compared with

TDF-based 3-drug ART; comparisons to TAF-based 3-drug ART are ongoing. Understanding the potential advantages of 2-drug maintenance ART over TAF-based standard regimens will help inform clinical decision-making around when to simplify to 2 drugs.

In the author's practice, he considers 2-drug maintenance ART for individuals who are stably suppressed on standard triple ART for an extended period (6 to 12 months minimum), who ideally need to avoid NRTIs due to intolerance or comorbidities and who have no resistance to the components of the 2-drug regimen. For example, the author would consider dolutegravir/rilpivirine for an individual with creatinine clearance less than 30 mL/min (thus ideally would not take TDF or TAF) who also has contraindications to abacavir (positive HLA-B*5701, ischemic cardiovascular disease, or Child-Pugh class B or C cirrhosis) and who has always had excellent adherence and a suppressed viral load. There may be benefits to switching other individuals to 2-drug maintenance therapy in order to avoid long-term exposure to NRTIs, but more research is needed to fully understand the benefits and risks.

Although 2-drug maintenance therapy may be effective for carefully selected individuals, ARV monotherapy should be avoided, even with potent, high-resistance barrier agents. Studies have demonstrated that dolutegravir monotherapy, for example, leads to unacceptably high risk of virologic failure and resistance.[37] Boosted PI monotherapy should also be avoided, as multiple investigations, including systematic reviews and meta-analyses, have demonstrated higher rates of virologic rebound as compared with combination ART.[38–40]

EXAMPLES OF SWITCH DECISIONS

Example 1: this individual started a regimen of emtricitabine/TDF + ritonavir-boosted darunavir 10 years ago, had no resistance on a genotype at entry into care, and has taken the regimen with excellent adherence. They started the boosted PI-based regimen because of a high baseline HIV RNA level, but the HIV RNA levels have been routinely suppressed since 4 months after initiation with no virologic failures.

Management: this person can safely switch to any recommended regimen, even if it has a lower barrier to resistance, because there is no resistance and the patient has demonstrated excellent adherence.

Example 2: this person started a regimen of zidovudine/lamivudine plus nevirapine approximately 15 years ago and viral loads from that period are unavailable. They switched to efavirenz/emtricitabine/TDF when it was approved but subsequently had virologic failure and a genotype resistance test done off ART demonstrated the K103N mutation. They switched to emtricitabine/TDF plus ritonavir-boosted darunavir and HIV RNA has been suppressed since, but they report chronic diarrhea and also want to take potent nasal corticosteroids for seasonal allergies.

Management: in this case, given past virologic failures, possible NRTI resistance, and absence of records from early years of ART, the author would only transition to a regimen with similar barrier to resistance, such as bictegravir/emtricitabine/TAF or dolutegravir plus emtricitabine/TAF. These options would avoid ritonavir or cobicistat pharmacokinetic boosting, which would allow for use of potent inhaled corticosteroids and hopefully reduce GI symptoms.

Example 3: this patient with long-standing HIV transferred to clinic taking emtricitabine/TDF plus twice-daily etravirine plus twice-daily raltegravir plus twice-daily maraviroc. They reported taking this regimen for years with excellent adherence. The exact prior regimens were unclear. The patient recognized zidovudine, zidovudine/lamivudine, and lopinavir/ritonavir on a pill chart. Multiple attempts to obtain prior records and laboratory results failed. The patient reported struggling with pill burden and requested a simpler regimen.

Management: this patient is on a regimen that implies a high degree of prior resistance. Given probable past virologic failures and desire to simplify a salvage regimen, a DNA ("archive") genotype was checked, which revealed the NRTI mutations M184V, M41L, and T215Y; the NNRTI mutations K103N, G190G/A, and V178V/I; multiple PI mutations but no darunavir resistance–associated mutations; and no INSTI mutations. The patient switched to darunavir/cobicistat/emtricitabine/TAF plus dolutegravir and did well.

SUMMARY AND FUTURE DIRECTIONS

In conclusion, an ART regimen switch for a person with routinely suppressed viral loads may be beneficial for various reasons. However, every ART change generates risk of new side effects or medication errors and certain factors must be considered to ensure the switch maintains viral suppression. Switches that require the most careful thought are those that involve a change from a regimen of high barrier to resistance to one of low barrier to resistance or one that reduces the number of active drugs in the regimen, especially in the setting of past virologic failures or resistance.

Growing data support 2-drug maintenance ART for carefully selected individuals, and we are likely to see more combinations approved for this in the future, including long-acting intramuscular combinations. Better understanding of the optimal candidates for switching to less than 3 active drugs, potential long-term benefits of making these switches empirically, and potential cost savings will help guide clinical decision-making.

The impact of generic formulations of commonly used ARVs, such as lamivudine and TDF, may influence insurance coverage and switch decisions and in the future clinicians may be tasked more with advising patients on whether generic TDF versus branded TAF-containing options are clinically safe. Clinicians should consider potential pros and cons of all ART regimen updates for patients with suppressed viral loads and make sure every switch includes a follow-up plan to address unforeseen issues and ensure ongoing viral suppression.

REFERENCES

1. Sabin CA. Do people with HIV infection have a normal life expectancy in the era of combination antiretroviral therapy? BMC Med 2013;11(1):1.
2. Ware D, Palella FJ, Chew KW, et al. Prevalence and trends of polypharmacy among HIV-positive and -negative men in the Multicenter AIDS Cohort Study from 2004 to 2016. PLoS One 2018;13(9):e0203890.
3. Moore HN, Mao L, Oramasionwu CU. Factors associated with polypharmacy and the prescription of multiple medications among persons living with HIV (PLWH) compared to non-PLWH. AIDS Care 2015;27(12):1443–8.
4. De Francesco D, Verboeket SO, Underwood J, et al. Patterns of co-occurring co-morbidities in people living with HIV. Open Forum Infect Dis 2018;5(11):ofy272.
5. Henrich TJ, Wood BR, Kuritzkes DR. Increased risk of virologic rebound in patients on antiviral therapy with a detectable HIV load <48 copies/mL. PLoS One 2012;7(11):1–5.
6. Saag MS, Benson CA, Gandhi RT, et al. Antiretroviral drugs for treatment and prevention of HIV infection in adults: 2018 recommendations of the international antiviral society-USA panel. JAMA 2018;320(4):379–96.

7. Department of Health and Human Services. The adult guidelines: panel on anti-retroviral guidelines for adults and adolescents. Guidelines for the use of antire-troviral agents in HIV-infected adults and adolescents. Available at: http://www.aidsinfo.nih.gov/ContentFiles/AdultandAdolescentsGL.pdf. Accessed December 30, 2018.

8. Department of Health and Human Services. Recommendations for the Use of An-tiretroviral Drugs in Pregnant Women with HIV Infection and Interventions to Reduce Perinatal HIV Transmission in the United States. Available at: https://aidsinfo.nih.gov/guidelines/html/3/perinatal/0. Accessed December 30, 2018.

9. Mollan KR, Smurzynski M, Eron JJ, et al. Association between efavirenz as initial therapy for HIV-1 infection and increased risk for suicidal ideation or attempted or completed suicide: an analysis of trial data. Ann Intern Med 2014;161(1):1–10.

10. Sinxadi PZ, McIlleron HM, Dave JA, et al. Plasma efavirenz concentrations are associated with lipid and glucose concentrations. Medicine (Baltimore) 2016; 95(2):1–7.

11. Nylén H, Habtewold A, Makonnen E, et al. Prevalence and risk factors for efavirenz-based antiretroviral treatment-Associated severe Vitamin D deficiency a prospective cohort study. Medicine (Baltimore) 2016;95(34). https://doi.org/10.1097/MD.0000000000004631.

12. Hakkers CS, Arends JE, van den Berk GE, et al. Objective and subjective improvement of cognition after discontinuing efavirenz in asymptomatic patients: a randomized controlled trial. J Acquir Immune Defic Syndr 2018;1. https://doi.org/10.1097/QAI.0000000000001876.

13. Hara M, Suganuma A, Yanagisawa N, et al. Atazanavir nephrotoxicity. Clin Kidney J 2015;8(2):137–42.

14. Jose S, Nelson M, Phillips A, et al. Improved kidney function in patients who switch their protease inhibitor from atazanavir or lopinavir to darunavir. AIDS 2017;31(4):485–92.

15. Beckman JA, Wood BR, Ard KL, et al. Conflicting effects of atazanavir therapy on atherosclerotic risk factors in stable HIV patients: a randomized trial of regimen switch to atazanavir. PLoS One 2017;12(10):1–14.

16. Muccini C, Galli L, Poli A, et al. Hyperbilirubinemia is associated with a decreased risk of carotid atherosclerosis in HIV-infected patients on virological suppression. J Acquir Immune Defic Syndr 2018;79(5):617–23.

17. Lafleur J, Bress AP, Rosenblatt L, et al. Cardiovascular outcomes among HIV-infected veterans receiving atazanavir. AIDS 2017;31(15):2095–106.

18. Lennox JL, Landovitz RJ, Ribaudo HJ, et al. Efficacy and tolerability of 3 nonnu-cleoside reverse transcriptase inhibitor–sparing antiretroviral regimens for treatment-naive volunteers infected with HIV-1. Ann Intern Med 2014;161(7):461.

19. Ofotokun I, Na LH, Landovitz RJ, et al. Comparison of the metabolic effects of ritonavir-boosted darunavir or atazanavir versus raltegravir, and the impact of ri-tonavir plasma exposure: ACTG 5257. Clin Infect Dis 2015;60(12):1842–51.

20. Molina JM, Clotet B, van Lunzen J, et al. Once-daily dolutegravir versus darunavir plus ritonavir for treatment-naive adults with HIV-1 infection (FLAMINGO): 96 week results from a randomised, open-label, phase 3b study. Lancet HIV 2015;2(4):e127–36.

21. Ucciferri C, Falasca K, VIgnale F, et al. Improved metabolic profile after switch to darunavir/ritonavir in HIV positive patients previously on protease inhibitor ther-apy. J Med Virol 2013;85(5):755–9.

22. Molina JM, Squires K, Sax PE, et al. Doravirine (DOR) versus ritonavir-boosted darunavir (DRV+r): 96-week results of the randomized, double-blind, phase 3

DRIVE FORWARD noninferiority trial. In: 22nd International AIDS Conference, Amsterdam, the Netherlands, July 2018.

23. Aloy B, Tazi I, Bagnis CI, et al. Is tenofovir alafenamide safer than tenofovir disoproxil fumarate for the kidneys? AIDS Rev 2016;18(4):184–92.

24. Gibson AK, Shah BM, Nambiar PH, et al. Tenofovir alafenamide: a review of its use in the treatment of HIV-1 infection. Ann Pharmacother 2016;50(11):942–52.

25. Goicoechea M, Liu S, Best B, et al. Greater tenofovir-associated renal function decline with protease inhibitor–based versus nonnucleoside reverse-transcriptase inhibitor–based therapy. J Infect Dis 2008;197(1):102–8.

26. Baxi SM, Greenblatt RM, Bacchetti P, et al. Common clinical conditions-age, low BMI, ritonavir use, mild renal impairment-affect tenofovir pharmacokinetics in a large cohort of HIV-infected women. AIDS 2014;28(1):59–66.

27. Mothobi NZ, Masters J, Marriott DJ. Fanconi syndrome due to tenofovir disoproxil fumarate reversed by switching to tenofovir alafenamide fumarate in an HIV-infected patient. Ther Adv Infect Dis 2018;5(5):91–5.

28. Eron JJ, Young B, Cooper DA, et al. Switch to a raltegravir-based regimen versus continuation of a lopinavir-ritonavir-based regimen in stable HIV-infected patients with suppressed viraemia (SWITCHMRK 1 and 2): two multicentre, double-blind, randomised controlled trials. Lancet 2010;375(9712):396–407.

29. Delaugerre C, Braun J, Charreau I, et al. Comparison of resistance mutation patterns in historical plasma HIV RNA genotypes with those in current proviral HIV DNA genotypes among extensively treated patients with suppressed replication. HIV Med 2012;13(9):517–25.

30. Derache A, Shin HS, Balamane M, et al. HIV drug resistance mutations in proviral DNA from a community treatment program. PLoS One 2015;10(1):1–14.

31. Corado KC, Caplan MR, Daar ES. Two-drug regimens for treatment of naïve HIV-1 infection and as maintenance therapy. Drug Des Devel Ther 2018;12:3731–40.

32. Llibre JM, Hung CC, Brinson C, et al. Efficacy, safety, and tolerability of dolutegravir-rilpivirine for the maintenance of virological suppression in adults with HIV-1: phase 3, randomised, non-inferiority SWORD-1 and SWORD-2 studies. Lancet 2018;391(10123):839–49.

33. Pulido F, Ribera E, Lagarde M, et al. Dual therapy with darunavir and ritonavir plus lamivudine vs triple therapy with darunavir and ritonavir plus tenofovir disoproxil fumarate and emtricitabine or abacavir and lamivudine for maintenance of human immunodeficiency virus type 1 viral suppressi. Clin Infect Dis 2017;65(12): 2112–8.

34. Taiwo BO, Marconi VC, Berzins B, et al. Dolutegravir plus lamivudine maintains human immunodeficiency virus-1 suppression through week 48 in a pilot randomized trial. Clin Infect Dis 2018;66(11):1794–7.

35. FDA. FDA News Release. FDA approves first two-drug regimen for certain patients with HIV. Available at: https://www.fda.gov/newsevents/newsroom/pressannouncements/ucm586305.htm. Accessed December 30, 2018.

36. Girouard MP, Sax PE, Parker RA, et al. The cost-effectiveness and budget impact of 2-drug dolutegravir-lamivudine regimens for the treatment of HIV infection in the United States. Clin Infect Dis 2015;62(6):784–91.

37. Wandeler G, Buzzi M, Anderegg N, et al. Virologic failure and HIV drug resistance on simplified, dolutegravir-based maintenance therapy: systematic review and meta-analysis. F1000Res 2018. https://doi.org/10.12688/f1000research.15995.1 [version 1; referees: 3 approved].

38. Bierman WFW, Van Agtmael MA, Nijhuis M, et al. HIV monotherapy with ritonavir-boosted protease inhibitors: a systematic review. AIDS 2009;23(3):279–91.

39. Arribas JR, Girard PM, Paton N, et al. Efficacy of protease inhibitor monotherapy vs. triple therapy: meta-analysis of data from 2303 patients in 13 randomized trials. HIV Med 2016;17(5):358–67.
40. Mathis S, Khanlari B, Pulido F, et al. Effectiveness of protease inhibitor monotherapy versus combination antiretroviral maintenance therapy: a meta-analysis. PLoS One 2011;6(7). https://doi.org/10.1371/journal.pone.0022003.

Management of Virologic Failure and HIV Drug Resistance

Suzanne M. McCluskey, MD[a],*, Mark J. Siedner, MD, MPH[a],
Vincent C. Marconi, MD[b]

KEYWORDS

- HIV-1 • Treatment failure • Virologic failure • HIV drug resistance
- Antiretroviral therapy

KEY POINTS

- Virologic failure can occur with or without drug resistance mutations, the latter being caused by poor adherence or low exposure to antiretroviral therapy (ART).
- Genotypic resistance testing is recommended as the preferred test to guide regimen choice following virologic failure and should be performed while the individual is on ART.
- Rule-based algorithms are available to aid in the interpretation of genotypic resistance results.
- ART regimens should include at least 2 to 3 active drugs when possible.
- ART should be continued, even if no active drugs are available.

INTRODUCTION

In 2014, the Joint United Nations Programme on HIV and AIDS established global targets such that 90% of people with HIV will be diagnosed, 90% of those diagnosed will be on antiretroviral therapy (ART), and 90% of those on ART will be virally suppressed by 2020.[1] However, in the United States, 20% of people with HIV who have linked to care or are on ART still remain virologically unsuppressed.[2,3] Thus, optimal management of treatment failure plays a critical role in the ability to improve viral suppression rates and to achieve epidemic control.

Disclosure: S.M. McCluskey is the recipient of a Gilead Sciences Research Scholars in HIV research award.
[a] Division of Infectious Diseases, Harvard Medical School, Massachusetts General Hospital, 55 Fruit Street, GRJ5, Boston, MA 02114, USA; [b] Division of Infectious Diseases, Department of Global Health, Emory University School of Medicine, Rollins School of Public Health, Health Sciences Research Building, 1760 Haygood Dr NE, Room W325, Atlanta, GA 30322, USA
* Corresponding author. 55 Fruit Street, GRJ 504, Boston, MA 02114.
E-mail address: smccluskey@mgh.harvard.edu

Infect Dis Clin N Am 33 (2019) 707–742
https://doi.org/10.1016/j.idc.2019.05.004
0891-5520/19/© 2019 Elsevier Inc. All rights reserved.

id.theclinics.com

IDENTIFYING VIROLOGIC FAILURE

Terminology regarding levels of human immunodeficiency virus (HIV)-1 viremia and virologic suppression are presented in **Table 1**.[4] In the United States, virologic suppression is typically defined as a confirmed HIV-1 RNA that is below the lower limit of detection for the assay, whereas virologic failure is defined as failure to achieve or sustain suppression of viral replication to an HIV-1 RNA level less than 200 copies/mL.[4] Modern polymerase chain reaction assays for HIV-1 RNA quantify detectable viral load less than 200 copies/mL. However, the clinical significance of low-level viremia and viral blips, as well as their optimal management, remain uncertain, with data from various sources showing both increased risk of future virologic failure[5–7] and that blips are of little clinical consequence.[8] For patients with viral load less than 200 copies/mL, current treatment guidelines suggest that the current ART regimen should be continued, along with frequent viral load monitoring.[4,8,9]

Resistance Testing

After identifying virologic failure, or in cases in which there is concern for incomplete virologic response, providers should obtain resistance testing to guide the next steps in management.[4] **Table 2** summarizes the literature regarding the clinical efficacy of resistance testing, stratified by testing method and time point. Most studies support the use of resistance testing, both to guide initial therapy and for selection of an optimal ART regimen following treatment failure.[10–21] Cost-effectiveness analyses of resistance testing are summarized in **Table 3**.[22–32] Overall, these studies conclude that standard genotypic resistance testing is cost-effective both before ART initiation and at the time of virologic failure. One notable exception is that pretreatment integrase gene sequencing for individuals taking integrase strand transfer inhibitors (INSTIs) is expected to increase costs and lead to poorer clinical outcomes, because results could lead providers away from selecting regimens based on dolutegravir (DTG) or bictegravir (BIC) that retain activity.[31]

Genotypic resistance tests involve direct sequencing of the viral genome and remain the preferred resistance testing method.[4,33] Currently available commercial assays use Sanger sequencing to sequence the HIV-1 reverse transcriptase–producing and protease (PR)-producing region of the *pol* gene,[33] which typically detects resistance mutations occurring in at least 20% of the viral population. In the United States, turnaround time for these tests is approximately 7 to 14 days. Of note, the integrase

Table 1 Virologic response	
Viral suppression	HIV-1 RNA <200 copies/mL
Virologic failure	HIV-1 RNA ≥200 copies/mL
Incomplete virologic response	Failure to achieve viral suppression to <200 copies/mL on 2 measurements after 24 wk on antiretroviral therapy
Virologic rebound	Sustained HIV-1 RNA ≥200 copies/mL on at least 2 HIV-1 RNA measurements after a previous period of viral suppression
Viral blips	Brief, isolated episode of detectable HIV-1 RNA, between 2 suppressed HIV-1 RNA measurements

Data from DHHS. Guidelines for the Use of Antiretroviral Agents in Adults and Adolescents Living with HIV. Accessed December 5, 2018.

Table 2
Studies of the clinical impact of resistance testing at the time of virologic failure

Study	Citation	Sample Size	Population	Outcome	Results
Randomized Controlled Trials Comparing Genotype with No Resistance Test					
VIRADAPT	Durant et al,[10] 1999	108	HIV-1 RNA >10,000 copies/mL; exposure to PIs	Change in VL	Favors use of resistance testing
CPCRA 046	Baxter et al,[11] 2000	153	Three-fold increase in HIV-1 RNA; exposure to PIs	Change in VL	Favors use of resistance testing
ARGENTA	Cingolani et al,[12] AIDS 2002	174	HIV-1 RNA >2000 copies/mL ×2 or incomplete virologic response to combination ART	Virologic suppression	Does not favor resistance testing
Havana	Tural et al,[13] 2002	326	HIV-1 RNA >1000 copies/mL; on combination ART	Virologic suppression	Favors use of resistance testing
PENTA 8	Green et al,[14] 2006	170	Children with HIV-1 RNA >2000 copies/mL; on combination ART	Virologic suppression	Does not favor resistance testing
Randomized Controlled Trials Comparing Phenotype with No Resistance Test					
VIRA3001	Cohen et al,[15] 2002	272	HIV-1 RNA >2000 copies/mL; exposure to PIs	Virologic suppression	Favors use of resistance testing
CCTG 575	Haubrich et al,[16] 2005	256	HIV-1 RNA >400 copies/mL; on combination ART	Virologic suppression	Does not favor resistance testing
Randomized Controlled Trials Comparing Genotype, Phenotype, and No Resistance Test					
NARVAL	Meynard et al,[17] 2002	591	HV RNA >1000 copies/mL; history of exposure to PIs	Virologic suppression	Does not favor resistance testing

(continued on next page)

Table 2
(continued)

Study	Citation	Sample Size	Population	Outcome	Results
CERT	Wegner et al,[18] 2004	450	On combination ART	Time to persistent treatment failure despite change in regimen	Favors resistance testing, but only for those with extensive treatment experience
Randomized Controlled Trials Comparing Modes of Resistance Tests					
GenFheRex	Mazzotta et al,[19] 2003	201	Virologic failure; exposure to at least 6 ART agents	Virologic suppression	No difference between real vs virtual phenotype
Realvirfen	Perez-Elias et al,[20] 2003	276	Virologic failure	Virologic suppression	Favors virtual phenotype more than real phenotype
ERA	Dunn et al,[21] 2005	311	Virologic failure	Virologic response	Favors genotype more than genotype + phenotype

Abbreviations: NNRTI, non-nucleoside reverse transcriptase inhibitor; PI, protease inhibitor; VL, viral load.

Table 3
Modeling studies evaluating cost-effectiveness of genotypic resistance testing

Study	Setting	Favors Pre-ART Resistance Testing	Favors Resistance Testing at Virologic Failure
Weinstein et al,[22] 2001	United States, Europe	Yes	Yes
Corzillius et al,[23] 2004	Central Europe	Yes	Yes
Sax et al,[24] 2005	United States	Yes	Not addressed
Yazdanpanah et al,[25] 2007	Europe	Not addressed	Yes
Sendi et al,[26] 2007	Switzerland	Not addressed	Yes
Rosen et al,[27] 2011	South Africa	Not addressed	Yes
Levison et al,[28] 2013	South Africa	Not addressed	Yes
Phillips et al,[29] 2014	Zimbabwe	Not addressed	No
Luz et al,[30] 2015	Brazil	Yes	Not addressed
Koullias et al,[31] 2017	United States	Pre-ART INSTI testing not favored	Not addressed
Phillips et al,[32] 2018	Sub-Saharan Africa	Yes (though less effective than a policy change to INSTI-based first-line ART)	Not addressed

Abbreviation: INSTI, integrase strand transfer inhibitor.

protein (IN) region sequencing is usually not included as part of standard testing and must be requested separately as another assay. Similarly, HIV-1 viral tropism assays and sequencing of the *env* gene to assess susceptibility to maraviroc and enfuvirtide, respectively, are also not included as part of standard resistance testing.

In contrast, phenotypic tests culture clinical HIV-1 virus in the presence of various antiretroviral agents and directly measure drug activity. These assays are less commonly used given higher costs and a longer turnaround time.[33] Thus, phenotypic tests are only recommended for new or investigational agents or for individuals with extensive ART exposure (especially involving protease inhibitors [PIs]) and/or complex resistance profiles.[4,33]

In addition, next-generation sequencing (NGS) is a newer technology for genotypic resistance testing. NGS differs from Sanger sequencing in that it uses high-throughput methods, which require less specialized personnel and reduce the costs per specimen.[33] In addition, NGS can detect minority variants at thresholds as low as 1%, thus capturing significantly more drug resistance mutations than traditional Sanger sequencing. An important unresolved challenge is to determine the optimal threshold for detection of mutations by NGS that correlates with clinically significant resistance.[33]

Use of Resistance Tests in Clinical Practice

The most clinically useful resistance testing results are yielded if resistance testing is performed while individuals are taking ART or within 4 weeks of treatment cessation.[4] If an individual has spent a longer duration without selective pressure from a failing ART regimen, it is possible that mutations in the HIV-1 viral population would revert to wild-type, whereas resistant strains could be circulating in lower numbers and/or archived, and therefore not detected.[34,35] However, relevant mutations (particularly to non-nucleoside reverse transcriptase inhibitors [NNRTIs]) can still frequently be identified even in patients who have stopped their ART.

Interpreting genotypic resistance test results can be complex. Algorithms that incorporate evidence from the literature and expert opinion to derive scores for predicted susceptibility to each of the antiretroviral agents are available to aid with interpretation. The Stanford HIV Drug Resistance Database, French National Agency for AIDS Research (ANRS), HIV Genotypic Resistance-Algorithm Deutschland (HIV-GRADE), and Rega are all widely recognized algorithms for this purpose.[36–40]

In addition, it is important to consider current and past resistance test results when choosing a new ART regimen.[4] If selective pressure from a prior agent is no longer present, resistance to that drug may not manifest on a current HIV genotype. However, if a mutation was present on a prior genotypic resistance test result, the mutation should still be considered as part of a cumulative genotype result.

VIROLOGIC FAILURE WITHOUT RESISTANCE
Causes of Virologic Failure Without Resistance

Some individuals with virologic failure have detectable viremia in the absence of detectable resistance mutations by standard genotype testing. Virologic failure without resistance is most often the result of inadequate drug levels caused by nonadherence. Other possible contributors include limited gastrointestinal absorption and drug-drug interactions.

Nonadherence to ART is a complex, multidimensional challenge. Psychosocial factors such as concurrent substance abuse, unstable housing or homelessness, financial challenges, and issues related to stigma and nondisclosure of HIV status should all be considered.[41–46] Medical comorbidities, including concurrent mental illness, may also increase risk of nonadherence to ART.[46,47] In addition, regimen factors may represent barriers to adherence, particularly if there is a high pill burden or if the regimen is poorly tolerated because of side effects.[46,48] In addition, system-level factors can also contribute to nonadherence, which is often most pronounced in resource-limited settings where medication stock-outs are common.[49]

Nearly all patients taking modern ART regimens are virologically suppressed. As a result, virologic failure without resistance mutations in the setting of high-level ART adherence is rare. Potential causes include drug interactions and errors either in pharmacy dispensing or patient misunderstanding of how to take ART correctly. In these settings, pharmacy refill records can be used to ensure accuracy and frequency of drug dispensing. Drug-drug interactions may be assessed with the assistance of online or other interaction review tools.[50] Furthermore, some antiretroviral medications, including atazanavir (ATV), darunavir (DRV), and rilpivirine, should be taken with food to achieve appropriate drug concentrations.[51–53] Medical and anatomic disorders of impaired absorption may also lead to decreased drug levels; thus, providers should carefully assess patient symptoms and review medical and surgical history in the evaluation of virologic failure.[54,55]

In scenarios of either nonadherence or poor drug absorption, genotypic resistance tests may fail to identify extant resistance-conferring mutations, if there is insufficient exposure to ART to create selective pressure on the sequenced viral population.[4,34,35] Consequently, it is important to repeat viral load testing in 2 to 4 weeks after adherence has improved or absorption issues have resolved to ensure response to ART.[4]

Management of Virologic Failure Without Resistance

The core management principles for treatment failure without resistance involve interventions to improve patient adherence to ART and to ensure therapeutic drug levels.

These interventions typically include patient-centered strategies to target barriers to adherence.[56] Providers can often address regimen-specific barriers through simplification of the ART regimen, regimens without a requirement for coadministration with food, and fixed dose combinations to decrease pill burden and scheduling complexity.[48,57] Providers may also need to substitute components of the ART regimen for agents with better side effect profiles if symptoms are responsible for poor adherence and cannot be otherwise managed. Pill boxes and text-message reminders have also proved effective at improving ART adherence in cases in which mnemonic aids are needed.[4] Interventions to address more complex factors, such as substance use disorders, concurrent mental illness, food, transportation or housing insecurity, and economic hardship, have also been shown to improve adherence to ART.[46] In addition, one-on-one individualized patient education, adherence assessment, and adherence counseling should be prioritized at every clinical visit for patients with, or at risk for, drug adherence challenges.[4,46]

VIROLOGICAL FAILURE WITH RESISTANCE

Virologic failure with drug resistance mutations can arise as a result of 2 scenarios: pretreatment HIV drug resistance and/or acquired drug resistance.

Pretreatment Human Immunodeficiency Virus Drug Resistance

Transmitted drug resistance (TDR) occurs when a treatment-naive individual is infected with a resistant strain of virus.[33] Globally, the term pretreatment drug resistance (PDR) refers to TDR, as well as any resistance mutations present before initiating or reinitiating first-line ART, including acquired mutations that resulted from prior treatment exposure or prevention of mother-to-child transmission practices.[33,58] With increasing numbers of people with HIV now on ART, rates of PDR are increasing worldwide, with the prevalence of PDR reaching 10% or greater in many regions.[33,58–61] PDR is driven primarily by resistance to NNRTIs, whereas PDR to other classes remains much less common.[58,60,62] PDR to INSTIs is extremely rare, with transmitted major INSTI mutations occurring in 0% to 0.8% in cohort studies from the United States and Europe[63–71] and in isolated case reports.[72–74]

Acquired Human Immunodeficiency Virus Drug Resistance

Acquired drug resistance refers to drug resistance mutations that are selected in individuals who are receiving ART.[33] The high rate of HIV-1 viral replication, combined with the high error rate of reverse transcriptase, allows the emergence of viral strains with resistance-conferring mutations when ART is used imperfectly.[75,76] Without selective pressure from ART, mutant strains typically comprise a minority of the viral population because many nonpolymorphic viral mutations lead to a reduction in viral fitness and replication capacity.[77,78] However, under selective pressure of ART, mutant strains can emerge as the dominant viral population if ART is not sufficiently potent for viral suppression, with potency being a factor of both susceptibility of the mutant virus to the ART regimen as well as the necessary therapeutic drug levels.[79] Imperfect adherence to ART is the most likely cause for ongoing viral replication.[80] Other possible explanations include incorrect dosing, poor absorption, or reduced drug levels caused by drug-drug interactions. In addition, some regimens may be particularly susceptible to selecting for drug resistance because of differences in the half-lives of component drugs, leading to unplanned monotherapy sometimes referred to as a pharmacokinetic tail.[81] With continued viral replication despite ART, emergence of resistant mutants is also related to the genetic barrier to resistance of the ART regimen, which is a factor of the number of mutations required to reduce viral susceptibility.[79] Thus, although nucleoside reverse transcriptase inhibitors (NRTIs), NNRTIs, and early-generation INSTIs are considered to have a low genetic barrier to resistance, PIs and later-generation INSTIs require multiple mutations before drug susceptibility is affected. In addition, mutations can continue to accumulate over time, leading to worsening resistance, which particularly occurs when mutations appear on the same virus through recombination, rather than being distributed throughout the quasispecies.

Human Immunodeficiency Virus Drug Resistance Mutations

Table 4 summarizes drug susceptibility information adapted from the Stanford HIVdb algorithm for common resistance mutations for the NRTIs, NNRTIs, PIs, and INSTIs, although it is not meant to be a comprehensive list.[36] The World Health Organization and IAS-USA also maintain a list of relevant mutations, which is freely available online.[82,83]

Nucleoside Reverse Transcriptase Inhibitor Mutations

NRTIs are nucleoside analogues that lead to chain termination when incorporated into viral DNA by the viral reverse transcriptase enzyme (see Table 4).[84] This drug class has a low genetic barrier to resistance, which occurs by one of 2 mechanisms: (1) decreasing the rate of NRTI binding versus natural nucleotides, or (2) increasing the rate of NRTI excision.[84] M184V/I, K65R, K70E, and L74V are examples of mutations in the discriminatory pathway, which require only single mutations to cause resistance and lead to a substantial reduction in viral fitness.[84] M184V is often the first mutation to arise and causes high-level resistance to lamivudine (3TC) and emtricitabine (FTC). This mutation also causes increased susceptibility to zidovudine (AZT) and tenofovir (TDF), which can act in opposition to thymidine analogue mutations (TAMs), as discussed later (see Table 4).[85] In clinical practice, either 3TC or FTC is typically maintained as part of ART regimens, even when M184V is present, to intentionally select for a less fit virus.[86] K65R, the signature mutation for TDF, also leads to a reduction in viral fitness and causes hypersusceptibility to AZT (see Table 4).[78,87]

In contrast, TAMs are selected by AZT and stavudine (d4T), and function through the excisional pathway. These mutations confer less of a viral fitness cost than discriminatory NRTI mutations.[79] Single TAMs have little impact on NRTI susceptibility[88]; however, the fold-change level, or decreased activity of the drug, is directly correlated with an increasing number of TAMs. In addition, although all TAMs confer resistance to AZT and d4T, the type I TAM pathway has a greater negative impact on tenofovir susceptibility than the type 2 TAM pathway (see Table 4).[84]

Non-nucleoside Reverse Transcriptase Inhibitors Mutations

NNRTIs bind to the hydrophobic pocket of reverse transcriptase, thus inhibiting viral replication (see Table 4).[84] Mutations conferring resistance to NNRTIs cause changes in the hydrophobic pocket, which decrease the ability of NNRTIs to bind.[84] Compared with the PIs and INSTIs, NNRTIs generally have a lower barrier to resistance. Cross-resistance among drugs within this class occurs with most NNRTI mutations.[84] However, etravirine (ETR) retains activity against isolates with K103N, allowing its use in salvage regimens (see Table 6).[89,90] Rilpivirine is also active in vitro against virus with the K103N mutation, and was effective in maintaining viral suppression in study participants who switched from boosted PI regimens and harbored this mutation.[91] In addition, doravirine (DOR), the newest agent in this class, is active against viral

Table 4
Common human immunodeficiency virus drug resistance mutations and impact on antiretroviral susceptibility

Mutation	Agents Leading to Mutation Selection	Reduced Susceptibility	Increased Susceptibility	Notes for Use
Nucleoside Reverse Transcriptase Inhibitor Mutations				
K65R	TDF/TAF, ABC, d4T, ddI	High-level resistance: TDF/TAF. Intermediate resistance: ABC, 3TC, FTC	AZT	—
K70E	TDF/TAF, ABC, d4T	Low-level resistance: TDF/TAF, ABC. Potential low-level resistance: 3TC, FTC	AZT	—
L74V	ABC, ddI	Intermediate resistance: ABC	—	—
M184V/I	3TC, FTC	High-level resistance: 3TC and FTC. Low-level resistance: ABC	TDF/TAF, AZT	Leads to reduced viral fitness; 3TC or FTC usually continued
Type 1 TAMs	AZT, d4T	—	—	Resistance to AZT increases with additional TAMs; greater negative impact on TDF and ABC than type 2 TAMs
M41L	AZT, d4T	Low-level resistance: AZT	—	—
L210W	AZT, d4T	Low-level resistance: AZT	—	—
T215Y	AZT, d4T	Intermediate resistance: AZT. Potential low-level resistance: ABC, TDF	—	—
Type 2 TAMs	AZT, d4T	—	—	Resistance increases with additional TAMs
D67N	AZT, d4T	Low-level resistance: AZT	—	—
K70R	AZT, d4T	Intermediate resistance: AZT	—	—
T215F	AZT, d4T	Intermediate resistance: AZT. Potential low-level resistance: ABC, TDF	—	—

(continued on next page)

Table 4
(continued)

Mutation	Agents Leading to Mutation Selection	Reduced Susceptibility	Increased Susceptibility	Notes for Use
K219Q/E	AZT, d4T	Potential low-level resistance: AZT	—	—
Non-nucleoside Reverse Transcriptase Inhibitor Mutations				
L100I	EFV, RPV, ETR	High-level resistance: EFV, NVP, RPV. Intermediate resistance: ETR	—	When K103N is present, leads to reduced DOR susceptibility
K101E	EFV, NVP, RPV, ETR	Intermediate resistance: EFV, RPV. Low-level resistance: NVP, ETR, DOR	—	—
K101ᴾ	EFV, NVP, RPV, ETR	High-level resistance: EFV, NVP, ETR, RPV	—	—
K103N/S	EFV, NVP	High-level resistance: EFV, NVP	—	—
Y181C	EFV, NVP, RPV	High-level resistance: NVP. Intermediate resistance: EFV, ETR, RPV	—	—
Y181I/V	NVP, ETR	High-level resistance: NVP, ETR, RPV. Intermediate resistance: EFV	—	—
Y188C/H	EFV, NVP	High-level resistance: NVP, EFV	—	—
Y188L	EFV, NVP	High-level resistance: EFV, NVP, RPV, DOR. Potential low-level resistance: ETR	—	—
G190A	EFV, NVP	High-level resistance: NVP. Intermediate resistance: EFV	—	—
G190S	EFV, NVP	High-level resistance: EFV, NVP. Intermediate resistance: DOR	—	—
G190E	EFV, ETR	High-level resistance: EFV, NVP, RPV, DOR. Intermediate resistance: ETR	—	—

Protease Inhibitor Mutations

Mutation	Drugs	Resistance interpretation		Notes
V32I	IDV, FPV, LPV, DRV	Low-level resistance: ATV/r, LPV/r, DRV/r	—	DRV/r should be given twice daily
I47V	IDV, FPV, LPV, DRV	Low-level resistance: LPV/r. Potential low-level resistance: ATV/r, DRV/r	—	—
G48V/M	SQV, IDV, LPV	Intermediate resistance: ATV/r. Low-level resistance: LPV/r	—	—
I50L	ATV	High-level resistance: ATV/r	LPV/r, DRV/r	—
I50V	DRV, LPV, FPV	Intermediate resistance: LPV/r Low-level resistance: DRV/r	—	DRV/r should be given twice daily
I54M/L	DRV, FPV	Low-level resistance: ATV/r, LPV/r, DRV/r	—	DRV/r should be given twice daily
L76V	IDV, LPV, DRV	Intermediate resistance: LPV/r. Low-level resistance: DRV/r	ATV	DRV/r should be given twice daily
V82A	IDV, LPV	Intermediate resistance: LPV/r. Low-level resistance: ATV/r	—	—
V82F	IDV, LPV	Intermediate resistance: LPV/r. Low-level resistance: ATV/r, DRV/r	—	DRV/r should be given twice daily
V82T/S	ATV, IDV, LPV, TPV	Intermediate resistance: LPV/r, ATV/r	—	—
I84V/C	All PIs	High-level resistance: ATV/r. Intermediate resistance: LPV/r. Low-level resistance: DRV/r	—	DRV/r should be given twice daily
I84A	All PIs	High-level resistance: ATV/r, LPV/r. Intermediate resistance: DRV/r	—	DRV/r should be given twice daily
N88S	ATV, NFV, IDV	High-level resistance: ATV/r	DRV/r	—
INSTI Mutations				
T66A	EVG, RAL	High-level resistance: EVG. Low-level resistance: RAL	—	—
T66I	EVG, RAL, DTG	High-level resistance: EVG. Low-level resistance: RAL	—	—

(continued on next page)

Table 4
(continued)

Mutation	Agents Leading to Mutation Selection	Reduced Susceptibility	Increased Susceptibility	Notes for Use
T66K	EVG, RAL	High-level resistance: EVG, RAL. Low-level resistance: DTG, BIC	—	DTG should be given twice daily
E92G	EVG, RAL	Intermediate resistance: EVG. Low-level resistance: RAL	—	—
E92Q	EVG, RAL, DTG	High-level resistance: EVG. Intermediate resistance: RAL. Potential low-level resistance: DTG	—	—
G118R	DTG	Intermediate resistance: EVG, RAL. Low-level resistance: DTG, BIC	—	DTG should be given twice daily
Y143C/R	RAL	High-level resistance: RAL	—	Synergistic with T97A; reduces EVG susceptibility with L74M, T97A, G163R, S230R
Y143A/G/K/S	RAL	High-level resistance: RAL	—	Reduces EVG susceptibility with accessory INSTI mutations
Q148H/R	EVG, RAL, DTG	High-level resistance: EVG, RAL. Low-level resistance: DTG, BIC	—	When combined with E138K and/or G140SA, susceptibility to DTG and BIC are affected. Effect is more pronounced with N155H, L74M, or T97A. DTG should be given twice daily
Q148K	EVG, RAL, DTG	High-level resistance: EVG, RAL. Intermediate resistance: DTG, BIC	—	When combined with E138 and G140 mutations, can lead to high-level resistance to DTG and BIC. DTG should be given twice daily
N155H	EVG, RAL, DTG	High-level resistance: EVG, RAL. Potential low-level resistance: DTG, BIC	—	—

| S230R | EVG, RAL, DTG | Low-level resistance: EVG, RAL, DTG Potential low-level resistance: BIC | — | DTG should be given twice daily |
| R263K | EVG, DTG, BIC | Intermediate resistance: EVG. Low-level resistance: RAL, DTG, BIC | — | DTG should be given twice daily |

Abbreviations: 3TC, lamivudine; ABC, abacavir; ATV, atazanavir; AZT, zidovudine; BIC, bictegravir; d4T, stavudine; ddI, didanosine; DOR, doravirine; DRV, daruna-vir; DTG, dolutegravir; EFV, efavirenz; ETR, etravirine; EVG, elvitegravir; FPV, fosamprenavir; FTC, emtricitabine; IDV, indinavir; LPV, lopinavir; NFV, nelfinavir; NVP, nevirapine; r, ritonavir; RAL, raltegravir; RPV, rilpivirine; SQV, saquinavir; TAF, tenofovir alafenamide; TAM, thymidine analog mutation; TDF, tenofovir disoproxil fumarate; TPV, tipranavir.

Adapted from Liu TF, Shafer RW. Web resources for HIV type 1 genotypic-resistance test interpretation. *Clinical infectious diseases : an official publication of the Infectious Diseases Society of America.* 2006;42(11):1608-1618; with permission.

strains with K103N or Y181C[92] (see **Table 4**). Data on the use of DOR in patients with NNRTI resistance are limited.

Protease Inhibitor Mutations

PIs bind competitively to the active site of PR, which prevents necessary cleaving of viral polypeptides required for formation of new HIV virions as well as maturation and cell budding (see **Table 4**).[84] At present, the most commonly used agents in this class include lopinavir (LPV), ATV, and DRV. LPV and DRV must be given with pharmacologic boosters, whereas doing so with ATV improves drug exposure and is generally recommended. Mutations conferring resistance to these PIs confer changes such that the PIs are unable to bind to the active site.[84] Unlike NRTIs and NNRTIs, pharmacologically boosted PIs have a higher barrier to resistance and usually require more than 1 major mutation to cause a reduction in susceptibility.[84] Thus, failure on PI-based regimens, particularly when given as part of initial therapy, is more often caused by nonadherence than resistance.[80,93,94] Cross-resistance within this class is variable. For example, I50L causes resistance to ATV alone, whereas other PIs retain full activity.[84] By contrast, mutations selected by unboosted indinavir, saquinavir, and sometimes nelfinavir can lead to broad resistance within this class. Similarly, prolonged failure on lopinavir/ritonavir in treatment-experienced patients can select for resistance to other PIs. In this setting, only DRV and tipranavir reliably retain activity (see **Table 6**).[95–97] Fosamprenavir (and its earlier formulation amprenavir) are structurally similar to DRV, and hence may compromise activity of DRV in future regimens. As a result, fosamprenavir is no longer recommended.

Integrase Strand Transfer Inhibitor Mutations

INSTIs bind the active site of IN, preventing viral DNA strand transfer (see **Table 4**). Mutations conferring resistance to INSTIs cause changes in the active site, which prevent binding of the drug.[84] Early-generation INSTIs, raltegravir (RAL) and elvitegravir (EVG), have a much lower genetic barrier to resistance than the later-generation INSTIs DTG and BIC, which require multiple mutations to lower susceptibility to a clinically significant degree.[79,84]

Resistance to RAL and EVG can develop quickly in the setting of suboptimal adherence. There is also significant cross-resistance between RAL and EVG, which prevents sequential use of these earlier-generation INSTIs.[84] Resistance to RAL can occur through any of 3 main pathways: (1) Y143C, (2) Q148H/K/R, or (3) N155H.[98] EVG shares the Q148 and N155 pathways, but resistance to EVG can also develop with the presence of T66A/I/K and E92Q.[99] Of these pathways, Q148 is the most significant INSTI mutation and reduces activity of DTG and BIC, especially when combined with additional mutations.[100]

Although DTG is active against many strains that are resistant to RAL and EVG, resistance to DTG has been documented.[100] Clinical trial data have shown emergence of DTG resistance through the Q148 pathway when other INSTI mutations are also present.[100] DTG resistance also emerges when DTG is used as monotherapy.[101,102] Although rare, additional DTG resistance pathways have been identified, which include G118R, R263K, and S230R.[103–105] Resistance patterns for BIC are considered to be similar[106]; however, there are currently no data for its use in treatment-experienced patients with INSTI resistance, and it is not included in US guidelines for this population.[4]

Management of Human Immunodeficiency Virus Drug Resistance

Many resistance mutations have important interactions with other mutations, and so it is vital to consider the resistance genotype as a whole. Many commercial resistance test reports have accompanying drug susceptibility summaries that can assist providers in selecting the best treatment regimen. In addition, rule-based algorithms such as the Stanford University HIV Database, as mentioned earlier, allow users to input resistance data or sequences and provide interpretation of results.[36] Providers should also consider an individual's entire resistance genotype history to construct a cumulative resistance profile, particularly for patients who are very treatment experienced,[4] because of the potential presence of archived and minority drug resistance viruses, as previously discussed.

When selecting active drugs for a new ART regimen, providers may select a new drug class and/or drugs from a class to which the individual has been exposed but has no evidence of cross-resistance on resistance test results. Regimens should include at least 2 active agents when possible, although 3 are preferred.[4] If 2 active drugs are not available, ART should still be continued, with inclusion of NRTIs because resistance to this class has been most clearly associated with reduced viral fitness, a phenomenon further discussed later.[4] Guidelines recommend against the addition of only 1 active agent to a failing regimen because of the risk of failure with functional monotherapy.[4]

Although resistance to NRTIs may be present, there is evidence that there may still be clinical benefit from residual activity. Numerous studies have shown a paradoxic outcome in which rates of viral suppression are inversely correlated with the number of active NRTIs, when used with both PIs and DTG.[107–109] However, NRTI-containing regimens still lead to better viral suppression rates than PI or DTG monotherapy.[110] Thus, NRTIs should be continued in salvage regimens when possible. Furthermore, as discussed earlier, 3TC or FTC are often continued despite the presence of M184V in order to select for a less fit virus. M184V has also been shown to delay (but not prevent) emergence of TAMs.[111,112] In addition, K65R and TAMs function via antagonistic pathways.[113] Thus, continuation of NRTIs to maintain K65R or TAMs can help to prevent new mutations of the opposing type.

Second-Line Regimens

Table 5 summarizes the results of clinical trials for second-line ART regimens.[110,114–117] Current US guidelines offer recommendations for second-line regimens based on the failed first-line regimen.[4] For patients failing an NNRTI-based first-line regimen, second-line options include 2 NRTIs (at least 1 of which should be active) with either a boosted PI or DTG, or a boosted PI combined with an INSTI.[110,115–117] The same strategy is recommended for those failing a PI-based first-line regimen with PI resistance, though a different boosted PI should be used.[4] If an individual is failing a regimen containing the early-generation INSTIs RAL or EVG, a regimen containing twice-daily DTG may be used in second line with either a boosted PI or 2 NRTIs (at least 1 active) if DTG remains susceptible.[100,118] A boosted PI with 2 NRTIs is also a reasonable option. Of note, there are no published data at present regarding optimal choice of second-line therapy for patients failing DTG-based or BIC-based first-line regimens.

Salvage Regimens

This article refers to salvage regimens as ART regimens that are used in ART-experienced individuals with limited treatment options. Virologic failure occurring on second-line and salvage regimens presents a challenge because of the amount of ART exposure and extensive resistance that is often present. **Table 6** summarizes the results of clinical trials for salvage ART regimens.[89,90,95–97,100,103,118–131] Dosing may differ for agents used in the setting of resistance. For example, both DRV/r and

Table 5
Clinical trials of second-line therapies for treatment-experienced patients

Study	Citation	Setting	Study Population	Arms	Outcome	Results
Second-line Studies						
HIV STAR	Bunupuradah et al,[114] 2012	Thailand	Virologic failure on 2 NRTIs + 1 NNRTI and PI naive	LPV/r monotherapy TDF/3TC/LPV/r	Viral suppression at 48 wk	Against LPV/r monotherapy P<.01
SECOND-LINE	SECOND-LINE Study Group,[115] 2013	Australia, Asia, Europe, Mexico, South America, Sub-Saharan Africa	Virologic failure on 2 NRTIs + 1 NNRTI and PI and INSTI naive	LPV/r + RAL BID Optimized NRTI background + LPV/r	Viral suppression at 48 wk	RAL + LPV/r noninferior to NRTIs + LPV/r
SELECT	La Rosa et al,[116] 2016	Asia, South America, Sub-Saharan Africa	Virologic failure on an NNRTI-based regimen	LPV/r + RAL BID optimized NRTI background + LPV/r	Time to virologic failure at or after week 24	RAL + LPV/r noninferior to NRTIs + LPV/r
EARNEST	Paton et al,[110] 2014	Sub-Saharan Africa	Virologic, immunologic, or clinical failure on 2 NRTIs + 1 NNRTI and PI naive	LPV/r monotherapy LPV/r + RAL BID 2 or 3 NRTIs + LPV/r	Good HIV control at 96 wk	RAL + LPV/r not superior to NRTIs + LPV/r; PI monotherapy inferior
DAWNING	Aboud et al,[117] 2017	Asia, Eastern Europe, Mexico, South America, Sub-Saharan Africa	Virologic failure on 2 NRTIs + 1 NNRTI	2 NRTIs ($\geq$1 active NRTI) + LPV/r 2 NRTIs ($\geq$1 active NRTI) + DTG	Viral suppression at 24 wk	Favors 2 NRTIs + DTG P<.001

Table 6
Clinical trials of salvage therapies for treatment-experienced patients

Study	Citation	Setting	Study Population	Arms	Outcome	Results
Studies of Nucleoside Reverse Transcriptase Inhibitors						
OPTIONS	Tashima et al,[119] 2015	United States	Virologic failure on a PI-based regimen and exposure or resistance to 3 drug classes	Optimized regimen without NRTIs optimized regimen with NRTIs	Regimen failure at 48 wk	Regimen without NRTIs is noninferior
Studies of Second-generation Non-nucleoside Reverse Transcriptase Inhibitors						
DUET 1	Madruga et al,[122] 2007	Asia, Central America, Mexico, South America, United States	Virologic failure and ≥3 primary PI mutations and ≥1 NNRTI mutations	NRTIs + DRV/r + ETV ± enfuvirtide NRTIs + DRV/r + placebo ± enfuvirtide	Viral suppression at 24 wk	Favors ETV P = .005
DUET 2	Lazzarin et al,[90] 2007	Australia, Canada, Europe, United States	Virologic failure and ≥3 primary PI mutations and ≥1 NNRTI mutations	NRTIs + DRV/r + ETV ± enfuvirtide NRTIs + DRV/r + placebo ± enfuvirtide	Viral suppression at 24 wk	Favors ETV P = .0003
Studies of Protease Inhibitors						
RESIST-1	Gathe et al,[120] 2006	Australia, Canada, United States	Virologic failure on a PI-based regimen and exposure to 3 classes (≥2 PIs) and ≥1 PI mutation	Optimized background + TPV/r optimized background + LPV/r, IDV/r, SQV/r, or APV/r	Reduction in HIV-1 RNA at 24 wk	Favors TPV/r P<.0001
RESIST-2	Cahn et al,[121] 2006	Europe, Latin America	Virologic failure on a PI-based regimen and exposure to 3 classes (≥2 PIs) and ≥1 PI mutation	Optimized background + TPV/r Optimized background + LPV/r, IDV/r, SQV/r, or APV/r	Reduction in HIV-1 RNA at 24 wk	Favors TPV/r P<.0001

(continued on next page)

Table 6
(continued)

Study	Citation	Setting	Study Population	Arms	Outcome	Results
POWER 1	Katlama et al,[95] 2007	Australia, Brazil, Canada, Europe	Virologic failure on a PI-based regimen and exposure to 3 drug classes and ≥1 PI mutation	Optimized background + DRV/r Optimized background + control PIs	Reduction in HIV-1 RNA at 24 wk	Favors DRV/r P<.001
POWER 2	Haubrich et al,[96] 2007	Argentina, United States	Virologic failure on a PI-based regimen and exposure to 3 drug classes and ≥1 PI mutation	Optimized background + DRV/r Optimized background + control PIs	Reduction in HIV-1 RNA at 24 wk	Favors DRV/r P≤.003
POWER 3	Molina et al,[97] 2007	Australia, Canada, Europe, South America, United States	Virologic failure on a PI-based regimen and exposure to 3 drug classes and ≥1 PI mutation	Single arm: optimized background + DRV/r BID	Reduction in HIV-1 RNA at 24 wk	Supports DRV/r BID
TITAN	Madruga et al,[122] 2007	Global	Virologic failure on combination ART and naive to LPV, DRV, TPV and naive to T-20	Optimized background + DRV/r BID optimized background + LPV/r BID	Viral suppression at 48 wk	DRV/r noninferior to LPV/r
ODIN	Cahn et al,[123] 2011	Asia, Australia, Central America, Europe, North America, South America	Virologic failure on combination ART and no DRV resistance mutations and no exposure to DRV, TPV, or enfuvirtide	Optimized background (≥2 NRTIs) + DRV/r daily optimized background (≥2 NRTIs) + DRV/r BID	Viral suppression at 48 wk	DRV/r daily noninferior to DRV/r BID without DRV resistance

Studies of Integrase Strand Transfer Inhibitors

BENCHMRK	Steigbigel et al,[124] 2008	Asia, Australia, Europe, North America, South America	Virologic failure and resistance to 3 drug classes and INSTI naive	Optimized background + RAL BID optimized background + placebo	Viral suppression at 48 wk	Favors RAL P<.001
Study 145	Molina et al,[125] 2012	Australia, Europe, North America	Virologic failure and resistance and/or exposure to 2 classes	Background with boosted PI + EVG/r PI-containing background + RAL	Viral suppression at 48 wk	EVG/r noninferior to RAL
SAILING	Cahn et al,[103] 2013	Australia, Canada, Europe, Latin America, Taiwan, South Africa, United States	Virologic failure and resistance to at least 2 classes and at least 1 active drug for background therapy	Background + DTG daily + placebo background + RAL BID + placebo	Viral suppression at 48 wk	DTG superior to RAL P = .03
VIKING	Eron et al,[118] 2013	Canada, France, Italy, Spain, United States	Virologic failure and resistance to RAL/EVG and 2 other classes and ≥1 available active agent	DTG daily (I) or BID (II) + 10d failing regimen followed by optimized background + DTG daily (I) or BID (II)	Reduction in HIV-1 RNA at 11 d	Favors DTG BID P = .017
VIKING-3	Castagna et al,[100] 2014	Canada, Europe, United States	Virologic failure and resistance to RAL/EVG and 2 other classes and ≥1 available active agent	Single arm: 7-d DTG BID functional monotherapy followed by optimized background + DTG BID	Reduction in HIV-1 RNA at 8 d, viral suppression at 24 wk	Supports DTG BID

Studies of Entry Inhibitors

TORO 1	Lalezari et al,[126] 2003	Brazil, Canada, Mexico, United States	Virologic failure and resistance and/or exposure to 3 drug classes (including ≥2 PIs)	Optimized background + enfuvirtide BID optimized background alone	Reduction in HIV-1 RNA at 24 wk	Favors enfuvirtide P<.001

(continued on next page)

Table 6
(continued)

Study	Citation	Setting	Study Population	Arms	Outcome	Results
TORO 2	Lazzarin et al,[127] 2003	Europe, Australia	Virologic failure and resistance and/or exposure to 3 drug classes	Optimized background + enfuvirtide BID optimized background alone	Reduction in HIV-1 RNA at 24 wk	Favors enfuvirtide P<.001
MOTIVATE 1 & 2	Gulick et al,[128] 2008	Australia, Europe, United States	Virologic failure and resistance and/or exposure to 3 classes and CCR5 tropic HIV-1	Optimized background + maraviroc daily optimized background + maraviroc BID optimized background + placebo	Reduction in HIV-1 RNA at 48 wk	Favors maraviroc
A4001029 Study	Saag et al,[129] 2009	Australia, Canada, Europe, United States	Virologic failure and resistance or exposure to multiple classes and dual/mixed-tropic HIV-1	Optimized background + maraviroc daily optimized background + maraviroc BID optimized background + placebo	Reduction in HIV-1 RNA at 24 wk	Against use of maraviroc for non-R5-tropic HIV-1
Studies of Post Attachment Inhibitors						
Ibalizumab	Emu et al,[132] 2018	North America, Taiwan	Virologic failure with multidrug-resistant HIV-1	Single arm: ibalizumab Control period: continued failing regimen for 7 d	Decrease in HIV-1 RNA of 0.5 log10 copies/mL by day 14	Supports Ibalizumab P<.001

Other						
ANRS 139 TRIO	Yazdanpanah et al,[130] 2009	France	Virologic failure, RAL, ETR, DRV naive and ≥3 PI and NRTI mutations and ≤3 DRV or NNRTI mutations	Single arm: DRV/r BID + RAL BID + ETR BID ± Optimized background (NRTIs or enfuvirtide)	Viral suppression at 24 wk	Supports DRV/r BID + RAL BID + ETR BID
MULTI-OCTAVE	Grinsztejn et al,[131] 2018	Africa, Asia, Caribbean, South America	Virologic failure on PI-containing second-line ART	2 NRTIs + PI NRTIs + RAL + DRV/r RAL + DRV/r + ETR	Viral suppression at 48 wk	Supports DRV/r + RAL ± ETR in cases of LPV resistance

Abbreviations: APV, amprenavir; BID, twice daily; ETV, etravirine.

DTG are advised to be given twice daily when certain PI and INSTI mutations are present, respectively.[97,100,118] For individuals who are extremely treatment experienced, additional agents, including maraviroc (a CCR5 antagonist), enfuvirtide (a fusion inhibitor), and ibalizumab (IBA), have shown benefit when added to an optimized background regimen.[126–128] Importantly, maraviroc may only be used in individuals who are found to have CCR5-tropic virus by tropism testing.[129] Recently, IBA, a monoclonal antibody, has shown efficacy in treatment-experienced mutations with extensive multiclass resistance, and is now approved for use in this patient population. IBA is a novel drug that is classified as a postattachment inhibitor that prevents viral entry. However, reduced susceptibility to this agent leading to virologic failure was shown to occur in a phase 3 clinical trial.[132] In addition, IBA must be administered via intravenous infusion, which may be challenging in some settings. Note that the treatment of patients with extensive drug resistance is a rapidly evolving field, owing to the pipeline of new HIV drugs[133] and classes, such as nucleoside reverse transcriptase translocation inhibitors,[134] maturation inhibitors,[135] and attachment inhibitors.[136] These new agents are likely to offer additional choices for the increasingly rare patients with multiclass resistance; whereas the principle of selecting at least 2 active agents from 2 separate classes is likely to continue to apply for the foreseeable future. Furthermore, continuation of ART is always preferred to treatment interruption or cessation, regardless of whether there any active agents available.[4,137]

MANAGING VIROLOGIC FAILURE IN SPECIAL POPULATIONS
Women of Childbearing Potential

There are preliminary data linking DTG use during conception and an increased risk of neural tube defects in babies born to these mothers.[138] As a result, treatment guidelines have recommended counseling women of childbearing potential about this risk, and strong consideration for use of alternative agents whenever possible.[4] However, where DTG is required for maintaining or achieving viral suppression, the authors advocate use of this agent despite these preliminary data. Virologic failure could worsen maternal outcomes and increase the risk of viral transmission to the newborn.

Coinfection with Tuberculosis

For individuals presenting concurrently with virologic failure and newly diagnosed active tuberculosis (TB), the authors favor an approach in which TB treatment initiation and ART regimen switch do not occur simultaneously, to avoid occurrence of toxicity without a clear cause. TB treatment should be initiated immediately.[139] Although current guidelines do not offer recommendations regarding the optimal timing of regimen switch relative to initiation of TB treatment, we favor waiting approximately 2 weeks to start a new HIV treatment, as is done for people presenting with co-occurring new diagnoses of HIV and pulmonary TB.

ART regimens in this scenario should be selected to achieve viral suppression, minimize side effects, and avoid drug-drug interactions with the TB treatment regimen.[139] Particular attention must be paid to the rifamycin component of standard TB treatment regimens. Rifamycins are strong inducers of cytochrome P3A4 enzymes (with the exception of rifabutin, a less potent inducer) and can lead to increased metabolism and decreased systemic levels of some antiretroviral agents.[140] Thus, when selecting ART regimens for individuals with treatment failure, drug interaction review is particularly important.[50,141] In general, rifabutin leads to fewer interactions than rifampin.[142] However, rifabutin is unavailable in many resource-limited settings with a high prevalence of TB.

NRTIs can be safely included in second-line and salvage regimens with rifamycin-containing TB treatment regimens without dose adjustment. As an exception, current guidelines do not recommend coadministration of tenofovir alafenamide (TAF) with any of the rifamycins given the potential for decreased plasma concentrations of TAF.[139] However, recent data show high intracellular concentrations of tenofovir diphosphate with coadministration of TAF and rifampin, which were greater than the intracellular levels achieved with administration of TDF alone.[143] Thus, although not currently recommended because of an absence of more robust outcomes data, coadministration of TAF and rifamycins still may prove efficacious.

Earlier-generation NNRTIs, efavirenz and nevirapine, are the most studied agents for use in TB/HIV coinfection. However, these agents are not often used in second-line and salvage regimens because of the high prevalence of drug resistance mutations. ETR is more often used in salvage regimens and may be coadministered with rifabutin. However, ETR should not be coadministered with rifampin because of an inability to achieve appropriate drug levels.[4,139] DOR, a newly approved NNRTI in 2018, is not yet discussed in US guidelines for TB/HIV coinfection. However, studies have shown that it can be coadministered at a double dose with rifabutin but should not be used with rifampin.[144]

If a boosted PI is used in the second-line or salvage ART regimen, rifabutin is the preferred rifamycin, given that dose adjustments of the boosted PI are not required.[145,146] However, all PIs increase drug levels of rifabutin, requiring downward dose adjustment of the rifabutin to avoid drug toxicities.[145] If rifampin must be used with a PI because of a lack of access to rifabutin, a dose increase in the boosted PI is required to achieve therapeutic levels. LPV/r is the only PI that has been well studied for concurrent administration with rifampin. Dosing options include either doubling the dose of LPV/r or increasing the dose of the ritonavir booster.[137,147,148] However, both of these strategies lead to markedly increased pill burden, risk of hepatoxicity, and significant gastrointestinal side effects.[149,150]

If an INSTI is chosen as part of the second-line or salvage ART regimen, dose adjustments are also required to achieve therapeutic INSTI levels. Specifically, DTG should be administered twice daily. RAL should be double dosed when coadministered with rifampin, although no adjustment is necessary when coadministered with rifabutin.[151–154] Coadministration of rifamycins with either BIC or elvitegravir/cobicistat should be avoided.[139,155]

In addition, enfuvirtide and rifamycins can be coadministered without dose adjustment. However, drug interactions do exist with maraviroc and rifamycins, and there are no clinical studies to guide use of this combination.[4]

Coinfection with Hepatitis B

For all patients coinfected with HIV-1 and hepatitis B virus (HBV), it is important to maintain agents with activity against HBV as part of the ART regimen. Although 3TC and FTC have activity against HBV, these agents readily select for HBV resistance and as a result are not recommended as the only agent with activity against HBV.[156–158] Even in the setting of HIV-1 drug resistance mutations to tenofovir, TDF or TAF should be included as part of the second-line or salvage ART regimen given that it is the first-line drug for HBV, has a high barrier to resistance, and is active against 3TC-resistant HBV strains.[159–164] In addition, patients are at risk of HBV DNA rebound and hepatitis flare if agents active against HBV are discontinued.[165] If a patient with HBV coinfection otherwise has contraindications to tenofovir, such as renal failure, entecavir can be added to a fully active ART regimen.[4]

Coinfection with Hepatitis C

With the introduction of direct-acting antivirals, there are many options for the treatment of hepatitis C virus (HCV). However, it is important to be aware of the drug-drug interactions between anti-HCV and ART regimens. Drug-drug interactions between HCV and HIV drugs have been published previously[166] and are available online. If an ART regimen change is required during the course of HCV treatment because of HIV virologic failure, providers should consult a drug interaction resource.[50,167–169] If virologic failure is diagnosed before the start of HCV treatment, then the ART regimen should be appropriately adjusted and viral suppression achieved before beginning the HCV treatment regimen.[168]

Infection with Human Immunodeficiency Virus 2

In contrast with HIV-1, there are currently no standard genotypic resistance tests available for HIV-2 to guide treatment decisions at the time of virologic failure.[4] However, knowledge of key features of HIV-2 can aid in the empiric selection of ART regimens at the time of treatment failure. In particular, HIV-2 is intrinsically resistant to both NNRTIs[170] and to enfuvirtide.[171] NRTIs have activity against HIV-2, but, as in HIV-1, they should be used in combination with another drug class. Select boosted PIs have shown activity against HIV-2, including DRV, LPV, and saquinavir; however, other PIs do not show equivalent activity and should be avoided.[172,173] All currently available INSTIs show potent activity against HIV-2,[174–178] although development of resistance has been shown, particularly with earlier generation INSTIs.[178–179] Although CCR5 antagonists may have activity against HIV-2, there are currently no standardized tropism assays for HIV-2.[180]

MANAGING VIROLOGIC FAILURE IN RESOURCE-LIMITED SETTINGS

In resource-limited settings, virologic failure is defined as 2 consecutive HIV-1 RNA levels greater than 1000 copies/mL despite interval intensive adherence counseling.[137] This higher HIV-1 RNA cutoff has been selected because of the widespread use of viral load monitoring using dried blood spots in many regions, and as a public health approach to minimize unnecessary switching to more costly and burdensome HIV regimens.[137] Notably, genotypic resistance testing is not routinely available or recommended for pretreatment resistance testing or resistance testing at the time of virologic failure on first-line ART.[137,181] Empiric first-line regimens recommended by the World Health Organization (WHO) are based on results of national pretreatment drug resistance surveillance studies.[58] Given the increasing rate of PDR to NNRTIs, as discussed earlier, ART programs are advised to now use a DTG-based regimen as the preferred first-line treatment, with the exception of women of childbearing age, for whom assessment of contraception access and risk-based stratification is recommended.[58,181] Similarly, empiric second-line regimens are recommended based on the first-line regimen that an individual has failed. Specifically, WHO recommends a boosted PI-containing regimen following failure on DTG-based first-line regimens and a DTG-containing regimen following failure on NNRTI-based first-line regimens.[181] The NRTI component of second-line regimens is also empirically recommended based on the most likely resistance mutations that would have been selected by the first-line regimen, thus requiring a switched NRTI backbone.[137] For example, an individual failing a TDF-containing first-line regimen should be switched to an AZT-containing second-line regimen, given the presumed presence of K65R, with the caveat that TDF should also be continued in the setting of chronic HBV coinfection. An individual failing an AZT-containing first-line regimen should be switched to a TDF-containing second-line regimen, given the presumed presence of TAMs.

In contrast with first-line treatment failure, WHO now recommends the use of genotypic resistance testing when feasible at the time of virologic failure on second-line ART.[181] Both boosted PIs and DTG have higher barriers to resistance than NNRTIs.[182,183] Thus, resistance testing allows the identification of individuals with second-line failure caused by poor adherence alone, as well as treatment optimization in those who are found to have second-line failure caused by drug resistance. In those who do require a switch to third-line ART, WHO currently recommends that salvage regimens include DRV/r, DTG, and an optimized NRTI background when possible.[181] Many countries use an expert panel or committee to review resistance results and approve the use of third-line regimens to ensure appropriate use and stewardship of these agents.[184,185] For individuals with no active drugs available, or in settings without access to salvage regimens, WHO recommends continuation rather than cessation of ART.[137]

SUMMARY

Although virologic failure can be a complex and clinically significant complication of HIV infection, advances in diagnostics and novel therapeutics have expanded treatment options even for those patients with extensive exposure to ART and multidrug-resistant virus. Principles of management for virologic failure include (1) conduct of genotypic resistance testing; (2) differentiating between adherence and resistance driven failure, which are not mutually exclusive; and (3) selection of optimized regimens with a minimum of 2 active drugs from 2 separate classes. As with treatment initiation, the goal of therapy after treatment failure is to select a regimen that is well tolerated, minimally burdensome, and rapidly and durably yields virologic suppression. Achieving this goal will improve health for people with HIV and prevent viral transmission.

ACKNOWLEDGMENTS

This work was supported by the National Institutes of Health (K23 AI143470 and 5T32 AI007387 to S.M.M., R01 AI124718 to M.J.S., R01 AI098558 to V.C.M.), the Harvard University Center for AIDS Research (P30 AI060354 to M.J.S.), the Emory Center for AIDS Research (P30 AI050409 to V.C.M.), and the Massachusetts General Hospital Executive Committee on Research Fund for Medical Discovery (Clinical Fellowship Award to S.M.M.). The contents are solely the responsibility of the authors and do not necessarily represent the official views of the NIH.

REFERENCES

1. Joint United Nations Programme on HIV/AIDS. 90-90-90: an ambitious treatment target to help end the AIDS epidemic. 2014.
2. Centers for Disease Control. HIV in the United States 2018. Available at: https://www.cdc.gov/hiv/images/library/infographics/continuum-infographic.png. Accessed December 7, 2018.
3. Bradley H, Hall HI, Wolitski RJ, et al. Vital Signs: HIV diagnosis, care, and treatment among persons living with HIV–United States, 2011. MMWR Morb Mortal Wkly Rep 2014;63(47):1113–7.
4. Panel on Antiretroviral Guidelines for Adults and Adolescents. Guidelines for the Use of Antiretroviral Agents in Adults and Adolescents Living with HIV. United States Department of Health and Human Services. Available at: http://www.aidsinfo.nih.gov/ContentFiles/AdultandAdolescentGL.pdf. Accessed December 4, 2018.

5. Hermans LE, Moorhouse M, Carmona S, et al. Effect of HIV-1 low-level viraemia during antiretroviral therapy on treatment outcomes in WHO-guided South African treatment programmes: a multicentre cohort study. Lancet Infect Dis 2018; 18(2):188–97.

6. Vandenhende MA, Perrier A, Bonnet F, et al. Risk of virological failure in HIV-1-infected patients experiencing low-level viraemia under active antiretroviral therapy (ANRS C03 cohort study). Antivir Ther 2015;20(6):655–60.

7. Laprise C, de Pokomandy A, Baril JG, et al. Virologic failure following persistent low-level viremia in a cohort of HIV-positive patients: results from 12 years of observation. Clin Infect Dis 2013;57(10):1489–96.

8. Nettles RE, Kieffer TL, Kwon P, et al. Intermittent HIV-1 viremia (Blips) and drug resistance in patients receiving HAART. JAMA 2005;293(7):817–29.

9. Sungkanuparph S, Overton ET, Seyfried W, et al. Intermittent episodes of detectable HIV viremia in patients receiving nonnucleoside reverse-transcriptase inhibitor-based or protease inhibitor-based highly active antiretroviral therapy regimens are equivalent in incidence and prognosis. Clin Infect Dis 2005; 41(9):1326–32.

10. Durant J, Clevenbergh P, Halfon P, et al. Drug-resistance genotyping in HIV-1 therapy: the VIRADAPT randomised controlled trial. Lancet 1999;353(9171): 2195–9.

11. Baxter JD, Mayers DL, Wentworth DN, et al. A randomized study of antiretroviral management based on plasma genotypic antiretroviral resistance testing in patients failing therapy. CPCRA 046 Study Team for the Terry Beirn Community Programs for Clinical Research on AIDS. AIDS 2000;14(9):F83–93.

12. Cingolani A, Antinori A, Rizzo MG, et al. Usefulness of monitoring HIV drug resistance and adherence in individuals failing highly active antiretroviral therapy: a randomized study (ARGENTA). AIDS 2002;16(3):369–79.

13. Tural C, Ruiz L, Holtzer C, et al. Clinical utility of HIV-1 genotyping and expert advice: the Havana trial. AIDS 2002;16(2):209–18.

14. Green H, Gibb DM, Compagnucci A, et al. A randomized controlled trial of genotypic HIV drug resistance testing in HIV-1-infected children: the PERA (PENTA 8) trial. Antivir Ther 2006;11(7):857–67.

15. Cohen CJ, Hunt S, Sension M, et al. A randomized trial assessing the impact of phenotypic resistance testing on antiretroviral therapy. AIDS 2002;16(4):579–88.

16. Haubrich RH, Kemper CA, Hellmann NS, et al. A randomized, prospective study of phenotype susceptibility testing versus standard of care to manage antiretroviral therapy: CCTG 575. AIDS 2005;19(3):295–302.

17. Meynard JL, Vray M, Morand-Joubert L, et al. Phenotypic or genotypic resistance testing for choosing antiretroviral therapy after treatment failure: a randomized trial. AIDS 2002;16(5):727–36.

18. Wegner SA, Wallace MR, Aronson NE, et al. Long-term efficacy of routine access to antiretroviral-resistance testing in HIV type 1-infected patients: results of the clinical efficacy of resistance testing trial. Clin Infect Dis 2004;38(5): 723–30.

19. Mazzotta F, Lo Caputo S, Torti C, et al. Real versus virtual phenotype to guide treatment in heavily pretreated patients: 48-week follow-up of the Genotipo-Fenotipo di Resistenza (GenPheRex) trial. J Acquir Immune Defic Syndr 2003; 32(3):268–80.

20. Perez-Elias MJ, Garcia-Arota I, Munoz V, et al. Phenotype or virtual phenotype for choosing antiretroviral therapy after failure: a prospective, randomized study. Antivir Ther 2003;8(6):577–84.

21. Dunn DT, Green H, Loveday C, et al. A randomized controlled trial of the value of phenotypic testing in addition to genotypic testing for HIV drug resistance: evaluation of resistance assays (ERA) trial investigators. J Acquir Immune Defic Syndr 2005;38(5):553–9.

22. Weinstein MC, Goldie SJ, Losina E, et al. Use of genotypic resistance testing to guide hiv therapy: clinical impact and cost-effectiveness. Ann Intern Med 2001; 134(6):440–50.

23. Corzillius M, Muhlberger N, Sroczynski G, et al. Cost effectiveness analysis of routine use of genotypic antiretroviral resistance testing after failure of antiretroviral treatment for HIV. Antivir Ther 2004;9(1):27–36.

24. Sax PE, Islam R, Walensky RP, et al. Should resistance testing be performed for treatment-naive HIV-infected patients? A cost-effectiveness analysis. Clin Infect Dis 2005;41(9):1316–23.

25. Yazdanpanah Y, Vray M, Meynard J, et al. The long-term benefits of genotypic resistance testing in patients with extensive prior antiretroviral therapy: a model-based approach. HIV Med 2007;8(7):439–50.

26. Sendi P, Gunthard HF, Simcock M, et al. Cost-effectiveness of genotypic antiretroviral resistance testing in HIV-infected patients with treatment failure. PLoS One 2007;2(1):e173.

27. Rosen S, Long L, Sanne I, et al. The net cost of incorporating resistance testing into HIV/AIDS treatment in South Africa: a Markov model with primary data. J Int AIDS Soc 2011;14:24.

28. Levison JH, Wood R, Scott CA, et al. The clinical and economic impact of genotype testing at first-line antiretroviral therapy failure for HIV-infected patients in South Africa. Clin Infect Dis 2013;56(4):587–97.

29. Phillips A, Cambiano V, Nakagawa F, et al. Cost-effectiveness of HIV drug resistance testing to inform switching to second line antiretroviral therapy in low income settings. PLoS One 2014;9(10):e109148.

30. Luz PM, Morris BL, Grinsztejn B, et al. Cost-effectiveness of genotype testing for primary resistance in Brazil. J Acquir Immune Defic Syndr 2015;68(2):152–61.

31. Koullias Y, Sax PE, Fields NF, et al. Should we be testing for baseline integrase resistance in patients newly diagnosed with human immunodeficiency virus? Clin Infect Dis 2017;65(8):1274–81.

32. Phillips AN, Cambiano V, Nakagawa F, et al. Cost-effectiveness of public-health policy options in the presence of pretreatment NNRTI drug resistance in sub-Saharan Africa: a modelling study. Lancet HIV 2018;5(3):e146–54.

33. Gunthard HF, Calvez V, Paredes R, et al. Human immunodeficiency virus drug resistance: 2018 recommendations of the International Antiviral Society-USA Panel. Clin Infect Dis 2019;68(2):177–87.

34. Devereux HL, Youle M, Johnson MA, et al. Rapid decline in detectability of HIV-1 drug resistance mutations after stopping therapy. AIDS 1999;13(18):F123–7.

35. Verhofstede C, Wanzeele FV, Van Der Gucht B, et al. Interruption of reverse transcriptase inhibitors or a switch from reverse transcriptase to protease inhibitors resulted in a fast reappearance of virus strains with a reverse transcriptase inhibitor-sensitive genotype. AIDS 1999;13(18):2541–6.

36. Liu TF, Shafer RW. Web resources for HIV type 1 genotypic-resistance test interpretation. Clin Infect Dis 2006;42(11):1608–18.

37. Camacho R, Van Laethem, Geretti AM, et al. Algorithm for the use of genotypic HIV-1 resistance data (version Rega v10.0.0) 2017. Available at: https://rega.kuleuven.be/cev/avd/software/rega-hiv1-rules-v10.pdf. Accessed January 4, 2019.

38. Agence National de Recerche sur le SIDA (ANRS). HIV-1 genotypic drug resistance interpretation's algorithms. Available at: http://www.hivfrenchresistance.org/index.html. Accessed January 4, 2019.

39. Obermeier M, Pironti A, Berg T, et al. HIV-GRADE: a publicly available, rules-based drug resistance interpretation algorithm integrating bioinformatic knowledge. Intervirology 2012;55(2):102–7.

40. Available at: https://www.iasusa.org/wp-content/uploads/2018/01/2017hiv-muta-article.pdf. Accessed January 4, 2019.

41. Murphy DA, Marelich WD, Hoffman D, et al. Predictors of antiretroviral adherence. AIDS Care 2004;16(4):471–84.

42. Aidala AA, Wilson MG, Shubert V, et al. Housing status, medical care, and health outcomes among people living with HIV/AIDS: a systematic review. Am J Public Health 2016;106(1):e1–23.

43. Zhang Y, Wilson TE, Adedimeji A, et al. The impact of substance use on adherence to antiretroviral therapy among HIV-infected women in the United States. AIDS Behav 2018;22(3):896–908.

44. Carr RL, Gramling LF. Stigma: a health barrier for women with HIV/AIDS. J Assoc Nurses AIDS Care 2004;15(5):30–9.

45. Stirratt MJ, Remien RH, Smith A, et al. The role of HIV serostatus disclosure in antiretroviral medication adherence. AIDS Behav 2006;10(5):483–93.

46. Thompson MA, Mugavero MJ, Amico KR, et al. Guidelines for improving entry into and retention in care and antiretroviral adherence for persons with HIV: evidence-based recommendations from an International Association of Physicians in AIDS Care panel. Ann Intern Med 2012;156(11):817–33. W-284, W-285, W-286, W-287, W-288, W-289, W-290, W-291, W-292, W-293, W-294.

47. Palmer NB, Salcedo J, Miller AL, et al. Psychiatric and social barriers to HIV medication adherence in a triply diagnosed methadone population. AIDS Patient Care STDS 2003;17(12):635–44.

48. Parienti JJ, Bangsberg DR, Verdon R, et al. Better adherence with once-daily antiretroviral regimens: a meta-analysis. Clin Infect Dis 2009;48(4):484–8.

49. World Health Organization. Global action plan on HIV drug resistance 2017-2012: 2018 progress report. Geneva (Switzerland): World Health Organization; 2018.

50. University of Liverpool. HIV drug interactions. Available at: https://www.hiv-druginteractions.org/checker. Accessed December 21, 2018.

51. Sekar V, Kestens D, Spinosa-Guzman S, et al. The effect of different meal types on the pharmacokinetics of darunavir (TMC114)/ritonavir in HIV-negative healthy volunteers. J Clin Pharmacol 2007;47(4):479–84.

52. Le Tiec C, Barrail A, Goujard C, et al. Clinical pharmacokinetics and summary of efficacy and tolerability of atazanavir. Clin Pharmacokinet 2005;44(10):1035–50.

53. Custodio JM, Yin X, Hepner M, et al. Effect of food on rilpivirine/emtricitabine/tenofovir disoproxil fumarate, an antiretroviral single-tablet regimen for the treatment of HIV infection. J Clin Pharmacol 2014;54(4):378–85.

54. Kamimura M, Watanabe K, Kobayakawa M, et al. Successful absorption of antiretroviral drugs after gastrojejunal bypass surgery following failure of therapy through a jejunal tube. Intern Med 2009;48(12):1103–4.

55. Brantley RK, Williams KR, Silva TM, et al. AIDS-associated diarrhea and wasting in Northeast Brazil is associated with subtherapeutic plasma levels of antiretroviral medications and with both bovine and human subtypes of Cryptosporidium parvum. Braz J Infect Dis 2003;7(1):16–22.

56. Mannheimer SB, Morse E, Matts JP, et al. Sustained benefit from a long-term antiretroviral adherence intervention. Results of a large randomized clinical trial. J Acquir Immune Defic Syndr 2006;43(Suppl 1):S41–7.

57. Nachega JB, Parienti JJ, Uthman OA, et al. Lower pill burden and once-daily antiretroviral treatment regimens for HIV infection: a meta-analysis of randomized controlled trials. Clin Infect Dis 2014;58(9):1297–307.

58. World Health Organization. HIV drug resistance report. Geneva (Switzerland): World Health Organization; 2017.

59. Rhee SY, Blanco JL, Jordan MR, et al. Geographic and temporal trends in the molecular epidemiology and genetic mechanisms of transmitted HIV-1 drug resistance: an individual-patient- and sequence-level meta-analysis. PLoS Med 2015;12(4):e1001810.

60. Gupta RK, Gregson J, Parkin N, et al. HIV-1 drug resistance before initiation or re-initiation of first-line antiretroviral therapy in low-income and middle-income countries: a systematic review and meta-regression analysis. Lancet Infect Dis 2018;18(3):346–55.

61. Ross LL, Shortino D, Shaefer MS. Changes from 2000 to 2009 in the prevalence of HIV-1 containing drug resistance-associated mutations from antiretroviral therapy-naive, HIV-1-infected patients in the United States. AIDS Res Hum Retroviruses 2018;34(8):672–9.

62. McCluskey SM, Lee GQ, Kamelian K, et al. Increasing prevalence of HIV pretreatment drug resistance in women but not men in rural uganda during 2005-2013. AIDS Patient Care STDS 2018;32(7):257–64.

63. Frange P, Assoumou L, Descamps D, et al. HIV-1 subtype B-infected MSM may have driven the spread of transmitted resistant strains in France in 2007-12: impact on susceptibility to first-line strategies. J Antimicrob Chemother 2015;70(7):2084–9.

64. Spertilli Raffaelli C, Rossetti B, Paglicci L, et al. Impact of transmitted HIV-1 drug resistance on the efficacy of first-line antiretroviral therapy with two nucleos(t)ide reverse transcriptase inhibitors plus an integrase inhibitor or a protease inhibitor. J Antimicrob Chemother 2018;73(9):2480–4.

65. Doyle T, Dunn DT, Ceccherini-Silberstein F, et al. Integrase inhibitor (INI) genotypic resistance in treatment-naive and raltegravir-experienced patients infected with diverse HIV-1 clades. J Antimicrob Chemother 2015;70(11):3080–6.

66. Stekler JD, McKernan J, Milne R, et al. Lack of resistance to integrase inhibitors among antiretroviral-naive subjects with primary HIV-1 infection, 2007-2013. Antivir Ther 2015;20(1):77–80.

67. Tostevin A, White E, Dunn D, et al. Recent trends and patterns in HIV-1 transmitted drug resistance in the United Kingdom. HIV Med 2017;18(3):204–13.

68. Scherrer AU, Yang WL, Kouyos RD, et al. Successful prevention of transmission of integrase resistance in the Swiss HIV Cohort Study. J Infect Dis 2016;214(3):399–402.

69. Casadella M, van Ham PM, Noguera-Julian M, et al. Primary resistance to integrase strand-transfer inhibitors in Europe. J Antimicrob Chemother 2015;70(10):2885–8.

70. De Francesco MA, Izzo I, Properzi M, et al. Prevalence of integrase strand transfer inhibitors resistance mutations in integrase strand transfer inhibitors-Naive and -experienced HIV-1 infected patients: a single center experience. AIDS Res Hum Retroviruses 2018;34(7):570–4.

71. McClung R, Ocfemia CB, Saduvala N, et al. Integrase and Other Transmitted HIV Drug Resistance: 23 US Jurisdictions, 2013-2016. Conference on Retroviruses and Opportunistic Infections. Seattle, WA, March 4–7, 2019.

72. McGee KS, Okeke NL, Hurt CB, et al. Canary in the coal mine? transmitted mutations conferring resistance to all integrase strand transfer inhibitors in a treatment-naive patient. Open Forum Infect Dis 2018;5(11):ofy294.

73. Boyd SD, Maldarelli F, Sereti I, et al. Transmitted raltegravir resistance in an HIV-1 CRF_AG-infected patient. Antivir Ther 2011;16(2):257–61.

74. Young B, Fransen S, Greenberg KS, et al. Transmission of integrase strand-transfer inhibitor multidrug-resistant HIV-1: case report and response to raltegravir-containing antiretroviral therapy. Antivir Ther 2011;16(2):253–6.

75. Wei X, Ghosh SK, Taylor ME, et al. Viral dynamics in human immunodeficiency virus type 1 infection. Nature 1995;373(6510):117–22.

76. Abram ME, Ferris AL, Shao W, et al. Nature, position, and frequency of mutations made in a single cycle of HIV-1 replication. J Virol 2010;84(19):9864–78.

77. Sufka SA, Ferrari G, Gryszowka VE, et al. Prolonged CD4+ cell/virus load discordance during treatment with protease inhibitor-based highly active antiretroviral therapy: immune response and viral control. J Infect Dis 2003;187(7):1027–37.

78. Weber J, Chakraborty B, Weberova J, et al. Diminished replicative fitness of primary human immunodeficiency virus type 1 isolates harboring the K65R mutation. J Clin Microbiol 2005;43(3):1395–400.

79. Clutter DS, Jordan MR, Bertagnolio S, et al. HIV-1 drug resistance and resistance testing. Infect Genet Evol 2016;46:292–307.

80. Bangsberg DR, Acosta EP, Gupta R, et al. Adherence-resistance relationships for protease and non-nucleoside reverse transcriptase inhibitors explained by virological fitness. AIDS 2006;20(2):223–31.

81. Ribaudo HJ, Haas DW, Tierney C, et al. Pharmacogenetics of plasma efavirenz exposure after treatment discontinuation: an Adult AIDS Clinical Trials Group Study. Clin Infect Dis 2006;42(3):401–7.

82. Bennett DE, Camacho RJ, Otelea D, et al. Drug resistance mutations for surveillance of transmitted HIV-1 drug-resistance: 2009 update. PLoS One 2009;4(3):e4724.

83. Wensing AM, Calvez V, Gunthard HF, et al. 2017 update of the drug resistance mutations in HIV-1. Top Antivir Med 2017;24(4):132–3.

84. Tang MW, Shafer RW. HIV-1 antiretroviral resistance: scientific principles and clinical applications. Drugs 2012;72(9):e1–25.

85. Whitcomb JM, Parkin NT, Chappey C, et al. Broad nucleoside reverse-transcriptase inhibitor cross-resistance in human immunodeficiency virus type 1 clinical isolates. J Infect Dis 2003;188(7):992–1000.

86. Campbell TB, Shulman NS, Johnson SC, et al. Antiviral activity of lamivudine in salvage therapy for multidrug-resistant HIV-1 infection. Clin Infect Dis 2005;41(2):236–42.

87. Boyer PL, Sarafianos SG, Arnold E, et al. The M184V mutation reduces the selective excision of zidovudine 5′-monophosphate (AZTMP) by the reverse transcriptase of human immunodeficiency virus type 1. J Virol 2002;76(7):3248–56.

88. Ross L, Parkin N, Chappey C, et al. Phenotypic impact of HIV reverse transcriptase M184I/V mutations in combination with single thymidine analog mutations on nucleoside reverse transcriptase inhibitor resistance. AIDS 2004;18(12):1691–6.

89. Madruga JV, Cahn P, Grinsztejn B, et al. Efficacy and safety of TMC125 (etravirine) in treatment-experienced HIV-1-infected patients in DUET-1: 24-week results from a randomised, double-blind, placebo-controlled trial. Lancet 2007; 370(9581):29–38.
90. Lazzarin A, Campbell T, Clotet B, et al. Efficacy and safety of TMC125 (etravirine) in treatment-experienced HIV-1-infected patients in DUET-2: 24-week results from a randomised, double-blind, placebo-controlled trial. Lancet 2007; 370(9581):39–48.
91. Porter DP, Toma J, Tan Y, et al. Clinical outcomes of virologically-suppressed patients with pre-existing HIV-1 drug resistance mutations switching to rilpivirine/emtricitabine/tenofovir disoproxil fumarate in the SPIRIT Study. HIV Clin Trials 2016;17(1):29–37.
92. Lai MT, Feng M, Falgueyret JP, et al. In vitro characterization of MK-1439, a novel HIV-1 nonnucleoside reverse transcriptase inhibitor. Antimicrob Agents Chemother 2014;58(3):1652–63.
93. Lathouwers E, De Meyer S, Dierynck I, et al. Virological characterization of patients failing darunavir/ritonavir or lopinavir/ritonavir treatment in the ARTEMIS study: 96-week analysis. Antivir Ther 2011;16(1):99–108.
94. Stockdale AJ, Saunders MJ, Boyd MA, et al. Effectiveness of protease inhibitor/nucleos(t)ide reverse transcriptase inhibitor-based second-line antiretroviral therapy for the treatment of human immunodeficiency virus type 1 infection in Sub-Saharan Africa: a systematic review and meta-analysis. Clin Infect Dis 2018;66(12):1846–57.
95. Katlama C, Esposito R, Gatell JM, et al. Efficacy and safety of TMC114/ritonavir in treatment-experienced HIV patients: 24-week results of POWER 1. AIDS 2007;21(4):395–402.
96. Haubrich R, Berger D, Chiliade P, et al. Week 24 efficacy and safety of TMC114/ritonavir in treatment-experienced HIV patients. AIDS 2007;21(6):F11–8.
97. Molina JM, Cohen C, Katlama C, et al. Safety and efficacy of darunavir (TMC114) with low-dose ritonavir in treatment-experienced patients: 24-week results of POWER 3. J Acquir Immune Defic Syndr 2007;46(1):24–31.
98. Fransen S, Gupta S, Frantzell A, et al. Substitutions at amino acid positions 143, 148, and 155 of HIV-1 integrase define distinct genetic barriers to raltegravir resistance in vivo. J Virol 2012;86(13):7249–55.
99. Abram ME, Hluhanich RM, Goodman DD, et al. Impact of primary elvitegravir resistance-associated mutations in HIV-1 integrase on drug susceptibility and viral replication fitness. Antimicrob Agents Chemother 2013;57(6):2654–63.
100. Castagna A, Maggiolo F, Penco G, et al. Dolutegravir in antiretroviral-experienced patients with raltegravir- and/or elvitegravir-resistant HIV-1: 24-week results of the phase III VIKING-3 study. J Infect Dis 2014;210(3):354–62.
101. Hocqueloux L, Raffi F, Prazuck T, et al. Dolutegravir monotherapy versus dolutegravir/abacavir/lamivudine for virologically suppressed people living with chronic HIV infection: the randomized non-inferiority MONCAY trial. Clin Infect Dis 2019. https://doi.org/10.1093/cid/ciy1132.
102. Wijting I, Rokx C, Boucher C, et al. Dolutegravir as maintenance monotherapy for HIV (DOMONO): a phase 2, randomised non-inferiority trial. Lancet HIV 2017;4(12):e547–54.
103. Cahn P, Pozniak AL, Mingrone H, et al. Dolutegravir versus raltegravir in antiretroviral-experienced, integrase-inhibitor-naive adults with HIV: week 48 results from the randomised, double-blind, non-inferiority SAILING study. Lancet 2013;382(9893):700–8.

104. Pham HT, Labrie L, Wijting IEA, et al. The S230R integrase substitution associated with virus load rebound during dolutegravir monotherapy confers low-level resistance to integrase strand-transfer inhibitors. J Infect Dis 2018;218(5): 698–706.

105. Brenner BG, Thomas R, Blanco JL, et al. Development of a G118R mutation in HIV-1 integrase following a switch to dolutegravir monotherapy leading to cross-resistance to integrase inhibitors. J Antimicrob Chemother 2016;71(7):1948–53.

106. Tsiang M, Jones GS, Goldsmith J, et al. Antiviral activity of Bictegravir (GS-9883), a novel potent HIV-1 integrase strand transfer inhibitor with an improved resistance profile. Antimicrob Agents Chemother 2016;60(12):7086–97.

107. Paton NI, Kityo C, Thompson J, et al. Nucleoside reverse-transcriptase inhibitor cross-resistance and outcomes from second-line antiretroviral therapy in the public health approach: an observational analysis within the randomised, open-label, EARNEST trial. Lancet HIV 2017;4(8):e341–8.

108. Boyd MA, Moore CL, Molina JM, et al. Baseline HIV-1 resistance, virological outcomes, and emergent resistance in the SECOND-LINE trial: an exploratory analysis. Lancet HIV 2015;2(2):e42–51.

109. Sension M, Cahn P, Domingo P, et al. Subgroup analysis of virological response rates with once- and twice-daily darunavir/ritonavir in treatment-experienced patients without darunavir resistance-associated mutations in the ODIN trial. HIV Med 2013;14(7):437–44.

110. Paton NI, Kityo C, Hoppe A, et al. Assessment of second-line antiretroviral regimens for HIV therapy in Africa. N Engl J Med 2014;371(3):234–47.

111. Kuritzkes DR, Shugarts D, Bakhtiari M, et al. Emergence of dual resistance to zidovudine and lamivudine in HIV-1-infected patients treated with zidovudine plus lamivudine as initial therapy. J Acquir Immune Defic Syndr 2000;23(1): 26–34.

112. Averbuch D, Schapiro JM, Lanier ER, et al. Diminished selection for thymidine-analog mutations associated with the presence of M184V in Ethiopian children infected with HIV subtype C receiving lamivudine-containing therapy. Pediatr Infect Dis J 2006;25(11):1049–56.

113. Parikh UM, Zelina S, Sluis-Cremer N, et al. Molecular mechanisms of bidirectional antagonism between K65R and thymidine analog mutations in HIV-1 reverse transcriptase. AIDS 2007;21(11):1405–14.

114. Bunupuradah T, Chetchotisakd P, Ananworanich J, et al. A randomized comparison of second-line lopinavir/ritonavir monotherapy versus tenofovir/lamivudine/lopinavir/ritonavir in patients failing NNRTI regimens: the HIV STAR study. Antivir Ther 2012;17(7):1351–61.

115. SECOND-LINE Study Group, Boyd MA, Kumarasamy N, Moore CL, et al. Ritonavir-boosted lopinavir plus nucleoside or nucleotide reverse transcriptase inhibitors versus ritonavir-boosted lopinavir plus raltegravir for treatment of HIV-1 infection in adults with virological failure of a standard first-line ART regimen (SECOND-LINE): a randomised, open-label, non-inferiority study. Lancet 2013;381(9883):2091–9.

116. La Rosa AM, Harrison LJ, Taiwo B, et al. Raltegravir in second-line antiretroviral therapy in resource-limited settings (SELECT): a randomised, phase 3, non-inferiority study. Lancet HIV 2016;3(6):e247–58.

117. Aboud M, Kaplan R, Lombaard J, et al. Superior efficacy of dolutegravir (DTG) plus 2 nucleoside reverse transcriptase inhibitors (NRTIs) compared with lopinavir/ritonavir (LPV/RTV) plus 2 NRTIs in second-line treatment: interim data

from the DAWNING study. 9th IAS Conference on HIV Science. Paris, France, July 25, 2017.

118. Eron JJ, Clotet B, Durant J, et al. Safety and efficacy of dolutegravir in treatment-experienced subjects with raltegravir-resistant HIV type 1 infection: 24-week results of the VIKING Study. J Infect Dis 2013;207(5):740–8.

119. Tashima KT, Smeaton LM, Fichtenbaum CJ, et al. HIV salvage therapy does not require nucleoside reverse transcriptase inhibitors: a randomized, controlled trial. Ann Intern Med 2015;163(12):908–17.

120. Gathe J, Cooper DA, Farthing C, et al. Efficacy of the protease inhibitors tipranavir plus ritonavir in treatment-experienced patients: 24-week analysis from the RESIST-1 trial. Clin Infect Dis 2006;43(10):1337–46.

121. Cahn P, Villacian J, Lazzarin A, et al. Ritonavir-boosted tipranavir demonstrates superior efficacy to ritonavir-boosted protease inhibitors in treatment-experienced HIV-infected patients: 24-week results of the RESIST-2 trial. Clin Infect Dis 2006;43(10):1347–56.

122. Madruga JV, Berger D, McMurchie M, et al. Efficacy and safety of darunavir-ritonavir compared with that of lopinavir-ritonavir at 48 weeks in treatment-experienced, HIV-infected patients in TITAN: a randomised controlled phase III trial. Lancet 2007;370(9581):49–58.

123. Cahn P, Fourie J, Grinsztejn B, et al. Week 48 analysis of once-daily vs. twice-daily darunavir/ritonavir in treatment-experienced HIV-1-infected patients. AIDS 2011;25(7):929–39.

124. Steigbigel RT, Cooper DA, Kumar PN, et al. Raltegravir with optimized background therapy for resistant HIV-1 infection. N Engl J Med 2008;359(4):339–54.

125. Molina JM, Lamarca A, Andrade-Villanueva J, et al. Efficacy and safety of once daily elvitegravir versus twice daily raltegravir in treatment-experienced patients with HIV-1 receiving a ritonavir-boosted protease inhibitor: randomised, double-blind, phase 3, non-inferiority study. Lancet Infect Dis 2012;12(1):27–35.

126. Lalezari JP, Henry K, O'Hearn M, et al. Enfuvirtide, an HIV-1 fusion inhibitor, for drug-resistant HIV infection in North and South America. N Engl J Med 2003; 348(22):2175–85.

127. Lazzarin A, Clotet B, Cooper D, et al. Efficacy of enfuvirtide in patients infected with drug-resistant HIV-1 in Europe and Australia. N Engl J Med 2003;348(22): 2186–95.

128. Gulick RM, Lalezari J, Goodrich J, et al. Maraviroc for previously treated patients with R5 HIV-1 infection. N Engl J Med 2008;359(14):1429–41.

129. Saag M, Goodrich J, Fatkenheuer G, et al. A double-blind, placebo-controlled trial of maraviroc in treatment-experienced patients infected with non-R5 HIV-1. J Infect Dis 2009;199(11):1638–47.

130. Yazdanpanah Y, Fagard C, Descamps D, et al. High rate of virologic suppression with raltegravir plus etravirine and darunavir/ritonavir among treatment-experienced patients infected with multidrug-resistant HIV: results of the ANRS 139 TRIO trial. Clin Infect Dis 2009;49(9):1441–9.

131. Grinsztejn B, Hughes M, Ritz J, et al. Results of ACTG A5288: a strategy study in RLS for 3rd-line ART candidates. Conference on Retroviruses and Opportunistic Infections. Boston, MA, March 4–7, 2018.

132. Emu B, Fessel J, Schrader S, et al. Phase 3 study of ibalizumab for multidrug-resistant HIV-1. N Engl J Med 2018;379(7):645–54.

133. Gulick RM. Investigational antiretroviral drugs: what is coming down the pipeline. Top Antivir Med 2018;25(4):127–32.

134. Takamatsu Y, Das D, Kohgo S, et al. The high genetic barrier of EFdA/MK-8591 stems from strong interactions with the active site of drug-resistant HIV-1 reverse transcriptase. Cell Chem Biol 2018;25(10):1268–78.e3.

135. Ray N, Li T, Lin Z, et al. The second-generation maturation inhibitor GSK3532795 maintains potent activity toward HIV protease inhibitor-resistant clinical isolates. J Acquir Immune Defic Syndr 2017;75(1):52–60.

136. Lalezari JP, Latiff GH, Brinson C, et al. Safety and efficacy of the HIV-1 attachment inhibitor prodrug BMS-663068 in treatment-experienced individuals: 24 week results of AI438011, a phase 2b, randomised controlled trial. Lancet HIV 2015;2(10):e427–37.

137. World Health Organization. Consolidated guidelines on the Use of antiretroviral drugs for treating and preventing HIV infection: recommendations for a public health approach. 2nd edition. Geneva (Switzerland): World Health Organization; 2016.

138. Zash R, Makhema J, Shapiro RL. Neural-tube defects with dolutegravir treatment from the time of conception. N Engl J Med 2018;379(10):979–81.

139. Guidelines for the prevention and treatment of opportunistic infections in HIV-infected adults and adolescents. United States Department of Health and Human Services; 2017. Services. Available at: https://aidsinfo.nih.gov/guidelines/html/4/adult-and-adolescent-opportunistic-infection/325/tb. Accessed December 26, 2018.

140. Baciewicz AM, Self TH. Rifampin drug interactions. Arch Intern Med 1984;144(8):1667–71.

141. University of California San Francisco Center for HIV Information. HIV insite: database of antiretroviral drug interactions. Available at: http://hivinsite.ucsf.edu/insite?page=ar-00-02&post=1. Accessed January 15, 2019.

142. Baciewicz AM, Chrisman CR, Finch CK, et al. Update on rifampin, rifabutin, and rifapentine drug interactions. Curr Med Res Opin 2013;29(1):1–12.

143. Cerrone M, Alfarisi O, Neary M, et al. Rifampin effect on tenofovir alafenamide (TAF) plasma/intracellular pharmacokinetics. Conference on Retroviruses and Opportunistic Infections. Boston, MA, March 4–7, 2018.

144. Yee KL, Khalilieh SG, Sanchez RI, et al. The effect of single and multiple doses of rifampin on the pharmacokinetics of doravirine in healthy subjects. Clin Drug Investig 2017;37(7):659–67.

145. Lan NT, Thu NT, Barrail-Tran A, et al. Randomised pharmacokinetic trial of rifabutin with lopinavir/ritonavir-antiretroviral therapy in patients with HIV-associated tuberculosis in Vietnam. PLoS One 2014;9(1):e84866.

146. Sekar V, Lavreys L, Van de Casteele T, et al. Pharmacokinetics of darunavir/ritonavir and rifabutin coadministered in HIV-negative healthy volunteers. Antimicrob Agents Chemother 2010;54(10):4440–5.

147. la Porte CJ, Colbers EP, Bertz R, et al. Pharmacokinetics of adjusted-dose lopinavir-ritonavir combined with rifampin in healthy volunteers. Antimicrob Agents Chemother 2004;48(5):1553–60.

148. Decloedt EH, McIlleron H, Smith P, et al. Pharmacokinetics of lopinavir in HIV-infected adults receiving rifampin with adjusted doses of lopinavir-ritonavir tablets. Antimicrob Agents Chemother 2011;55(7):3195–200.

149. Nijland HM, L'Homme RF, Rongen GA, et al. High incidence of adverse events in healthy volunteers receiving rifampicin and adjusted doses of lopinavir/ritonavir tablets. AIDS 2008;22(8):931–5.

150. Murphy RA, Marconi VC, Gandhi RT, et al. Coadministration of lopinavir/ritonavir and rifampicin in HIV and tuberculosis co-infected adults in South Africa. PLoS One 2012;7(9):e44793.

151. Dooley KE, Sayre P, Borland J, et al. Safety, tolerability, and pharmacokinetics of the HIV integrase inhibitor dolutegravir given twice daily with rifampin or once daily with rifabutin: results of a phase 1 study among healthy subjects. J Acquir Immune Defic Syndr 2013;62(1):21–7.
152. Dooley KE, Kaplan R, Mwelase N, et al. Safety and efficacy of dolutegravir-based ART in TB/HIV coinfected adults at week 24. Conference on Retroviruses and Opportunistic Infections. Boston, MA, March 4–7, 2018.
153. Wenning LA, Hanley WD, Brainard DM, et al. Effect of rifampin, a potent inducer of drug-metabolizing enzymes, on the pharmacokinetics of raltegravir. Antimicrob Agents Chemother 2009;53(7):2852–6.
154. Brainard DM, Kassahun K, Wenning LA, et al. Lack of a clinically meaningful pharmacokinetic effect of rifabutin on raltegravir: in vitro/in vivo correlation. J Clin Pharmacol 2011;51(6):943–50.
155. Custodio JM, West SK, Collins S, et al. Pharmacokinetics of bictegravir administered twice daily in combination with rifampin. Conference on Retroviruses and Opportunistic Infections. Boston, MA, March 4–7, 2018.
156. Hoff J, Bani-Sadr F, Gassin M, et al. Evaluation of chronic hepatitis B virus (HBV) infection in coinfected patients receiving lamivudine as a component of anti-human immunodeficiency virus regimens. Clin Infect Dis 2001;32(6):963–9.
157. Matthews GV, Bartholomeusz A, Locarnini S, et al. Characteristics of drug resistant HBV in an international collaborative study of HIV-HBV-infected individuals on extended lamivudine therapy. AIDS 2006;20(6):863–70.
158. Benhamou Y, Bochet M, Thibault V, et al. Long-term incidence of hepatitis B virus resistance to lamivudine in human immunodeficiency virus-infected patients. Hepatology 1999;30(5):1302–6.
159. Benhamou Y, Tubiana R, Thibault V. Tenofovir disoproxil fumarate in patients with HIV and lamivudine-resistant hepatitis B virus. N Engl J Med 2003;348(2):177–8.
160. Dore GJ, Cooper DA, Pozniak AL, et al. Efficacy of tenofovir disoproxil fumarate in antiretroviral therapy-naive and -experienced patients coinfected with HIV-1 and hepatitis B virus. J Infect Dis 2004;189(7):1185–92.
161. Nunez M, Perez-Olmeda M, Diaz B, et al. Activity of tenofovir on hepatitis B virus replication in HIV-co-infected patients failing or partially responding to lamivudine. AIDS 2002;16(17):2352–4.
162. Nelson M, Portsmouth S, Stebbing J, et al. An open-label study of tenofovir in HIV-1 and Hepatitis B virus co-infected individuals. AIDS 2003;17(1):F7–10.
163. Ristig MB, Crippin J, Aberg JA, et al. Tenofovir disoproxil fumarate therapy for chronic hepatitis B in human immunodeficiency virus/hepatitis B virus-coinfected individuals for whom interferon-alpha and lamivudine therapy have failed. J Infect Dis 2002;186(12):1844–7.
164. Bihl F, Martinetti G, Wandeler G, et al. HBV genotypes and response to tenofovir disoproxil fumarate in HIV/HBV-coinfected persons. BMC Gastroenterol 2015;15:79.
165. Dore GJ, Soriano V, Rockstroh J, et al. Frequent hepatitis B virus rebound among HIV-hepatitis B virus-coinfected patients following antiretroviral therapy interruption. AIDS 2010;24(6):857–65.
166. Garrison KL, German P, Mogalian E, et al. The drug-drug interaction potential of antiviral agents for the treatment of chronic hepatitis C infection. Drug Metab Dispos 2018;46(8):1212–25.
167. Panel on Antiretroviral Guidelines for Adults and Adolescents. Table 13. Concomitant Use of Selected Antiretroviral Drug and Hepatitis C Virus Direct-Acting Antiviral Drugs for Treatment of Hepatitis C Virus in Adults with HIV. Guidelines for the Use of Antiretroviral Agents in Adults and Adolescents Living

with HIV. United States Department of Health and Human Services. Available at: http://www.aidsinfo.nih.gov/ContentFiles/AdultandAdolescentGL.pdf. Accessed December 21, 2018.

168. HCV guidance: recommendations for testing, managing, and treating hepatitis C. Available at: https://www.hcvguidelines.org/unique-populations/hiv-hcv. Accessed December 21, 2018.

169. HEP drug interactions. Available at: https://www.hep-druginteractions.org/checker. Accessed January 21, 2019.

170. Tuaillon E, Gueudin M, Lemee V, et al. Phenotypic susceptibility to nonnucleoside inhibitors of virion-associated reverse transcriptase from different HIV types and groups. J Acquir Immune Defic Syndr 2004;37(5):1543–9.

171. Poveda E, Rodes B, Toro C, et al. Are fusion inhibitors active against all HIV variants? AIDS Res Hum Retroviruses 2004;20(3):347–8.

172. Desbois D, Roquebert B, Peytavin G, et al. In vitro phenotypic susceptibility of human immunodeficiency virus type 2 clinical isolates to protease inhibitors. Antimicrob Agents Chemother 2008;52(4):1545–8.

173. Brower ET, Bacha UM, Kawasaki Y, et al. Inhibition of HIV-2 protease by HIV-1 protease inhibitors in clinical use. Chem Biol Drug Des 2008;71(4):298–305.

174. Descamps D, Peytavin G, Visseaux B, et al. Dolutegravir in HIV-2-infected patients with resistant virus to first-line integrase inhibitors from the French named patient program. Clin Infect Dis 2015;60(10):1521–7.

175. Roquebert B, Damond F, Collin G, et al. HIV-2 integrase gene polymorphism and phenotypic susceptibility of HIV-2 clinical isolates to the integrase inhibitors raltegravir and elvitegravir in vitro. J Antimicrob Chemother 2008;62(5):914–20.

176. Xu L, Anderson J, Ferns B, et al. Genetic diversity of integrase (IN) sequences in antiretroviral treatment-naive and treatment-experienced HIV type 2 patients. AIDS Res Hum Retroviruses 2008;24(7):1003–7.

177. Smith RA, Raugi DN, Pan C, et al. In vitro activity of dolutegravir against wild-type and integrase inhibitor-resistant HIV-2. Retrovirology 2015;12:10.

178. Le Hingrat Q, Collin G, Le M, et al. A new mechanism of resistance of HIV-2 to integrase inhibitors: a 5 amino-acids insertion in the integrase C-terminal domain. Clin Infect Dis 2018. https://doi.org/10.1093/cid/ciy940.

179. Ni XJ, Delelis O, Charpentier C, et al. G140S/Q148R and N155H mutations render HIV-2 Integrase resistant to raltegravir whereas Y143C does not. Retrovirology 2011;8:68.

180. Visseaux B, Charpentier C, Hurtado-Nedelec M, et al. In vitro phenotypic susceptibility of HIV-2 clinical isolates to CCR5 inhibitors. Antimicrob Agents Chemother 2012;56(1):137–9.

181. World Health Organization. Updated recommendations on first-line and second-line antiretroviral regimens and post-exposure prophylaxis and recommendation on early infant diagnosis of HIV. Geneva (Switzerland): World Health Organization; 2018.

182. von Wyl V, Yerly S, Boni J, et al. Emergence of HIV-1 drug resistance in previously untreated patients initiating combination antiretroviral treatment: a comparison of different regimen types. Arch Intern Med 2007;167(16):1782–90.

183. Walmsley SL, Antela A, Clumeck N, et al. Dolutegravir plus abacavir-lamivudine for the treatment of HIV-1 infection. N Engl J Med 2013;369(19):1807–18.

184. Meintjes G, Moorhouse MA, Carmona S, et al. Adult antiretroviral therapy guidelines 2017. South Atr J HIV Med 2017;18(1):776.

185. Consolidated guidelines for prevention and treatment of HIV in Uganda. In: Health Mo, editor 2018.

Management of Advanced HIV Disease

Nathan A. Summers, MD, Wendy S. Armstrong, MD*

KEYWORDS

- HIV • AIDS • Opportunistic infections • OI
- Immune reconstitution inflammatory syndrome • IRIS

KEY POINTS

- Despite great progress in human immunodeficiency virus (HIV) care, a significant proportion of persons with HIV (PWH) continue to present with advanced disease.
- Close observation is paramount because these individuals are at high risk for opportunistic infections and immune reconstitution inflammatory syndrome.
- Although limited, there are increasing data about optimal management of immune reconstitution inflammatory syndrome.

INTRODUCTION

The human immunodeficiency virus (HIV) care continuum describes the steps a person with HIV (PWH) must achieve after HIV acquisition to achieve virologic suppression, including diagnosis, linkage to care, retention, and receipt of antiretroviral therapy (ART).[1,2] Significant efforts have been made to improve progression along the HIV care continuum since it was first described, and the rates of PWH who are virally suppressed have increased from approximately 30% in 2011 to 51% in 2015.[2,3] However, there is still a large proportion of individuals who initially present or reenter care with advanced disease. Despite efforts to increase testing in hopes of diagnosing HIV earlier in the disease course, more than 20% of newly diagnosed individuals in the United States in 2015 had a CD4 cell count of less than 200 cells/mm^3. At our center, an urban safety net hospital in the South, approximately half of patients diagnosed in routine screening in our emergency room and outpatient clinics have a CD4 count less than 200 cells/mm^3 (B. Shah, personal communication, 2017).[4,5] As such, it is

Disclosure: The authors have no competing financial incentives to disclose.
Department of Medicine, Division of Infectious Diseases, Emory University School of Medicine, 341 Ponce de Leon Avenue, Atlanta, GA 30308, USA
* Corresponding author.
E-mail address: wsarmst@emory.edu

Infect Dis Clin N Am 33 (2019) 743–767
https://doi.org/10.1016/j.idc.2019.05.005
0891-5520/19/© 2019 Elsevier Inc. All rights reserved.

important that HIV providers become aware of unique treatment considerations when caring for individuals with advanced HIV disease.

LINKAGE AND RETENTION IN CARE

The most important treatment outcome for any person living with HIV is achieving long-term viral suppression. Success requires linkage to and retention in care. Patients who are retained in care usually achieve viral suppression even with advanced HIV; however, delayed presentation to care is associated with other barriers, including stigma, limited access to care, poverty, food insecurity, unstable housing, and substance use. These same factors lead to poor long-term engagement in care.[6–8] Clinic systems must be adapted to enhance linkage and retention in care. Patient navigators, trained professionals who focus on an individual patients' needs, have been shown to improve linking recently diagnosed individuals into HIV care.[9,10] Rapid initiation of HIV care at the time of diagnosis essentially leads to immediate linkage and reduces the time to viral suppression. Whether or not rapid-start programs improve retention in all clinic settings remains to be seen.[11] Evidence-based interventions that improve retention in care are limited.[11] Despite serving more vulnerable patients socioeconomically, Ryan White–funded clinics have excellent rates of viral suppression, suggesting that the supportive services that are bundled into these clinic systems may be critical to long-term success.[12] Providing a welcoming clinic environment, addressing social determinants of health, ensuring continuous access to ART, and providing holistic treatment are important factors in caring for all PWH and particularly for those with advanced HIV. Additional interventions tailored to the specific needs of the local population must be determined on a regional level if not at the city or county level. These tailored approaches will be key to ending the US epidemic and require more than ensuring access to medications alone.

ANTIRETROVIRAL THERAPY SELECTION

Current guidelines recommend starting ART immediately for most patients, including those with advanced HIV.[13–16] This recommendation remains true for patients with a concurrently diagnosed opportunistic infection (OI), despite concern for immune reconstitution inflammatory syndrome (IRIS), drug interactions, polypharmacy, and the risk of poor adherence, with rare exceptions, such as cryptococcal meningitis,[17] which are detailed later. Regardless, the choice of ART in treatment-naive individuals with advanced disease remains straightforward, because the current US Department of Health and Human Services–recommended initial regimens are the same as for patients with a high CD4 count. Most first-line ART regimens consist of 1 or 2 pills with minimal side effects.[13] In treatment-experienced patients, it is important to review all available HIV genotypic and phenotypic results before selecting an ART regimen. The management of drug-resistant HIV is addressed in detail Suzanne M. McCluskey and colleagues' article, "Management of Virologic Failure and HIV Drug Resistance," elsewhere in this issue.[13,15]

Some ART regimens are not recommended in patients with CD4 cell counts less than 200 cells/mm^3 or high viral loads, and these are important to avoid (**Table 1**). Specifically, rilpivirine, the combination of boosted darunavir and raltegravir as dual therapy, and lamivudine with dolutegravir as dual therapy should not be used in patients with CD4 cell counts less than 200 cells/mm^3.[18–21] Higher rates of virologic failure in those with viral loads more than 100,000 copies/ml were seen with use of rilpivirine, boosted darunavir and raltegravir as dual therapy, and the combination therapy of abacavir and lamivudine combined with either efavirenz or boosted

Table 1
Antiretroviral therapy selection in the patient with advanced human immunodeficiency virus

Setting	Drug/Regimen to Avoid	Reason
CD4<200 cells/mL	Rilpivirine	Higher rate of virologic failure
	Darunavir/r + raltegravir as dual therapy	Higher rate of virologic failure
	Lamivudine + dolutegravir as dual therapy	Lower response rate at 48 wk, not virologic failure
HIV VL >100,000 copies/mL	Rilpivirine	Higher rate of virologic failure
	Darunavir/r + raltegravir as dual therapy	Higher rate of virologic failure
	Abacavir/ lamivudine + efavirenz or atazanavir/r	Higher rate of virologic failure
HIV VL >500,000 copies/mL	Lamivudine + dolutegravir as dual therapy	Those with a VL >500,000 copies/mL were excluded from the study

Abbreviations: r, ritonavir; VL, viral load.

atazanavir.[18–20,22,23] Data are lacking about the use of lamivudine and dolutegravir dual therapy in treatment-naive individuals with an HIV viral load more than 500,000 copies/mL.[21] Drug-drug interactions and overlapping toxicities must also be taken into account for those patients concurrently initiating therapy for OIs, particularly in those with mycobacterial disease, who may require use of a rifamycin.

An important limitation of recent clinical trials in treatment-naive patients is that they enrolled few participants with advanced HIV disease. Furthermore, these studies exclude patients with active HIV-related complications or those with anticipated poor adherence, both of which are commonly encountered in newly diagnosed people with severe immunosuppression. Among recent studies, only those conducted in resource-limited settings include a high proportion of people with low CD4 cell counts and high viral loads.[24,25] An important finding from one of these studies is that viral suppression rates were substantially lower than in licensing studies,[24] supporting the greater difficulty of treating real-world patients with advanced disease.

IMMUNE RECONSTITUTION INFLAMMATORY SYNDROME

IRIS is characterized by an exuberant inflammatory response that occurs after starting ART in response to an underlying infection, neoplasm (eg, Kaposi sarcoma), or inflammatory state (eg, Graves disease). There are 2 primary IRIS presentations. The first, known as unmasking IRIS, describes the discovery of a previously undiagnosed disease after starting ART. The second, known as paradoxic IRIS, describes the worsening of a previously diagnosed condition after starting ART. Risk factors for the development of IRIS include a low CD4 count, high HIV viral load, and high antigenic burden of disease at the time of ART initiation, and possibly the use of integrase strand transfer inhibitors (INSTIs).[26,27] Although increased metabolic activity on PET–computed tomography (CT) before ART initiation was recently shown to be associated with an increased risk for the development of IRIS, the clinical application of PET-CT is limited by cost and availability.[28] A rapid decrease in HIV viral load is typically seen at the time of IRIS presentation, which characteristically occurs between 2 and 6 weeks after initiating ART, but can present within days or as long as months after ART initiation.[26,29]

The presenting signs and symptoms for IRIS vary greatly depending on the underlying infection, and are described in more detail for specific infections later. The treatment and prevention of IRIS are also poorly understood at this time. Nonsteroidal antiinflammatory medications and corticosteroids are often used to allay symptoms of IRIS, although the dosing, duration, and efficacy are not well described except for tuberculosis (TB).[30,31] In a randomized clinical trial, maraviroc added to standard ART did not reduce the incidence of IRIS, although the overall incidence of IRIS in this study was low.[32–34]

OPPORTUNISTIC INFECTIONS

The risk factors, presentation, treatment, and preventive measures for several OIs are described in **Table 2**. The presenting signs and symptoms may vary depending on the individual's degree of immunosuppression. Furthermore, patients with advanced HIV may have multiple concurrent OIs.[35] A few of the most commonly encountered OIs in the United States are described, with targeted discussions of presentation, treatment, and considerations for IRIS.

Any CD4 Count

Mycobacterium tuberculosis
Although TB is the leading infectious cause of death and is among the top 10 causes of death worldwide, surpassing HIV, TB incidence is highly variable depending on geographic area.[36] In many areas of the United States, TB is infrequently seen except among individuals originating from highly endemic areas, whereas in other areas it is more commonly encountered. PWH are uniquely susceptible to TB. Although use of ART reduces an individual's risk for the development of TB, PWH retain a higher risk than HIV-negative individuals for active TB regardless of CD4 count.[36–38] As such, TB remains an important consideration when providing care for PWH.

All PWH should be screened for latent TB infection (LTBI) at the time of HIV diagnosis, with repeat testing performed once the CD4 count increases to more than 200 cells/mm^3 if initial testing was negative, followed by annual testing for those at high risk for repeated exposure.[30,39] PWH who have LTBI have an annual risk of reactivation between 3% and 16%, approximating the lifetime risk for HIV-negative individuals.[40] Although diagnosis of LTBI was classically made with a tuberculin skin test (TST) measuring more than 5 mm of induration among PWH, interferon-gamma

Table 2	
Opportunistic infections and their associated CD4 counts	
Opportunistic Infection	**CD4 (Cells/mm^3) at Risk**
Mycobacterium tuberculosis	Any
PCP	<200
Toxoplasmosis	<100
Cryptococcus	<100
MAC	<50
CMV	<50
JCV/PML	<50
Cryptosporidium and microsporidia	<50

Abbreviations: CMV, cytomegalovirus; JCV, JC virus; MAC, *Mycobacterium avium* complex; PCP, *Pneumocystis jiroveci* pneumonia; PML, progressive multifocal leukoencephalopathy.

release assays (IGRA) are increasingly used, and these tests are compared with TST in **Table 3**.[41–44] The agreement between TST and IGRA test results is inconsistent and studies do not definitively suggest which of the 2 strategies is superior.[45–47] The sensitivity of TST and IGRAs in patients with advanced HIV is even lower, further limiting their reliability when negative. Ultimately, the decision of which testing modality to use often comes down to the higher cost associated with IGRA versus the barriers associated with returning for a second visit for TST. All PWH in higher prevalence settings, regardless of results, should be evaluated to rule out active disease with symptom screening and a chest radiograph. Those who are diagnosed with LTBI should be offered treatment with approved regimens, as outlined in **Table 4**.[30,48] For those at high risk of exposure and advanced HIV disease, assessment for latent TB can be difficult. In this setting, treatment of latent TB, regardless of the result of the screening test, is warranted only in circumstances in which exposure to an infectious case of TB is confirmed or highly suspected.

PWH with pulmonary TB often present with typical symptoms, including cough, hemoptysis, fevers, night sweats, and weight loss. Radiographic imaging varies depending on the level of immunosuppression: among PWH with CD4 counts greater than 200 cells/mm^3, imaging resembles that of reactivation disease in HIV-negative individuals, with a predilection for upper lobes and cavity formation; however, among PWH with CD4 counts less than 200 cells/mm^3, the predilection for upper lobes is lost and cavity formation is less common.[49,50] Clinicians should therefore have a low threshold to evaluate for active pulmonary TB in individuals presenting with signs or symptoms that could be consistent with TB. Patients with advanced HIV can even have unremarkable chest radiographs with active disease, and symptom evaluation is critical to identify the appropriate disease process and treatment strategy. Although it is common for sputum smear microscopy to be negative, particularly with very low CD4 counts and non–cavity-forming disease, mycobacterial culture sensitivity is unaffected by the degree of immunosuppression.[30,51] Use of polymerase chain reaction (PCR) testing is recommended on at least 1 sputum sample and can aid in the diagnosis as well as providing rapid results, but sensitivity and specificity are slightly lower among PWH and in smear-negative samples.[52,53] Bronchoscopy should be considered when initial testing is unrevealing, both to diagnose TB as well as to rule out other

Table 3		
Tuberculin skin test and interferon-gamma release assay comparison among people with human immunodeficiency virus		
	TST	**IGRA**
Affected by low CD4 level	Yes	Yes, potentially less so
Affected by recent live virus vaccines	Yes	Yes, but less well studied
Affected by prior BCG vaccine	Yes	Minimally
Requires second visit	Yes	No
Cost	Inexpensive	Varies, generally more expensive
Interpretation	Varies depending on immune status (positive if induration >5 mm in PWH)	Based on manufacturer's cutoff points, no adjustment for immune suppression

Abbreviation: BCG, bacille Calmette-Guérin.

Table 4
Latent tuberculosis infection treatment regimens

Regimen	Duration
INH 300 mg daily[a]	9 mo
INH 900 mg twice weekly[b]	9 mo
Weekly INH + rifapentine[b]	3 mo (12 wk)
Rifampin 600 mg daily	4 mo
Rifabutin (dose adjusted for ART)	4 mo

Preferred therapy: INH daily for 9 months.
Abbreviation: INH, isoniazid.
[a] INH should always be supplemented with pyridoxine 25 to 50 mg daily.
[b] Given as directly observed therapy.

possible infections or malignancy.[54] Extrapulmonary and disseminated TB are increasingly common with lower CD4 counts, and presenting signs and symptoms are similar to those in HIV-negative individuals.[55] In addition, granuloma formation may be partially formed or absent with increased levels of immune suppression.[49]

The treatment of TB among PWH is similar to that of individuals without HIV. First-line recommended therapy consists of rifampin, isoniazid, pyrazinamide, and ethambutol as directly observed therapy (DOT).[56] Because of the increased risk for treatment failure and relapse with rifamycin resistance, daily DOT rather than intermittent dosing is recommended for both the 2-month intensive treatment phase[57,58] and the consolidation phase.[59] Adjuvant therapy with corticosteroids is recommended for TB meningitis/central nervous system (CNS) disease and pericarditis.[60,61]

The timing of ART initiation has been well studied in PWH with TB. Multiple trials have shown markedly improved mortality with early (ART 2–4 weeks after initiation of anti-TB therapy) rather than delayed ART in the subset of PWH with CD4 counts less than 50 cells/mm^3 despite an increased risk of IRIS in these individuals.[62,63] A potential exception is TB meningitis, for which a single study observed more severe and more frequent adverse events but similar mortality among PWH started on ART immediately.[64] These data have led to the current recommendation to initiate ART within 2 weeks after TB initiation if the CD4 count is less than 50 cells/mm^3 and within 8 weeks if the CD4 count is higher, with caution and careful monitoring advised in cases of CNS disease.[30] Drug-drug interactions are important to consider when starting treatment, particularly between the rifamycins and ART, and are summarized in **Table 5**.[13]

TB-IRIS is a common complication observed in coinfected individuals starting on ART. Symptoms vary and depend on the site of TB infection, but often include fevers, lymphadenopathy, and inflammatory changes at the site of infection.[65] Paradoxic IRIS, a worsening of TB-related symptoms after starting ART, has been estimated to occur in nearly one-fifth of cases, but death attributed to TB-IRIS was rare.[65,66] Clinicians must monitor for fevers, lymphadenopathy, worsening respiratory symptoms, and new or enlarging pulmonary infiltrates on imaging, which may be suggestive of paradoxic IRIS in the correct setting. Use of prednisone for the first 4 weeks after starting ART was recently shown to reduce the risk of paradoxic TB-IRIS without increasing risk for severe infections or malignancies.[67] Unmasking IRIS, or the presentation of TB in PWH without suspected disease shortly after starting ART, is uncommon in most areas but typically has an accelerated onset, progression, and severity of symptoms.[68] Treatment of TB-IRIS typically involves a prolonged course of corticosteroids, often for more than 4 weeks, followed by a gradual taper over several months.[30,31]

Table 5
Tuberculosis and human immunodeficiency virus drug-drug interactions

ART Class	ART Adjustment
Rifampin	
NRTIs	TAF: use alternative ART agent (eg, TDF)
NNRTIs	EFV: avoid 400-mg dose (use 600 mg instead) NVP, ETR, RPV, DOR: use alternative ART agent
INSTIs	BIC, ELV: use alternative ART agent DTG: use BID dosing RAL: use 600 mg BID rather than 300 mg BID (do not use 1200 mg once-daily dosing)
PIs	All PIs: use alternative ART agent (unable to achieve therapeutic ART concentrations)
Maraviroc	Dose 600 mg BID (if given with a strong 3A4 inhibitor then dose 300 mg BID)
Rifabutin	
NRTIs	TAF: use alternative agent (eg, TDF)
NNRTIs	EFV: increase rifabutin dose to 450–600 mg/d or 600 mg 3×/wk (if not given with PI) NVP: no ART dose adjustment necessary, use with caution (Cmin decr 16%) ETR: use rifabutin 300 mg/d (if not given with PI), avoid rifabutin if also on a PI RPV: increase RPV to 50 mg daily, no adjustment of rifabutin DOR: increase DOR to 100 mg daily, no adjustment of rifabutin
INSTIs	BIC, ELV: use alternative ART agent DTG, RAL: no dose adjustment necessary
PIs	All PIs: no dose adjustment of ART necessary, but dose rifabutin 150 mg daily or 300 mg 3×/wk
Maraviroc	No dose adjustment necessary (if given with a strong 3A4 inhibitor, dose 150 mg BID)
Rifapentine	
NRTIs	TAF: use alternative agent (eg, TDF)
NNRTIs	EFV: no dose adjustment necessary NVP, ETR, RPV, DOR: use alternative ART agent
INSTIs	BIC, ELV, DTG: use alternative ART agent RAL: no dose adjustment necessary (not to be used with daily rifapentine dosing)
PIs	All PIs: use alternative ART agent (unable to achieve therapeutic ART concentrations)
Maraviroc	Use alternative agent
Clarithromycin	
NRTIs	No dose adjustments necessary
NNRTIs	EFV, NVP, ETR, RPV: no dose adjustment of ART necessary, but consider use of alternative macrolide (eg, azithromycin)
INSTIs	BIC, DTG, RAL: no dose adjustment necessary ELV: reduce clarithromycin dose by 50% if CrCl 50–60 mL/min, avoid use if CrCl <50 mL/min
PIs	All PIs: consider use of alternative macrolide (eg, azithromycin) CrCl 30–60 mL/min: reduce clarithromycin dose by 50% CrCl <30 mL/min: reduce clarithromycin dose by 75%
Maraviroc	Dose 150 mg BID

Abbreviations: BIC, bictegravir; BID, twice a day; Cmin, minimum blood plasma concentration of drug; CrCl, creatinine clearance; DOR, doravirine; DTG, dolutegravir; EFV, efavirenz; ELV, elvitegravir; ETR, etravirine; INSTI, integrase strand transfer inhibitors; NNRTI, non-nucleotide reverse transcriptase inhibitors; NRTI, nucleotide reverse transcriptase inhibitors; NVP, nevirapine; PI, protease inhibitors; RAL, raltegravir; RPV, rilpivirine; TAF, tenofovir alafenamide; TDF, tenofovir disoproxil fumarate.

Corticosteroid use is of particular importance for TB-IRIS involving the CNS, which can have particularly severe outcomes.[69] Close follow-up is important to monitor both the response to therapy as well as worsening of symptoms while tapering the dose of corticosteroids.

CD4 Count Less than 200 Cells/mm³

Pneumocystis jiroveci pneumonia

The typical presentation of *Pneumocystis jiroveci* pneumonia (PCP) in PWH is the slowly progressive onset of dyspnea, fevers, and nonproductive cough that worsens over days to weeks. Physical examination may vary but tachycardia, tachypnea, and desaturation with ambulation are often present.[70,71] Like other interstitial pneumonias, lung auscultation may be normal and underestimates the degree of disease. Laboratory studies usually reveal increased serum lactate dehydrogenase and (1-3)-β-D-glucan levels, although these findings are not specific.[72] However, because (1–3)-β-D-glucan testing is highly sensitive in the appropriate clinical settings, some centers find this test more useful to guide therapy than induced sputum or invasive testing.[72] Chest radiograph findings range from normal findings to a classic diffuse interstitial pattern. CT chest is more sensitive and typically reveals bilateral, patchy ground-glass opacities.[73]

Because the organism cannot be routinely cultured, histopathologic or cytopathologic testing is required for definitive diagnosis using direct fluorescence antibody (DFA), Giemsa, Grocott-Gomori methenamine silver, and toluidine blue stains.[30] Reported sensitivities vary depending on the specimen quality, pathogen load, staining modality, and experience of the microbiologist, but in general specimens from bronchoalveolar lavage (BAL) or lung biopsy are more sensitive (>90%) than induced sputum samples (40%–90%), and expectorated sputum samples are of minimal benefit.[30,74] DFA staining is preferred to other staining methods at some centers because of less interuser variability, but there is no clear benefit favoring one staining technique compared with another.[30,75] Although PCR testing on BAL specimens has been shown to have improved sensitivity (>95%), specificity decreases because of concern for detection of asymptomatic colonization; nevertheless, PCR use is becoming more widespread.[76,77] Compared with other immunosuppressed populations, PWH with PCP often have very high pathogen loads, which increases the ease of diagnosis and the yield of samples regardless of the modality used for evaluation.

Treatment of PCP depends on the severity of illness (**Table 6**). First-line therapy is trimethoprim-sulfamethoxazole (TMP-SMX).[30] Prednisone should be added for moderate/severe disease to diminish the risk of acute decompensation after initiation of therapy caused by the inflammatory response from lysis of the organism.[78,79] Alternative treatment regimens are listed in **Table 6**. Although TMP-SMX is the preferred regimen regardless of illness severity, all regimens are considered to have equivalent efficacy apart from atovaquone, which was found to be less effective than TMP-SMX.[80–82] Regardless of the selected regimen, it is recommended to continue therapy for a 21-day course before de-escalating to secondary prophylaxis.[30] Although most patients improve on appropriate therapy, some patients fail to improve or even deteriorate. Although development of acute respiratory distress syndrome is one important cause, treatment failure is also a concern, and PCP IRIS has been reported.[83,84] Because PCP often responds slowly, it is recommended to wait 4 to 8 days before deciding to change regimens, with some data supporting clindamycin and primaquine as preferred salvage therapy.[30,85]

Table 6
Pneumocystis jiroveci pneumonia treatment

Severity	Treatment[a]	Common Side Effects
Moderate/severe[b]	TMP-SMX 15 mg/kg/d IV 8 h, switch to PO when improved	Hyperkalemia and AKI
	Pentamidine 4 mg/kg IV q 24 h (infuse over 60 min; can reduce to 3 mg/kg if toxicities occur)	Azotemia, pancreatitis, hypoglycemia and hyperglycemia, leukopenia, electrolyte abnormalities, and cardiac arrhythmias
	Primaquine 30 mg PO daily + clindamycin IV, 600 mg q 6 h or 900 mg q 8 h or PO, 450 mg q 6 h or 600 mg q 8 h	Methemoglobinemia and hemolysis (primaquine) Nausea and diarrhea (clindamycin)
Mild/moderate	TMP-SMX 15 mg/kg/d PO given TID, or TMP-SMX DS 2 tablets TID	Hyperkalemia and AKI
	Dapsone 100 mg PO daily + TMP 15/mg/kg/d PO TID	Rash, fever, methemoglobinemia, and hemolysis (dapsone)
	Primaquine 30 mg PO daily + clindamycin PO (450 mg q 6 h or 600 mg q 8 h)	Methemoglobinemia and hemolysis (primaquine) Nausea and diarrhea (clindamycin)
	Atovaquone 750 mg PO BID (given with fatty foods)	Headache, nausea, rash, and transaminase increases
Adjunctive steroids[b]	Prednisone taper: Days 1–5: 40 mg PO BID Days 6–10: 40 mg PO daily Days 11–21: 20 mg PO daily (can give methylprednisolone IV in place of prednisone at 75% of the prednisone dose)	Hyperglycemia

Abbreviations: AKI, acute kidney injury; DS, double strength; IV, intravenous; PO, by mouth; q, every; TID, 3 times a day; TMP-SMX, trimethoprim-sulfamethoxazole.
[a] TMP-SMX is the preferred treatment of both moderate/severe disease as well as mild/moderate disease.
[b] Use of steroids is recommended for moderate to severe disease, defined as Pao$_2$ less than 70 mm Hg or an alveolar-arterial O$_2$ gradient of greater than or equal to 35 mm Hg.

All PWH with a CD4 count of less than 200 cells/mm^3 should receive routine PCP prophylaxis. First-line therapy is daily TMP-SMX double strength (DS) or single strength (SS). Alternative regimens include TMP-SMX DS by mouth 3 times a week, daily dapsone, daily atovaquone, or monthly aerosolized pentamidine.[30] Importantly, compared with TMP-SMX, aerosolized pentamidine was not only found to be less effective but apical lung disease or extrapulmonary PCP was observed with higher frequency.[86] Because it induces cough, aerosolized pentamidine may also contribute to nosocomial spread of respiratory infections, most notably TB. Prophylaxis should be continued until the CD4 count is greater than 200 cells/mm^3 for longer than 3 months. Discontinuation of prophylaxis can be considered if the CD4 count is between 100 and 200 cells/mm^3 and the HIV RNA viral load remains less than the limit of detection for at least 3 to 6 months.[30,87]

CD4 Count Less than 100 Cells/mm^3

Toxoplasma gondii
Primary exposure to *Toxoplasma gondii*, the protozoan responsible for toxoplasma encephalitis (TE), typically occurs after ingestion of either undercooked meat

containing tissue cysts or oocysts shed in cat feces. Seroprevalence varies by region but ranges from near 10% in the United States to more than 50% in parts of Europe, Latin America, and Africa.[88,89] Although disease primarily occurs from reactivation of latent tissue cysts in the setting of immunosuppression, rarely TE can occur in seronegative individuals, which is more likely a result of insensitive serologic testing or poor antibody response than acute infection.[88] Close to half of all patients infected with *Toxoplasma* fail to identify a risk factor for exposure, therefore overreliance on history or serology is cautioned.[90]

Although *T gondii* can present as disseminated disease, multifocal lymphadenopathy, or pneumonia, these syndromes are rare among PWH.[89] Toxoplasma chorioretinitis is an important consideration in immunosuppressed individuals presenting with vision loss. Because findings on funduscopic examination can vary with *Toxoplasma*, referral to a retina specialist for a dilated examination is paramount.[91] Most commonly, toxoplasmosis in patients with advanced HIV presents with CNS disease with focal neurologic deficits, encephalopathy, headache, and fevers. The primary diagnostic concern in PWH with CD4 counts less than 100 cells/mm^3 is to differentiate TE from primary CNS lymphoma (PCNSL), although many other infectious and neoplastic processes can have similar findings. Both TE and PCNSL typically present with solitary or multiple lesions in the CNS that are ring enhancing with gadolinium on MRI, and can be accompanied by focal neurologic deficits. PCR testing of the cerebrospinal fluid (CSF) for *Toxoplasma* can assist in diagnosing TE, as can single-photon emission CT (SPECT), but availability and cost limit widespread use of the latter.[92,93] It is common, therefore, to initiate treatment with a presumptive diagnosis of TE in seropositive patients with findings consistent with TE in the absence of a confirmed diagnosis. In these cases, improvement in neurologic symptoms as well as MRI findings should be monitored closely. Biopsy should be reserved for seronegative patients or those seropositive patients who fail to improve radiologically or symptomatically after 10 to 14 days of appropriate treatment given the inherent risks associated with this procedure.[30,94]

First-line therapy for TE is with pyrimethamine plus sulfadiazine plus leucovorin dosed according to weight. Alternative regimens include pyrimethamine plus clindamycin plus leucovorin, TMP-SMX, and atovaquone plus pyrimethamine/leucovorin or clindamycin, as shown in **Box 1**. Although some studies found better outcomes with pyrimethamine/sulfadiazine compared with pyrimethamine/clindamycin,[95] other studies showed no difference.[96] However, drug shortages and high prices have limited the availability of pyrimethamine in the United States, leading practitioners to seek alternative therapies. Multiple small studies have shown TMP-SMX to be as effective as pyrimethamine/sulfadiazine, leading to TMP-SMX being the preferred regimen in patients unable to afford or obtain pyrimethamine.[97,98] Treatment failure is a rare occurrence, and should raise concern for an alternative diagnosis. In biopsy-confirmed cases that fail to improve, switching to an alternative regimen can be considered.[30] TE-associated IRIS is a rare event, often presenting with inflammatory changes on MRI and worsening neurologic symptoms. Because of its rarity, no treatment recommendations are available.[99] Induction therapy should be continued for at least 6 weeks but can be extended if the clinical or radiographic extent of disease is severe or if only a partial response is observed at 6 weeks of therapy.[95,96]

To reduce risk for recurrence, all patients should then be switched to chronic maintenance therapy for secondary prophylaxis, as shown in **Box 1**, until the CD4 count is greater than 200 cells/mm^3 for 6 months.[100,101] Primary prophylaxis typically consists of TMP-SMX DS daily, but alternative options are shown in **Box 1**. Primary prophylaxis should be continued until the CD4 counts is greater than 100 to 200 cells/mm^3 for 3 to

---

Box 1
***Toxoplasma gondii* prevention and treatment**

Primary prophylaxis[a]

TMP-SMX DS 1 tablet daily

TMP-SMX SS 1 tablet daily

Dapsone 50 mg daily + (pyrimethamine 50 mg and leucovorin 25 mg) weekly

Dapsone 200 mg + pyrimethamine 75 mg + leucovorin 25 mg weekly

Atovaquone 1500 mg daily

Acute treatment of TE

Pyrimethamine 200 mg PO ×1, then:
- Weight less than 60 kg: pyrimethamine 50 mg PO daily + sulfadiazine 1000 mg PO q 6 h + leucovorin 10 to 25 mg PO daily
- Weight greater than 60 kg: pyrimethamine 75 mg PO daily + sulfadiazine 1500 mg PO q 6 h + leucovorin 10 to 25 mg PO daily

Pyrimethamine (dosed as above) + clindamycin 600 mg IV or PO q 6 h + leucovorin 10 to 25 mg PO daily

TMP-SMX (dosed TMP 5 mg/kg, SMX 25 mg/kg) IV or PO BID

Atovaquone 1500 mg PO BID ± (pyrimethamine + leucovorin) or (sulfadiazine)

Chronic maintenance/secondary prophylaxis

Pyrimethamine 25 to 50 mg daily + sulfadiazine 2000 to 4000 mg divided 2 to 4×/d + leucovorin 10 to 25 mg daily

Pyrimethamine 25 to 50 mg daily + clindamycin 600 mg q 8 h + leucovorin 10 to 25 mg daily[b]

TMP-SMX DS 1 tablet BID or daily

Atovaquone 750 to 1500 mg BID ± (pyrimethamine 25 mg + leucovorin 10 mg daily) or (sulfadiazine 2000–4000 mg divided 2–4×/d)

Abbreviations: BID, twice a day; DS, double strength; IV, intravenous; PO, by mouth; q, every; SS, single strength; TMP-SMX, trimethoprim-sulfamethoxazole.
  [a] TMP-SMX DS 1 tablet daily is the preferred regimen for primary prophylaxis.
  [b] Additional agent for PCP prophylaxis is required.

---

6 months, although PCP prophylaxis should remain a consideration, as detailed previously.[101]

Cryptococcosis *Cryptococcus neoformans* and less commonly *Cryptococcus gattii* are the two predominant species responsible for cryptococcosis in the HIV population. Exposure occurs from inhalation and can lead to latency or active disease. Although cryptococcosis commonly presents with meningitis, it can also present with a lobar or nodular multifocal pneumonia, umbilicated skin eruptions, and prostatic inflammation. Cryptococcal meningitis most often presents with fevers, headache, and altered mental status, with meningismus occurring infrequently.[102]

Diagnosis of cryptococcal meningitis often requires a high index of suspicion. Cryptococcal antigen assays can be rapidly performed on the serum or CSF and have a high sensitivity and specificity.[103] The antigen assays can be performed via latex agglutination, enzyme immunoassays, or lateral flow assays (LFAs). However, caution is advised with the interpretation of low titers from LFA testing because false-positive results may occur.[104] Lumbar puncture is mandatory in all PWH with a CD4 count less than 200 cells/mm^3 and a positive serum cryptococcal antigen assay or neurologic symptoms. CSF pleocytosis may be absent in patients with advanced HIV disease despite active infection. The lumbar puncture opening pressure must be measured and trended to monitor for prognosis.[105,106] In addition to CSF cryptococcal antigen studies, fungal cultures from blood and CSF should be obtained for diagnostic reasons to aid in species identification, to monitor response to therapy, and to allow susceptibility testing when needed. India ink staining of CSF carries more interuser variability as well as lower sensitivity; although once widely used in the United States, it is now rarely performed.[102] The only role for India ink staining is in facilitating a rapid diagnosis in settings in which there is delay in processing cryptococcal antigen testing.

Cryptococcal meningitis is treated in 3 phases: induction, consolidation, and maintenance. Combination antifungal treatment is recommended for induction when available. Liposomal amphotericin B and flucytosine is preferred because of improved survival with this regimen.[107] Alternative induction regimens are shown in **Box 2**.[30] Induction therapy should be continued for 2 weeks, but increased to 4 weeks in the case of amphotericin B monotherapy. Many experts recommend obtaining a CSF fungal culture at the end of induction to document clearance of viable organisms, continuing induction therapy until the cultures have cleared. Adjunctive dexamethasone is not routinely recommended.[108] Consolidation therapy is typically fluconazole 400 mg by mouth or intravenous (IV) daily for 8 weeks, although some experts argue that fluconazole 800 mg daily should be considered.[109] At least 1 year of maintenance therapy with fluconazole 200 mg daily is recommended but can then be discontinued if the CD4 count is greater than or equal to 100 cells/mm^3 for at least 3 months, the patient has completed at least 1 year of maintenance therapy, and the patient is asymptomatic.[110] In patients with increased intracranial pressure, daily lumbar punctures to reduce the opening pressure by half are recommended, with consideration of a lumbar drain or CSF shunt for individuals with persistent symptoms despite several days of serial lumbar punctures.[106] The CSF ventricles are often not enlarged despite increased intracranial pressure and should not be used as a proxy to determine whether CSF diversion is required. Initiation of ART within 1 to 2 weeks after diagnosis

---

Box 2
Cryptococcal meningitis induction therapy regimens

Preferred regimen

Liposomal amphotericin B 3 to 4 mg/kg IV q 24 h + flucytosine 25 mg/kg PO q 6 h

Amphotericin B deoxycholate 0.7 to 1.0 mg/kg IV q 24 h + flucytosine 25 mg/kg PO q 6 h[a]

Alternative regimens

Amphotericin B lipid complex 5 mg/kg IV q 24 h + flucytosine 25 mg/kg PO q 6 h

Amphotericin B (liposomal or deoxycholate, dosed as above) + fluconazole 800 mg PO or IV q 24 h

Amphotericin B (liposomal or deoxycholate, dosed as above) monotherapy[b]

Fluconazole (400 mg or 800 mg PO or IV q 24 h) + flucytosine 25 mg/kg PO q 6 h

Fluconazole 1200 mg PO or IV daily monotherapy

    [a] Alternative if cost of liposomal amphotericin is an issue.
    [b] Extend induction period to 4 weeks if unable to tolerate flucytosine or fluconazole.

of cryptococcal meningitis in patients not on ART has been shown to have higher risk for mortality compared with starting ART 5 weeks after diagnosis (45% vs 30% mortality at 26 weeks).[17] As a result, initiation of ART is usually delayed until 2 to 5 weeks after starting induction therapy. Treatment of cryptococcosis without meningitis depends on the severity of illness. In severe cases or those with diffuse pulmonary disease, treatment is as for meningitis, whereas mild to moderate cases can be treated with fluconazole 400 mg daily for 12 months.

Although failure caused by antimicrobial resistance is a rare occurrence, clinical failure and persistence or worsening of symptoms despite prolonged therapy is common. Antimicrobial susceptibility testing should be considered if cultures become positive while on fluconazole, and amphotericin B should be continued until cultures are cleared.[30,111] In cases of antimicrobial failure caused by fluconazole resistance, use of a newer triazole (eg, voriconazole or posaconazole) may be considered after induction therapy because of potentially improved susceptibility patterns, although clinical data are limited.[112] Cryptococcal meningitis–associated IRIS is common, occurring in up to 30% of individuals after starting ART. Cultures in cryptococcal IRIS are usually negative, which helps differentiate it from antimicrobial failure. Risk factors for IRIS include individuals with high opening pressures and positive CSF cultures at the time of initiation of ART.[113] Management of cryptococcal IRIS can be extremely difficult and prolonged. The exuberant inflammatory response that is typical of IRIS syndromes can lead to persistent high intracranial pressure, neurologic symptoms, and CSF inflammation with symptoms of meningitis. Management of intracranial pressure may require a lumbar drain or ventriculoperitoneal shunt placement. However, shunt malfunction with high CSF protein levels can occur and complicate therapy. Clinicians are often left uncertain about how long to treat with intensive antifungal therapy, and it is common in clinical practice to prolong the induction course of amphotericin when recovery is delayed in the setting of IRIS or ongoing infection. In addition, corticosteroids are often added, although the dosing and duration are not well studied.[30]

CD4 Count Less than 50 Cells/mm^3

Mycobacterium avium complex
Acquisition of *Mycobacterium avium* complex (MAC), a ubiquitous organism in the environment and found in tap water, typically occurs through inhalation or ingestion.[114] The greatest risk factor for developing MAC disease is a CD4 count less than or equal to 50 cells/mm^3.[115] In PWH, MAC often presents as disseminated disease rather than localized disease, with symptoms including fevers, night sweats, weight loss, abdominal pain, and diarrhea. Laboratory evaluation often reveals cytopenias and increased alkaline phosphatase levels caused by infiltrative disease of the bone marrow and liver.[116]

Diagnosis of MAC can often be made with blood cultures, but cultures of bone marrow aspirate, lymph node tissue, and liver tissue can be helpful when signs or symptoms suggest disease involvement in those organs. Macrolides are the mainstay of therapy, and susceptibility testing to macrolides is recommended and correlates with clinical outcomes. The clinical significance of drug susceptibility testing to other agents is unclear. Combination therapy with a macrolide and ethambutol with or without rifabutin is recommended.[117,118] Although clinical response is similar with or without the addition of rifabutin, time to clearance of cultures and development of macrolide resistance was reduced with the 3-drug regimen, leading some experts to prefer this in severe cases. For individuals not already on ART, initiation of ART need not be delayed nor should treatment be discontinued in those with disease on ART. At least 12 months of antimycobacterial therapy is recommended for those with disseminated disease but can be discontinued after that time if symptoms have resolved and the CD4 count is greater than 100 cells/mm^3 for at least 6 months.[119]

PWH with treatment failure often have persistent positive blood cultures. In these cases, susceptibility testing is critical, and loss of macrolide susceptibility is ominous. When changing therapy, at least 2 new agents should be added at once.[120] Alternative therapeutics include amikacin, streptomycin, and fluoroquinolones (particularly moxifloxacin and levofloxacin), with anecdotal support for linezolid and bedaquiline.[30,120] The benefit of continuation of macrolide therapy in the case of resistance is not clear, although some experts support continued macrolide dosing regardless of susceptibility testing.

IRIS often presents with focal disease with sterile blood cultures, and unmasking presentations are common. Typical presentations for MAC IRIS are outlined in **Table 7** but include peripheral suppurative lymphadenitis with draining sinus tracts, pulmonary/thoracic disease or intra-abdominal disease with necrotic adenopathy, and bone and joint infections.[121] Involved areas show an exuberant inflammatory response driven by the antigenic load. Less frequently, PWH with poor immune recovery despite ART can have disease that shows features of both active disseminated disease and IRIS and are clinically particularly difficult to manage. Evidence-based recommendations for the management of MAC IRIS are limited, but nonsteroidal anti-inflammatory drugs for fever and symptom management are often mainstays of therapy, reserving the use of corticosteroids for more severe cases.[30] Intra-abdominal disease in particular can have prolonged and more severe symptoms, including severe postprandial abdominal pain, and often requires prolonged corticosteroids with a slow taper.[121]

With more rapidly effective ART and declining rates of MAC, the utility of primary prophylaxis for all PWH with CD4 counts less than or equal to 50 cells/mm^3 has come into question.[122] The incidence of MAC is exceedingly low among virally suppressed individuals on ART, with no reduction in incidence of MAC among individuals receiving prophylaxis.[122,123] As a result, recent updates to current guidelines have removed the recommendation for routine prophylaxis for MAC in PWH starting effective ART that results in viral suppression.[30,124]

Table 7
Presentations of *Mycobacterium avium* complex immune reconstitution inflammatory syndrome

Classification	Signs and Symptoms
Peripheral lymphadenitis	Regional and localized lymphadenitis Suppurative lymph nodes creating sinus tracts
Pulmonary/thoracic disease	Endobronchial lesions Mediastinal/hilar lymphadenitis Rare cavities
Intraabdominal disease	Bulky retroperitoneal and intraabdominal lymphadenitis Postprandial abdominal pain Small bowel ulcers Peritonitis
Miscellaneous	Vertebral osteomyelitis Bursitis and tenosynovitis Cutaneous abscesses Prostatic abscesses

Cytomegalovirus

Cytomegalovirus (CMV) is a double-stranded DNA virus in the human herpes virus family that can reactivate to cause disease in severely immunosuppressed individuals. Incidence of CMV disease has dramatically decreased with the advent of effective ART, but PWH with positive serology and persistently low CD4 counts less than or equal to 50 cells/mm^{3}remain at risk.[125] CMV retinitis is the most common presentation of CMV among PWH, accounting for up to 80% of all CMV disease.[126] CMV retinitis may be asymptomatic initially, but can present with an increase in number or frequency of floaters, peripheral or central visual defects, and decreased visual acuity. Urgent ophthalmologic referral is encouraged, with funduscopic examination revealing fluffy yellow or white lesions often with intraretinal hemorrhage.[127] CMV colitis accounts for 5% to 10% of CMV disease among PWH, and can present with abdominal pain, weight loss, and diarrhea. Colonoscopy may reveal ulcerations, and biopsies often stain positively for CMV. Massive hematochezia and bowel perforation are rare but potentially fatal presentations.[128] Less common manifestations of CMV disease among PWH include CNS disease (encephalitis, ventriculitis) and peripheral neuropathy (painful motor/sensory neuropathy, sacral/lumbar radiculopathy).[129] Although commonly isolated from the lungs, CMV pneumonia is rare and should not be assumed to be the cause of pulmonary disease without ruling out other infectious causes.[30,125]

Diagnosis of CMV disease is often made clinically. Positive serologies can aid in diagnosis, but negative results do not reliably rule out disease. Quantitative serum PCR can assist with diagnosis but can be positive in asymptomatic viremic patients, limiting its utility among PWH. Instead, CMV disease is more commonly diagnosed by demonstration of end-organ disease with characteristic findings on funduscopy or colonoscopy or with positive CSF PCR and neurologic disease, which is more sensitive than serum PCR.[30] Treatment of CMV disease varies depending on the clinical presentation, but optimization of ART with immune recovery is the cornerstone for all regimens. CMV retinitis is best treated in conjunction with ophthalmology. Systemic anti-CMV therapy with valganciclovir by mouth is preferred to intravitreal therapy alone, because the former is associated with lower rates of vision loss, contralateral eye involvement, and systemic CMV disease.[130] Induction therapy should be continued for 2 to 3 weeks followed by maintenance therapy. CMV colitis is typically treated with induction therapy for 3 to 6 weeks, followed by maintenance therapy. Ganciclovir IV is preferred initially for CMV colitis given issues with absorption in patients with CMV-associated diarrhea, with transition to valganciclovir by mouth once the individual is able to tolerate oral medications. Treatment of CNS and peripheral nerve disease is less well established, with prolonged courses of monotherapy or even dual therapy followed by maintenance therapy.[30] Maintenance therapy for CMV disease is recommended until CD4 counts increase to more than 100 cells/mm^3 in response to ART to reduce risk for recurrence. Primary prophylaxis for individuals with low CD4 counts and positive serology without evidence of end-organ disease is not recommended.

Response to treatment should be monitored closely for both treatment failure and IRIS. Treatment failure is most often caused by inadequate dosing or inadequate drug penetrance, because drug resistance is rare.[131] Resistance to ganciclovir typically occurs through mutations in the UL97 phosphotransferase gene, with resistance to cidofovir and foscarnet developing with mutations in the UL54 DNA polymerase gene. Management of CMV disease with a UL54 mutation is not extensively studied within the HIV population. Foscarnet may retain partial activity against CMV despite the UL54 mutation, and some experts recommend its use.[30] In addition to treatment failure, it is important to monitor closely for IRIS as a cause for clinical worsening in this population. When it occurs, CMV IRIS most often presents as immune reconstitution uveitis (IRU), an ocular form of CMV IRIS. Large retinal lesions are associated with increased risk for IRU, which is estimated to occur in close to 10% of PWH with CMV retinitis. IRU most often presents with cellular debris in the anterior chamber, vitreous haze, and worsening visual acuity.[132] Corticosteroids with or without anti-CMV therapy are often used, but the route of administration, dose, and duration of corticosteroids are not well defined.[30,132]

Progressive multifocal leukoencephalopathy

JC virus (JCV), a ubiquitous double-stranded DNA polyoma virus, is the causative agent for progressive multifocal leukoencephalopathy (PML), which is characterized by focal areas of demyelination in the CNS typically without edema or mass effect. The presenting signs and symptoms for PML depend largely on the location of the white matter lesions, but most often include the progressive onset of focal neurologic deficits, ataxia, aphasia, and tremors. Rarely, cranial nerve deficits, seizures, and vison loss may occur.[133]

The diagnosis of PML is primarily based on clinical suspicion from history and physical examination with support from radiographic imaging and laboratory data. MRI is more sensitive than CT, and classically shows hyperintense lesions on T2-weighted images and fluid-attenuated inversion recovery images.[134] It is important to differentiate PML from HIV encephalopathy, which can present with similar findings on MRI, by testing for JCV in the CSF, which has a high sensitivity.[133] The most important therapy for PML is reversal of the immunosuppression with effective ART. Several adjunctive therapies have been evaluated, including cytarabine, cidofovir, brincidofovir (CMX001), 5-hydroxytryptamine 2a inhibitors, and mefloquine, but all have failed to show any clinical benefit to date.[30,133] No preventive measures or prophylaxis exist beyond ART.

Careful monitoring for clinical response to ART is recommended. No formal recommendations exist, but close symptom monitoring is strongly encouraged, with repeat MRI 4 to 8 weeks after diagnosis or with clinical deterioration.[133] It is common for PWH to worsen initially after ART, and differentiating progressive disease from PML IRIS can prove difficult. Although both progression of PML and PML IRIS present with worsening neurologic symptoms, PML IRIS can be identified by inflammatory changes seen on pathology or more commonly imaging in the setting of HIV viral suppression. MRI often reveals enhancement, edema, and/or mass effect.[135] There are limited data for the treatment of PML IRIS. Corticosteroids are frequently used, although the dose and duration are not well defined, and the data supporting corticosteroid use are limited.[135,136] Maraviroc may be useful in treating or preventing PML IRIS, but most of the supportive literature comes from the multiple sclerosis population and is anecdotal, so use is not routinely recommended at this time.[33,137] Whether the development of PML IRIS in response to initiating ART portends a favorable outcome is debated, with observational studies finding contradictory results.[138,139] Although outcomes have improved with effective ART, they remain poor for both PML and PML IRIS, with a mortality near 70% and median survival time of less than 2 years.[139,140]

SUMMARY

Despite the many significant successes in improving HIV care outcomes and the push for earlier detection and diagnosis, a significant proportion of PWH continue to present with advanced disease. Areas of uncertainty abound in this population, because much of the literature is limited to small observational studies, many of which originate from the pre-ART or early-ART eras. It is important for HIV providers to be familiar with the unique aspects in caring for these individuals and how to monitor for and manage common infectious complications.

REFERENCES

1. Gardner EM, McLees MP, Steiner JF, et al. The spectrum of engagement in HIV care and its relevance to test-and-treat strategies for prevention of HIV infection. Clin Infect Dis 2011;52(6):793–800.
2. Centers for Disease Control and Prevention. Understanding the HIV care continuum 2018. Available at: https://www.cdc.gov/hiv/pdf/library/factsheets/cdc-hiv-care-continuum.pdf. Accessed September 28, 2018.
3. Centers for Disease Control and Prevention. Understanding the HIV care continuum 2014. Available at: https://www.cdc.gov/hiv/pdf/DHAP_Continuum.pdf. Accessed September 28, 2018.
4. Althoff KN, Gange SJ, Klein MB, et al. Late presentation for human immunodeficiency virus care in the United States and Canada. Clin Infect Dis 2010;50(11):1512–20.
5. Centers for Disease Control and Prevention. Monitoring selected national HIV prevention and care objectives by using HIV surveillance data—United States and 6 dependent areas, 2015. HIV surveillance supplemental report 2017. 22(2). Available at: https://www.cdc.gov/hiv/pdf/library/reports/surveillance/cdc-hiv-surveillance-supplemental-report-vol-22-2.pdf. Accessed September 28, 2018.
6. Sprague C, Simon SE. Understanding HIV care delays in the US South and the role of the social-level in HIV care engagement/retention: a qualitative study. Int J Equity Health 2014;13:28.
7. Walcott M, Kempf MC, Merlin JS, et al. Structural community factors and suboptimal engagement in HIV care among low-income women in the Deep South of the USA. Cult Health Sex 2016;18(6):682–94.
8. Colasanti J, Stahl N, Farber EW, et al. An exploratory study to assess individual and structural level barriers associated with poor retention and re-engagement in care among persons living with HIV/AIDS. J Acquir Immune Defic Syndr 2017; 74(Suppl 2):S113–20.
9. Craw JA, Gardner LI, Marks G, et al. Brief strengths-based case management promotes entry into HIV medical care: results of the antiretroviral treatment access study-II. J Acquir Immune Defic Syndr 2008;47(5):597–606.
10. Gardner LI, Metsch LR, Anderson-Mahoney P, et al. Efficacy of a brief case management intervention to link recently diagnosed HIV-infected persons to care. AIDS 2005;19(4):423–31.
11. Higa DH, Crepaz N, Mullins MM. Identifying best practices for increasing linkage to, retention, and re-engagement in HIV medical care: findings from a systematic review, 1996-2014. AIDS Behav 2016;20(5):951–66.
12. Health Resources and Services Administration. Ryan white HIV/AIDS program annual client-level data report 2017. 2018. Available at: http://hab.hrsa.gov/data/data-reports. Accessed May 13, 2019.
13. Panel on antiretroviral guidelines for adults and adolescents. Guidelines for the use of antiretroviral agents in adults and adolescents living with HIV. Department of Health and Human Services. Available at: http://aidsinfo.nih.gov/contentfiles/lvguidelines/AdultandAdolescentGL.pdf. Accessed September 28, 2018.
14. Guidelines for managing advanced HIV disease and rapid initiation of antiretroviral therapy. Geneva (Switzerland): World Health Organization; 2017. Licence:

CC BY-NC-SA 3.0 IGO. Available at: https://apps.who.int/iris/bitstream/handle/ 10665/255884/9789241550062-eng.pdf?sequence=1. Accessed June 17, 2019.

15. Wilson LE, Gallant JE. HIV/AIDS: the management of treatment-experienced HIV-infected patients: new drugs and drug combinations. Clin Infect Dis 2009; 48(2):214–21.

16. Ford N, Migone C, Calmy A, et al. Benefits and risks of rapid initiation of antiretroviral therapy. AIDS 2018;32(1):17–23.

17. Boulware DR, Meya DB, Muzoora C, et al. Timing of antiretroviral therapy after diagnosis of cryptococcal meningitis. N Engl J Med 2014;370(26):2487–98.

18. Cohen CJ, Andrade-Villanueva J, Clotet B, et al. Rilpivirine versus efavirenz with two background nucleoside or nucleotide reverse transcriptase inhibitors in treatment-naive adults infected with HIV-1 (THRIVE): a phase 3, randomised, non-inferiority trial. Lancet 2011;378(9787):229–37.

19. Lambert-Niclot S, George EC, Pozniak A, et al. Antiretroviral resistance at virological failure in the NEAT 001/ANRS 143 trial: raltegravir plus darunavir/ritonavir or tenofovir/emtricitabine plus darunavir/ritonavir as first-line ART. J Antimicrob Chemother 2016;71(4):1056–62.

20. Molina JM, Cahn P, Grinsztejn B, et al. Rilpivirine versus efavirenz with tenofovir and emtricitabine in treatment-naive adults infected with HIV-1 (ECHO): a phase 3 randomised double-blind active-controlled trial. Lancet 2011;378(9787): 238–46.

21. Cahn P, Madero JS, Arribas JR, et al. Dolutegravir plus lamivudine versus dolutegravir plus tenofovir disoproxil fumarate and emtricitabine in antiretroviral-naive adults with HIV-1 infection (GEMINI-1 and GEMINI-2): week 48 results from two multicentre, double-blind, randomised, non-inferiority, phase 3 trials. Lancet 2019;393(10167):143–55.

22. Post FA, Moyle GJ, Stellbrink HJ, et al. Randomized comparison of renal effects, efficacy, and safety with once-daily abacavir/lamivudine versus tenofovir/emtricitabine, administered with efavirenz, in antiretroviral-naive, HIV-1-infected adults: 48-week results from the ASSERT study. J Acquir Immune Defic Syndr 2010;55(1):49–57.

23. Sax PE, Tierney C, Collier AC, et al. Abacavir-lamivudine versus tenofovir-emtricitabine for initial HIV-1 therapy. N Engl J Med 2009;361(23):2230–40.

24. Cournil A, Kouanfack C, Eymard-Duvernay S, et al. Dolutegravir versus an efavirenz 400 mg based regimen for the initial treatment of HIV-infected patients in Cameroon: 48-week efficacy results of the NAMSAL ANRS 12313 trial. HIV. Glasgow, Scotland, UK, October 28–31, 2018. In.

25. Hakim J, Musiime V, Szubert AJ, et al. Enhanced prophylaxis plus antiretroviral therapy for advanced HIV infection in Africa. N Engl J Med 2017;377(3):233–45.

26. Chang CC, Sheikh V, Sereti I, et al. Immune reconstitution disorders in patients with HIV infection: from pathogenesis to prevention and treatment. Curr HIV/ AIDS Rep 2014;11(3):223–32.

27. Dutertre M, Cuzin L, Demonchy E, et al. Initiation of antiretroviral therapy containing integrase inhibitors increases the risk of IRIS requiring hospitalization. J Acquir Immune Defic Syndr 2017;76(1):e23–6.

20. Hammoud DA, Boulougoura A, Papadakis GZ, et al. Increased metabolic activity on 18F-fluorodeoxyglucose positron emission tomography-computed tomography in human immunodeficiency virus-associated immune reconstitution inflammatory syndrome. Clin Infect Dis 2019;68(2):229–38.

29. Walker NF, Scriven J, Meintjes G, et al. Immune reconstitution inflammatory syndrome in HIV-infected patients. HIV/AIDS 2015;7:49–64.
30. Panel on Opportunistic Infections in HIV-Infected Adults and Adolescents. Guidelines for the prevention and treatment of opportunistic infections in HIV-infected adults and adolescents: recommendations from the Centers for Disease Control and Prevention, the National Institutes of Health, and the HIV Medicine Association of the Infectious Diseases Society of America. Available at: http://aidsinfo.nih.gov/contentfiles/lvguidelines/adult_oi.pdf. Accessed September 28, 2018.
31. Meintjes G, Wilkinson RJ, Morroni C, et al. Randomized placebo-controlled trial of prednisone for paradoxical tuberculosis-associated immune reconstitution inflammatory syndrome. AIDS 2010;24(15):2381–90.
32. Sierra-Madero JG, Ellenberg SS, Rassool MS, et al. Effect of the CCR5 antagonist maraviroc on the occurrence of immune reconstitution inflammatory syndrome in HIV (CADIRIS): a double-blind, randomised, placebo-controlled trial. Lancet HIV 2014;1(2):e60–7.
33. Giacomini PS, Rozenberg A, Metz I, et al. Maraviroc and JC virus-associated immune reconstitution inflammatory syndrome. N Engl J Med 2014;370(5):486–8.
34. Steiner I, Benninger F. Maraviroc in PML-IRIS: a separate ball game under HIV infection and natalizumab? Neurol Neuroimmunol Neuroinflamm 2017;4(2):e331.
35. Armstrong WS, Katz JT, Kazanjian PH. Human immunodeficiency virus-associated fever of unknown origin: a study of 70 patients in the United States and review. Clin Infect Dis 1999;28(2):341–5.
36. Available at: https://apps.who.int/iris/bitstream/handle/10665/274453/9789241565646-eng.pdf. Accessed June 17, 2019.
37. Jones JL, Hanson DL, Dworkin MS, et al. HIV-associated tuberculosis in the era of highly active antiretroviral therapy. The Adult/Adolescent Spectrum of HIV Disease Group. Int J Tuberc Lung Dis 2000;4(11):1026–31.
38. Sonnenberg P, Glynn JR, Fielding K, et al. How soon after infection with HIV does the risk of tuberculosis start to increase? A retrospective cohort study in South African gold miners. J Infect Dis 2005;191(2):150–8.
39. Fisk TL, Hon HM, Lennox JL, et al. Detection of latent tuberculosis among HIV-infected patients after initiation of highly active antiretroviral therapy. AIDS 2003;17(7):1102–4.
40. Selwyn PA, Hartel D, Lewis VA, et al. A prospective study of the risk of tuberculosis among intravenous drug users with human immunodeficiency virus infection. N Engl J Med 1989;320(9):545–50.
41. Huebner RE, Schein MF, Bass JB Jr. The tuberculin skin test. Clin Infect Dis 1993;17(6):968–75.
42. Lee LM, Lobato MN, Buskin SE, et al. Low adherence to guidelines for preventing TB among persons with newly diagnosed HIV infection, United States. Int J Tuberc Lung Dis 2006;10(2):209–14.
43. Menzies D, Pai M, Comstock G. Meta-analysis: new tests for the diagnosis of latent tuberculosis infection: areas of uncertainty and recommendations for research. Ann Intern Med 2007;146(5):340–54.
44. Raby E, Moyo M, Devendra A, et al. The effects of HIV on the sensitivity of a whole blood IFN-gamma release assay in Zambian adults with active tuberculosis. PLoS One 2008;3(6):e2489.
45. Ayubi E, Doosti-Irani A, Sanjari Moghaddam A, et al. The clinical usefulness of tuberculin skin test versus interferon-gamma release assays for diagnosis of

latent tuberculosis in HIV patients: a meta-analysis. PLoS One 2016;11(9): e0161983.

46. Chkhartishvili N, Kempker RR, Dvali N, et al. Poor agreement between interferon-gamma release assays and the tuberculin skin test among HIV-infected individuals in the country of Georgia. BMC Infect Dis 2013;13:513.

47. Rangaka MX, Wilkinson KA, Seldon R, et al. Effect of HIV-1 infection on T-Cell-based and skin test detection of tuberculosis infection. Am J Respir Crit Care Med 2007;175(5):514–20.

48. Borisov AS, Bamrah Morris S, Njie GJ, et al. Update of recommendations for use of once-weekly isoniazid-rifapentine regimen to treat latent mycobacterium tuberculosis infection. MMWR Morb Mortal Wkly Rep 2018;67(25):723–6.

49. Jones BE, Young SM, Antoniskis D, et al. Relationship of the manifestations of tuberculosis to CD4 cell counts in patients with human immunodeficiency virus infection. Am Rev Respir Dis 1993;148(5):1292–7.

50. Perlman DC, el-Sadr WM, Nelson ET, et al. Variation of chest radiographic patterns in pulmonary tuberculosis by degree of human immunodeficiency virus-related immunosuppression. The Terry Beirn Community Programs for Clinical Research on AIDS (CPCRA). The AIDS Clinical Trials Group (ACTG). Clin Infect Dis 1997;25(2):242–6.

51. Elliott AM, Halwiindi B, Hayes RJ, et al. The impact of human immunodeficiency virus on presentation and diagnosis of tuberculosis in a cohort study in Zambia. J Trop Med Hyg 1993;96(1):1–11.

52. Centers for Disease Control and Prevention (CDC). Updated guidelines for the use of nucleic acid amplification tests in the diagnosis of tuberculosis. MMWR Morb Mortal Wkly Rep 2009;58(1):7–10.

53. Boehme CC, Nabeta P, Hillemann D, et al. Rapid molecular detection of tuberculosis and rifampin resistance. N Engl J Med 2010;363(11):1005–15.

54. Lewinsohn DM, Leonard MK, LoBue PA, et al. Official American Thoracic Society/Infectious Diseases Society of America/Centers for Disease Control and Prevention Clinical Practice Guidelines: Diagnosis of Tuberculosis in Adults and Children. Clin Infect Dis 2017;64(2):111–5.

55. Leeds IL, Magee MJ, Kurbatova EV, et al. Site of extrapulmonary tuberculosis is associated with HIV infection. Clin Infect Dis 2012;55(1):75–81.

56. Nahid P, Dorman SE, Alipanah N, et al. Official American Thoracic Society/Centers for Disease Control and Prevention/Infectious Diseases Society of America Clinical Practice Guidelines: Treatment of Drug-Susceptible Tuberculosis. Clin Infect Dis 2016;63(7):e147–95.

57. Narendran G, Menon PA, Venkatesan P, et al. Acquired rifampicin resistance in thrice-weekly antituberculosis therapy: impact of HIV and antiretroviral therapy. Clin Infect Dis 2014;59(12):1798–804.

58. Nettles RE, Mazo D, Alwood K, et al. Risk factors for relapse and acquired rifamycin resistance after directly observed tuberculosis treatment: a comparison by HIV serostatus and rifamycin use. Clin Infect Dis 2004;38(5):731–6.

59. Burman W, Benator D, Vernon A, et al. Acquired rifamycin resistance with twice-weekly treatment of HIV-related tuberculosis. Am J Respir Crit Care Med 2006; 173(3):350–6.

60. Mayosi BM, Ntsekhe M, Bosch J, et al. Prednisolone and mycobacterium indicus pranii in tuberculous pericarditis. N Engl J Med 2014;371(12):1121–30.

61. Thwaites GE, Nguyen DB, Nguyen HD, et al. Dexamethasone for the treatment of tuberculous meningitis in adolescents and adults. N Engl J Med 2004; 351(17):1741–51.

62. Abdool Karim SS, Naidoo K, Grobler A, et al. Timing of initiation of antiretroviral drugs during tuberculosis therapy. N Engl J Med 2010;362(8):697–706.

63. Havlir DV, Kendall MA, Ive P, et al. Timing of antiretroviral therapy for HIV-1 infection and tuberculosis. N Engl J Med 2011;365(16):1482–91.

64. Torok ME, Yen NT, Chau TT, et al. Timing of initiation of antiretroviral therapy in human immunodeficiency virus (HIV)–associated tuberculous meningitis. Clin Infect Dis 2011;52(11):1374–83.

65. Namale PE, Abdullahi LH, Fine S, et al. Paradoxical TB-IRIS in HIV-infected adults: a systematic review and meta-analysis. Future Microbiol 2015;10(6): 1077–99.

66. Lawn SD, Myer L, Bekker LG, et al. Tuberculosis-associated immune reconstitution disease: incidence, risk factors and impact in an antiretroviral treatment service in South Africa. AIDS 2007;21(3):335–41.

67. Meintjes G, Stek C, Blumenthal L, et al. Prednisone for the prevention of paradoxical tuberculosis-associated IRIS. N Engl J Med 2018;379(20):1915–25.

68. Meintjes G, Lawn SD, Scano F, et al. Tuberculosis-associated immune reconstitution inflammatory syndrome: case definitions for use in resource-limited settings. Lancet Infect Dis 2008;8(8):516–23.

69. Pepper DJ, Marais S, Maartens G, et al. Neurologic manifestations of paradoxical tuberculosis-associated immune reconstitution inflammatory syndrome: a case series. Clin Infect Dis 2009;48(11):e96–107.

70. Kovacs JA, Hiemenz JW, Macher AM, et al. Pneumocystis carinii pneumonia: a comparison between patients with the acquired immunodeficiency syndrome and patients with other immunodeficiencies. Ann Intern Med 1984;100(5): 663–71.

71. Selwyn PA, Pumerantz AS, Durante A, et al. Clinical predictors of Pneumocystis carinii pneumonia, bacterial pneumonia and tuberculosis in HIV-infected patients. AIDS 1998;12(8):885–93.

72. Sax PE, Komarow L, Finkelman MA, et al. Blood (1->3)-beta-D-glucan as a diagnostic test for HIV-related Pneumocystis jirovecii pneumonia. Clin Infect Dis 2011;53(2):197–202.

73. Richards PJ, Riddell L, Reznek RH, et al. High resolution computed tomography in HIV patients with suspected Pneumocystis carinii pneumonia and a normal chest radiograph. Clin Radiol 1996;51(10):689–93.

74. Baughman RP, Dohn MN, Frame PT. The continuing utility of bronchoalveolar lavage to diagnose opportunistic infection in AIDS patients. Am J Med 1994; 97(6):515–22.

75. Procop GW, Haddad S, Quinn J, et al. Detection of Pneumocystis jiroveci in respiratory specimens by four staining methods. J Clin Microbiol 2004;42(7): 3333–5.

76. Hauser PM, Bille J, Lass-Florl C, et al. Multicenter, prospective clinical evaluation of respiratory samples from subjects at risk for Pneumocystis jirovecii infection by use of a commercial real-time PCR assay. J Clin Microbiol 2011;49(5): 1872–8.

77. Torres J, Goldman M, Wheat LJ, et al. Diagnosis of Pneumocystis carinii pneumonia in human immunodeficiency virus-infected patients with polymerase chain reaction: a blinded comparison to standard methods. Clin Infect Dis 2000;30(1):141–5.

78. Bozzette SA, Sattler FR, Chiu J, et al. A controlled trial of early adjunctive treatment with corticosteroids for Pneumocystis carinii pneumonia in the acquired

immunodeficiency syndrome. California Collaborative Treatment Group. N Engl J Med 1990;323(21):1451–7.

79. Nielsen TL, Eeftinck Schattenkerk JK, Jensen BN, et al. Adjunctive corticosteroid therapy for Pneumocystis carinii pneumonia in AIDS: a randomized European multicenter open label study. J Acquir Immune Defic Syndr 1992;5(7):726–31.

80. Hughes W, Leoung G, Kramer F, et al. Comparison of atovaquone (566C80) with trimethoprim-sulfamethoxazole to treat Pneumocystis carinii pneumonia in patients with AIDS. N Engl J Med 1993;328(21):1521–7.

81. Safrin S, Finkelstein DM, Feinberg J, et al. Comparison of three regimens for treatment of mild to moderate Pneumocystis carinii pneumonia in patients with AIDS. A double-blind, randomized, trial of oral trimethoprim-sulfamethoxazole, dapsone-trimethoprim, and clindamycin-primaquine. ACTG 108 Study Group. Ann Intern Med 1996;124(9):792–802.

82. Toma E, Thorne A, Singer J, et al. Clindamycin with primaquine vs. Trimethoprim-sulfamethoxazole therapy for mild and moderately severe Pneumocystis carinii pneumonia in patients with AIDS: a multicenter, double-blind, randomized trial (CTN 004). CTN-PCP Study Group. Clin Infect Dis 1998;27(3):524–30.

83. Achenbach CJ, Harrington RD, Dhanireddy S, et al. Paradoxical immune reconstitution inflammatory syndrome in HIV-infected patients treated with combination antiretroviral therapy after AIDS-defining opportunistic infection. Clin Infect Dis 2012;54(3):424–33.

84. Grant PM, Komarow L, Andersen J, et al. Risk factor analyses for immune reconstitution inflammatory syndrome in a randomized study of early vs. deferred ART during an opportunistic infection. PLoS One 2010;5(7):e11416.

85. Smego RA Jr, Nagar S, Maloba B, et al. A meta-analysis of salvage therapy for Pneumocystis carinii pneumonia. Arch Intern Med 2001;161(12):1529–33.

86. Schneider MM, Hoepelman AI, Eeftinck Schattenkerk JK, et al. A controlled trial of aerosolized pentamidine or trimethoprim-sulfamethoxazole as primary prophylaxis against Pneumocystis carinii pneumonia in patients with human immunodeficiency virus infection. The Dutch AIDS Treatment Group. N Engl J Med 1992;327(26):1836–41.

87. Furrer H, Egger M, Opravil M, et al. Discontinuation of primary prophylaxis against Pneumocystis carinii pneumonia in HIV-1-infected adults treated with combination antiretroviral therapy. Swiss HIV Cohort Study. N Engl J Med 1999;340(17):1301–6.

88. Abgrall S, Rabaud C, Costagliola D. Incidence and risk factors for toxoplasmic encephalitis in human immunodeficiency virus-infected patients before and during the highly active antiretroviral therapy era. Clin Infect Dis 2001;33(10):1747–55.

89. Israelski DM, Chmiel JS, Poggensee L, et al. Prevalence of Toxoplasma infection in a cohort of homosexual men at risk of AIDS and toxoplasmic encephalitis. J Acquir Immune Defic Syndr 1993;6(4):414–8.

90. Boyer KM, Holfels E, Roizen N, et al. Risk factors for Toxoplasma gondii infection in mothers of infants with congenital toxoplasmosis: Implications for prenatal management and screening. Am J Obstet Gynecol 2005;192(2):564–71.

91. Park YH, Nam HW. Clinical features and treatment of ocular toxoplasmosis. Korean J Parasitol 2013;51(4):393–9.

92. Antinori A, Ammassari A, De Luca A, et al. Diagnosis of AIDS-related focal brain lesions: a decision-making analysis based on clinical and neuroradiologic

characteristics combined with polymerase chain reaction assays in CSF. Neurology 1997;48(3):687–94.

93. Skiest DJ, Erdman W, Chang WE, et al. SPECT thallium-201 combined with Toxoplasma serology for the presumptive diagnosis of focal central nervous system mass lesions in patients with AIDS. J Infect 2000;40(3):274–81.

94. Luft BJ, Hafner R, Korzun AH, et al. Toxoplasmic encephalitis in patients with the acquired immunodeficiency syndrome. Members of the ACTG 077p/ANRS 009 Study Team. N Engl J Med 1993;329(14):995–1000.

95. Katlama C, De Wit S, O'Doherty E, et al. Pyrimethamine-clindamycin vs. pyrimethamine-sulfadiazine as acute and long-term therapy for toxoplasmic encephalitis in patients with AIDS. Clin Infect Dis 1996;22(2):268–75.

96. Dannemann B, McCutchan JA, Israelski D, et al. Treatment of toxoplasmic encephalitis in patients with AIDS. A randomized trial comparing pyrimethamine plus clindamycin to pyrimethamine plus sulfadiazine. The California Collaborative Treatment Group. Ann Intern Med 1992;116(1):33–43.

97. Beraud G, Pierre-Francois S, Foltzer A, et al. Cotrimoxazole for treatment of cerebral toxoplasmosis: an observational cohort study during 1994-2006. Am J Trop Med Hyg 2009;80(4):583–7.

98. Torre D, Casari S, Speranza F, et al. Randomized trial of trimethoprim-sulfamethoxazole versus pyrimethamine-sulfadiazine for therapy of toxoplasmic encephalitis in patients with AIDS. Italian Collaborative Study Group. Antimicrob Agents Chemother 1998;42(6):1346–9.

99. Martin-Blondel G, Alvarez M, Delobel P, et al. Toxoplasmic encephalitis IRIS in HIV-infected patients: a case series and review of the literature. J Neurol Neurosurg Psychiatry 2011;82(6):691–3.

100. Bertschy S, Opravil M, Cavassini M, et al. Discontinuation of maintenance therapy against toxoplasma encephalitis in AIDS patients with sustained response to anti-retroviral therapy. Clin Microbiol Infect 2006;12(7):666–71.

101. Miro JM, Lopez JC, Podzamczer D, et al. Discontinuation of primary and secondary Toxoplasma gondii prophylaxis is safe in HIV-infected patients after immunological restoration with highly active antiretroviral therapy: results of an open, randomized, multicenter clinical trial. Clin Infect Dis 2006;43(1):79–89.

102. Sloan DJ, Parris V. Cryptococcal meningitis: epidemiology and therapeutic options. Clin Epidemiol 2014;6:169–82.

103. Huang HR, Fan LC, Rajbanshi B, et al. Evaluation of a new cryptococcal antigen lateral flow immunoassay in serum, cerebrospinal fluid and urine for the diagnosis of cryptococcosis: a meta-analysis and systematic review. PLoS One 2015;10(5):e0127117.

104. Dubbels M, Granger D, Theel ES. Low cryptococcus antigen titers as determined by lateral flow assay should be interpreted cautiously in patients without prior diagnosis of cryptococcal infection. J Clin Microbiol 2017;55(8):2472–9.

105. Graybill JR, Sobel J, Saag M, et al. Diagnosis and management of increased intracranial pressure in patients with AIDS and cryptococcal meningitis. The NIAID Mycoses Study Group and AIDS Cooperative Treatment Groups. Clin Infect Dis 2000;30(1):47–54.

106. Fessler RD, Sobel J, Guyot L, et al. Management of elevated intracranial pressure in patients with Cryptococcal meningitis. J Acquir Immune Defic Syndr Hum Retrovirol 1998;17(2):137–42.

107. Day JN, Chau TTH, Wolbers M, et al. Combination antifungal therapy for cryptococcal meningitis. N Engl J Med 2013;368(14):1291–302.

108. Beardsley J, Wolbers M, Kibengo FM, et al. Adjunctive Dexamethasone in HIV-associated cryptococcal meningitis. N Engl J Med 2016;374(6):542–54.
109. Murphy RA, Hatlen TJ, Moosa MS. High-dose fluconazole consolidation therapy for cryptococcal meningitis in Sub-Saharan Africa: much to gain, little to lose. AIDS Res Hum Retroviruses 2018;34(5):399–403.
110. Powderly WG, Saag MS, Cloud GA, et al. A controlled trial of fluconazole or amphotericin B to prevent relapse of cryptococcal meningitis in patients with the acquired immunodeficiency syndrome. The NIAID AIDS Clinical Trials Group and Mycoses Study Group. N Engl J Med 1992;326(12):793–8.
111. Brandt ME, Pfaller MA, Hajjeh RA, et al. Trends in antifungal drug susceptibility of Cryptococcus neoformans isolates in the United States: 1992 to 1994 and 1996 to 1998. Antimicrob Agents Chemother 2001;45(11):3065–9.
112. Govender NP, Patel J, van Wyk M, et al. Trends in antifungal drug susceptibility of Cryptococcus neoformans isolates obtained through population-based surveillance in South Africa in 2002-2003 and 2007-2008. Antimicrob Agents Chemother 2011;55(6):2606–11.
113. Shelburne SA 3rd, Darcourt J, White AC Jr, et al. The role of immune reconstitution inflammatory syndrome in AIDS-related Cryptococcus neoformans disease in the era of highly active antiretroviral therapy. Clin Infect Dis 2005;40(7):1049–52.
114. Thomson R, Tolson C, Carter R, et al. Isolation of nontuberculous mycobacteria (NTM) from household water and shower aerosols in patients with pulmonary disease caused by NTM. J Clin Microbiol 2013;51(9):3006–11.
115. Nightingale SD, Byrd LT, Southern PM, et al. Incidence of Mycobacterium avium-intracellulare complex bacteremia in human immunodeficiency virus-positive patients. J Infect Dis 1992;165(6):1082–5.
116. Gordin FM, Cohn DL, Sullam PM, et al. Early manifestations of disseminated Mycobacterium avium complex disease: a prospective evaluation. J Infect Dis 1997;176(1):126–32.
117. Benson CA, Williams PL, Currier JS, et al. A prospective, randomized trial examining the efficacy and safety of clarithromycin in combination with ethambutol, rifabutin, or both for the treatment of disseminated Mycobacterium avium complex disease in persons with acquired immunodeficiency syndrome. Clin Infect Dis 2003;37(9):1234–43.
118. Gordin FM, Sullam PM, Shafran SD, et al. A randomized, placebo-controlled study of rifabutin added to a regimen of clarithromycin and ethambutol for treatment of disseminated infection with Mycobacterium avium complex. Clin Infect Dis 1999;28(5):1080–5.
119. El-Sadr WM, Burman WJ, Grant LB, et al. Discontinuation of prophylaxis against Mycobacterium avium complex disease in HIV-infected patients who have a response to antiretroviral therapy. Terry Beirn Community Programs for Clinical Research on AIDS. N Engl J Med 2000;342(15):1085–92.
120. Griffith DE, Aksamit T, Brown-Elliott BA, et al. An official ATS/IDSA statement: diagnosis, treatment, and prevention of nontuberculous mycobacterial diseases. Am J Respir Crit Care Med 2007;175(4):367–416.
121. Phillips P, Bonner S, Gataric N, et al. Nontuberculous mycobacterial immune reconstitution syndrome in HIV-infected patients: spectrum of disease and long-term follow-up. Clin Infect Dis 2005;41(10):1483–97.
122. Jung Y, Song KH, Choe PG, et al. Incidence of disseminated Mycobacterium avium-complex infection in HIV patients receiving antiretroviral therapy with use of Mycobacterium avium-complex prophylaxis. Int J STD AIDS 2017;28(14):1426–32.

123. Yangco BG, Buchacz K, Baker R, et al. Is primary mycobacterium avium complex prophylaxis necessary in patients with CD4 <50 cells/muL who are virologically suppressed on cART? AIDS Patient Care STDs 2014;28(6):280–3.

124. Saag MS, Benson CA, Gandhi RT, et al. Antiretroviral drugs for treatment and prevention of HIV infection in adults: 2018 recommendations of the international antiviral society-USA panel. JAMA 2018;320(4):379–96.

125. Schwarcz L, Chen MJ, Vittinghoff E, et al. Declining incidence of AIDS-defining opportunistic illnesses: results from 16 years of population-based AIDS surveillance. AIDS 2013;27(4):597–605.

126. Jabs DA, Van Natta ML, Kempen JH, et al. Characteristics of patients with cytomegalovirus retinitis in the era of highly active antiretroviral therapy. Am J Ophthalmol 2002;133(1):48–61.

127. Holland GN. AIDS and ophthalmology: the first quarter century. Am J Ophthalmol 2008;145(3):397–408.

128. Dieterich DT, Rahmin M. Cytomegalovirus colitis in AIDS: presentation in 44 patients and a review of the literature. J Acquir Immune Defic Syndr 1991;4(Suppl 1):S29–35.

129. Arribas JR, Clifford DB, Fichtenbaum CJ, et al. Level of cytomegalovirus (CMV) DNA in cerebrospinal fluid of subjects with AIDS and CMV infection of the central nervous system. J Infect Dis 1995;172(2):527–31.

130. Jabs DA, Ahuja A, Van Natta M, et al. Comparison of treatment regimens for cytomegalovirus retinitis in patients with AIDS in the era of highly active antiretroviral therapy. Ophthalmology 2013;120(6):1262–70.

131. Martin BK, Ricks MO, Forman MS, et al. Change over time in incidence of ganciclovir resistance in patients with cytomegalovirus retinitis. Clin Infect Dis 2007; 44(7):1001–8.

132. Kempen JH, Min YI, Freeman WR, et al. Risk of immune recovery uveitis in patients with AIDS and cytomegalovirus retinitis. Ophthalmology 2006;113(4): 684–94.

133. Cinque P, Koralnik IJ, Gerevini S, et al. Progressive multifocal leukoencephalopathy in HIV-1 infection. Lancet Infect Dis 2009;9(10):625–36.

134. Berger JR, Aksamit AJ, Clifford DB, et al. PML diagnostic criteria: consensus statement from the AAN Neuroinfectious Disease Section. Neurology 2013; 80(15):1430–8.

135. Fournier A, Martin-Blondel G, Lechapt-Zalcman E, et al. Immune reconstitution inflammatory syndrome unmasking or worsening AIDS-related progressive multifocal leukoencephalopathy: a literature review. Front Immunol 2017;8:577.

136. Tan K, Roda R, Ostrow L, et al. PML-IRIS in patients with HIV infection: clinical manifestations and treatment with steroids. Neurology 2009;72(17):1458–64.

137. Martin-Blondel G, Brassat D, Bauer J, et al. CCR5 blockade for neuroinflammatory diseases–beyond control of HIV. Nat Rev Neurol 2016;12(2):95–105.

138. Sainz-de-la-Maza S, Casado JL, Perez-Elias MJ, et al. Incidence and prognosis of immune reconstitution inflammatory syndrome in HIV-associated progressive multifocal leucoencephalopathy. Eur J Neurol 2016;23(5):919–25.

139. Summers NA, Kelley CF, Armstrong W, et al. Not a disease of the past: a case series of progressive multifocal leukoencephalopathy in the established antiretroviral era. AIDS Res Hum Retroviruses 2019;35(6):544–52.

140. Engsig FN, Hansen AB, Omland LH, et al. Incidence, clinical presentation, and outcome of progressive multifocal leukoencephalopathy in HIV-infected patients during the highly active antiretroviral therapy era: a nationwide cohort study. J Infect Dis 2009;199(1):77–83.

HIV and Aging
Reconsidering the Approach to Management of Comorbidities

Kristine M. Erlandson, MD, MS[a],*, Maile Y. Karris, MD[b]

KEYWORDS

- HIV • Aging • Frailty • Comprehensive geriatric assessment • Polypharmacy
- Multimorbidity

KEY POINTS

- Adherence to general screening and management recommendations in addition to human immunodeficiency virus-specific guidelines is challenging and overwhelming for providers and patients.
- The 6Ms approach is a starting point to address the health issues impacting older adults with human immunodeficiency virus.
- This approach acknowledges the multicomplexity of older adults with human immunodeficiency virus, simplifies geriatric principles for non–geriatrics-trained providers, and minimizes training/specialized screening tests or tools that may add to administrative burden.
- Successful and sustainable implementation of novel approaches to care will require support at local and national levels and depend on changes to the standards of care used to measure the quality of human immunodeficiency virus clinics.

Over the past 30 years, human immunodeficiency virus (HIV) has transformed from a near uniformly fatal infection to a chronic condition, fueled in part by the tremendous efforts of advocates, dedication of scientists, and determination of providers and patients. Today, those who survived the early epidemic of HIV are now living well into their 50s, 60s, 70s, and beyond. The Centers for Disease Control and Prevention estimate that nearly 50% of persons with HIV in the United States are aged 50 years and older[1] (referred to herein as older adults with HIV). Estimates from some European countries predict a "silver tsunami" within the HIV community mirroring that of the

Funded by: National Institutes of Health, National Institute on Aging (NIH NIA), Grant number(s): AG054366.
[a] University of Colorado, Anschutz Medical Campus, 12700 East 19th Avenue, Mail Stop B168, Aurora, CO 80045, USA; [b] University of California San Diego, 200 West Arbor Drive #8208, San Diego, CA 92103-8208, USA
* Corresponding author.
E-mail address: Kristine.Erlandson@ucdenver.edu

Infect Dis Clin N Am 33 (2019) 769–786
https://doi.org/10.1016/j.idc.2019.04.005
0891-5520/19/© 2019 Elsevier Inc. All rights reserved.

id.theclinics.com

general population, with those aged 50 or older accounting for nearly 70% of people with HIV by 2030.[2] Although many of these survivors now have well-controlled HIV infection, they may have experienced marked immune suppression, toxic early antiretroviral therapy (ART) regimens, and profound loss through the untimely death of partners, close friends, and community members. In addition to these long-term survivors, many older people with HIV were diagnosed after the advent of effective ART, or acquired HIV at an older age, and were never exposed to early toxic ART or profound immune suppression. Thus, the health status of older people with HIV today is highly heterogeneous based on differences in exposure to ART, immunosuppression, trauma, and stigma, all of which are hypothesized to impact the aging progress.

The increasing effectiveness and lower toxicity of ART contributed to significant decreases in AIDS-associated conditions, although the prevalence of chronic end organ diseases has increased.[3] World-wide, more than two-thirds of deaths among people with HIV are now attributable to non–HIV-associated diseases.[4–8] Some noninfectious comorbidities, such as heart disease, malignancy, and cognitive decline,[9–13] occur in excess and at chronologically younger ages among people with HIV[14] (roughly 10 years before HIV-uninfected persons).[12,15] In fact, 83% of people with HIV aged 50 and older and 63% aged 18 to 49 have at least 1 comorbidity other than HIV.[16] All people with HIV 75 years and older have at least 1 comorbidity apart from HIV and more than two-thirds have multimorbidity (more than 2 comorbidities).[17] Recent literature in middle-aged HIV cohorts also describes the presence of geriatric syndromes such as frailty, falls, and cognitive decline.[18]

The accumulating burden of medical and psychiatric multimorbidities of people with HIV[19] contributes to impairments in physical, social, and mental health function, and higher levels of stress and depression.[20–22] Multimorbidity also contributes to very high costs of care. In California, the mean estimated cost of caring for 1 person with HIV with no comorbidities per year is an estimated $30,312, but this incrementally increases with each comorbidity to $219,000 for persons with 11 comorbidities or more.[23] People with HIV also experience social isolation, loneliness, stress, and stigma from HIV and age (internal and perceived external),[24–27] in part owing to losses during the AIDS epidemic.[28] This lack of informal support and other barriers to seeking support from family and peers[29] (ie, fear of disclosure of HIV status,[30] stigma[31,32]) drive many people with HIV to pursue professional care provision (ie, home care) when they can no longer care for themselves.[33,34] Professional care further increases costs for people with HIV and does not ensure they receive care free of discrimination, rejection, or abuse.[35,36]

CONSIDERATIONS IN COMORBIDITY SCREENING AND MANAGEMENT OF OLDER ADULTS WITH HUMAN IMMUNODEFICIENCY VIRUS

The HIV Primary Care guidelines[37] provide recommendations for routine screening and preventive care in people with HIV, much of which applies to older adults with HIV. Recommendations for specific comorbidity management and considerations in older adults with HIV are also published and regularly updated at HIV-Age.org.[38] Several factors, including system barriers, a lack of HIV-specific recommendations, and differing epidemiology of some comorbidities, may impact the implementation of comorbidity management. Furthermore, the high comorbidity burden of many older adults with HIV, transportation difficulties, navigation of complex medical systems, and competing priorities make adherence to these guidelines difficult. Thus, it is not surprising that many studies demonstrate low or only moderate adherence with published recommendations.[39–41] For example, although people with HIV have a markedly elevated cardiovascular disease risk in comparison with the general population, adherence to risk assessment and management of risk factors remains low.[39,41,42] Studies have shown that fewer than 1 in 5 eligible people with HIV receive aspirin prevention.[43] The use of antiplatelet therapy (5%) and statins (24%) are significantly lower in people with HIV compared with uninfected controls (14% and 36%, respectively), and smoking cessation advice or pharmacotherapy was provided to only 19% of people with HIV.[42]

Multilevel system barriers (knowledge of recommendations, availability/affordability, varying efficacy of the test/treatment in HIV, patient compliance) contribute to poor real-world guideline adherence. For example, bone density screening in people with HIV is recommended for all postmenopausal women and men aged 50 years or older, owing to high fracture risk.[37,44,45] Yet screening remains markedly low[46]: a national audit of the British HIV Association found that among older adults with HIV, only 17% of men aged 70 and older or women aged 65 and older had their bone density measured.[40] In the United States, Medicare, a primary insurer for many older adults with HIV, only covers densitometry for postmenopausal women, for men taking osteoporosis therapy or corticosteroids, or in persons with osteoporosis or stress fractures.[47] Furthermore, although some studies demonstrate that low bone density is associated with an increased fracture risk in people with HIV,[48] other studies report that measurement of bone density and use of estimation indices (ie, Fracture Risk Assessment score) insufficiently assesses fracture risk.[49–52]

Other comorbidity screening or preventive care recommendations are limited by a lack of guidelines for older adults with HIV, such as the Advisory Committee on Immunization Practices guidelines for immunization against herpes zoster (HZ).[53] Although risk for HZ remains higher in people with HIV, even with suppressed HIV-1 and a normal CD4 T lymphocyte count,[54] older adults with HIV are considerably less likely to receive HZ vaccination than their uninfected peers.[54,55] Despite several studies demonstrating safety of both the live HZ vaccine[56,57] and the newly licensed recombinant, adjuvanted HZ subunit vaccine in people with HIV,[58] the 2018 Advisory Committee on Immunization Practices guidelines, the Infectious Diseases Society of America guideline for immunocompromised hosts,[59] and primary care guidelines[37] fail to provide a formal recommendation. This lack of formal guideline recommendations seems to contribute, in part, to low rates of immunization.[55]

Finally, some comorbidities, such as cancer, have anticipated shifts in epidemiology with the changing age and immunosuppression of today's older adults with HIV. Compared with uninfected populations, people with HIV are at greater risk of some cancers (anal, lung, liver, and oral cavity/pharyngeal cancers),[60,61] and lower risk of others (breast, prostate, and colorectal cancers).[62] Current cancer screening guidelines do not differ from the general population, with the exception of anal and cervical cancers. Although the cancer burden among adults with HIV is estimated to decrease with continued improvement in immunosuppression,[63] cancer-attributable deaths have steadily increased over the past decade[64] and the combination of HIV and cancer is associated with greater than expected mortality than either condition alone.[65] Indeed, evidence suggests lower survival among people with HIV and with a cancer diagnosis[66] and emphasizes the importance of ongoing cancer screening for early diagnosis and management.

As we learn more about aging among people with HIV, considerations for the evaluation for many other comorbidities and conditions have been proposed, including routine evaluation of neurocognitive function, falls risk, presence of frailty or physical function impairment, and other geriatric syndromes. Completing the screening and management of the general population in addition to HIV-specific recommendations is increasingly challenging, with visit length limitations, feasibility of completion of recommendations, and patient burden/adherence to recommendations. As detailed in **Table 1**,[37,45,67–73] the recommended comorbidity screening and management of older adults with HIV has become overwhelming for providers and patients.

HOW DOES THE BUSY HUMAN IMMUNODEFICIENCY VIRUS PROVIDER MANAGE AND PRIORITIZE THE CARE OF OLDER ADULTS WITH HUMAN IMMUNODEFICIENCY VIRUS?

The care for people with HIV is often provided within the context of prioritizing goals unique to HIV infection (ART adherence and toxicity).[74] Yet it is steadily becoming clear that the management of other comorbidities is paramount to ensuring that older adults with HIV age well. Most HIV care providers have undergone training in the management of individual chronic diseases (internal medicine, family practice), and have used strategies that allow them to optimize the management of comorbidities through small to modest changes to current HIV practices. These changes may include additional appointments, health maintenance reminders in the electronic medical record, and collaborative care with general providers to allow HIV specialists to focus only on HIV. However, the question remains if it is appropriate and beneficial for HIV care providers to apply aggressive screening and treatment guidelines (see **Table 1**) developed in a population without complex chronic disease to a population with multimorbidity (ie, HIV).[75] Instead, should HIV providers embrace the approach of geriatricians and prioritize care based on individual morbidity and mortality risk, factors that are feasibly modifiable, and personal goals?[76,77]

The geriatric approach to care focuses less on optimizing individual comorbidities and more on geriatric syndromes (multifactorial conditions that result from deficits in multiple domains) that impact an individual's ability to function, with a focus on quality of life.[78] The goals of geriatricians can be summarized into 5 Ms: mind, mobility, medications, multicomplexity, and matters most[79] (**Table 2**). We propose emphasizing a sixth M—of modifiable factors within the context of the aging HIV epidemic. Integrating these concepts into HIV care has the potential to improve care for older adults with HIV and multimorbidity without overwhelming or overworking HIV providers and patients.

The mind goes beyond HIV-associated neurocognitive diseases, and other emerging causes of dementia, to incorporate mental health as well.[80] Depression and other mood disorders are more prevalent in older adults with HIV compared with uninfected persons; 27% report recent thoughts about taking their own life.[81–83] Ongoing depression clearly contributes to higher levels of emotional distress and poorer health-related quality of life[83,84] and is associated with loneliness and HIV stigma.[24,82] Thus, social prescriptions may be an adjunctive approach to depression management, particularly if loneliness is a key component.

Mobility is a cornerstone of older adult evaluation and one of the most important factors in maintaining independence with aging.[85] Older adults with HIV have greater than expected impairment in mobility measures such as gait speed[86] and seem to experience a more rapid decline in mobility with age than uninfected controls.[87] Frailty, a vulnerable physical state that impacts mobility,[88] is still relatively uncommon in older adults with HIV. However, prefrailty occurs in 40% to 60% of middle-aged or older adults with HIV.[18,86,89,90] Moreover, mobility impairments contribute to the high risk of falls observed in older adults with HIV.[18,91–93] In 1 study, 30% of middle-aged

Table 1
Recommended routine health care maintenance for the older adult with HIV

Screening/Prevention	Frequency	Comments
HIV-specific monitoring		
Retention	Regularly	
Adherence	Regularly	
Tolerability	Regularly	Regular monitoring of bone, kidney, metabolic, cardiovascular, and liver health
CD4 count	See comment	Every 3–6 mo during the first 2 y of care, if viremic while on ART, or if CD4 count <300 cells/μL; every 12 mo if CD4 300–500 cells/μL; optional if CD4 >500 cells/μL
HIV-1 RNA	Every 3–6 mo	
OI prophylaxis	See comment	If CD4 count <200 cells/μL or history of OI
Safer sex	Every visit	
Immunizations		
Influenza	Annually[a]	Live attenuated vaccine contraindicated; consider high-dose in those ≥65 y
Pneumonia (PCV13)	Once	
Pneumonia (PPSV23)	>8 wk after PCV13 (preferred)	Second dose >5 y after the first dose; if given before age 65, administer another dose after age 65 and >5 y after most recent dose
Tdap/Td	Once, then every 10 y	1 dose Tdap, then Td booster
MenACQY	2 doses, >8 wk apart	Booster every 5 y
Hepatitis A	If not immune	Among men who have sex with men, intravenous drug use, travel to endemic area, chronic liver disease, hepatitis B or C
Hepatitis B	A 2-, 3-, or 4-dose schedule, depending on vaccine used	Confirm antibody response 1–2 mo after completion, or subsequent visit
Recombinant zoster	2 doses, 2–6 mo apart ≥50 y[a]	ACIP provides no recommendation for HIV; should be administered even if prior receipt of live zoster vaccine
Varicella	See comments	If CD4 ≥200 cells/μL and no evidence of varicella infection
MMR	2 doses, ≥28 d apart	If CD4 ≥200 cells/μL for >6 mo and no evidence of immunity
Infection screening		
Hepatitis C antibody	Annually if risk[b]	
Interferon-γ release assay/tuberculin skin test	Annually/biannually if risk	At least once on entry into care
Treponemal antibody	Annually if risk[b]	

(continued on next page)

Table 1
(*continued*)

Screening/Prevention	Frequency	Comments
GC/chlamydia amplified DNA probe	Annually if risk[b]	Testing should include all sites of risk
Trichomoniasis screening	Annually in women[b]	
General screening		
Smoking	Regularly	USPSTF recommendation: ask and advise all adults regarding tobacco use; provide behavioral interventions and FDA–approved pharmacotherapy
Alcohol	Regularly	USPSTF recommendation: screen and provide brief behavioral counseling for persons engaged in risky or hazardous drinking
Marijuana use	Regularly	
Chronic pain	As needed	Pain contract, regularly toxicology, clinical evaluation every 3 months
Other substance use	Regularly	
Domestic violence	See comment	Highest risk among women of reproductive age
Gun safety	At least once	
Seat belt, helmet use	At least once	
Comorbidity screening		
Weight/height	At least annually	USPSTF recommendation: offer or refer adults with a body mass index of $\geq$30 to intensive, multicomponent behavioral interventions
Waist circumference	Annually	
Blood pressure	At least annually[a]	
Physical activity	Every visit	
Nutrition/food security	At least annually	
Depression screen	At least annually	
Glucose/A1c	Every 6–12 mo	USPSTF recommendation: offer or refer patients with abnormal blood glucose to intensive behavioral counseling interventions to promote a healthful diet and physical activity
Complete blood count with differential	Every 6 mo	
Complete metabolic panel	Every 3-6 mo	
Lipid panel	Every 6–12 mo	
Calculate cardiovascular disease risk	At least annually	

(*continued on next page*)

Table 1
(continued)

Screening/Prevention	Frequency	Comments
Statin need	At least annually	Per American College of Cardiology/American Heart Association risk assessment
25-OH vitamin D	See comment	If laboratory values suggestive of deficiency, or other risk (low bone density, fragility fracture, high risk of falls, chronic kidney disease); consider screening in all HIV owing to increased risk of osteoporosis
Consider vitamin D and calcium	See comment	In patients with known low vitamin D, chronic kidney disease, osteopenia/osteoporosis, or tenofovir disoproxil fumarate/tenofovir alafenamide based therapy
DXA scan/Fracture Risk Assessment score if DXA not available	$\geq$50 in all men; after menopause in women	
Urinalysis	Every 6–12 mo	Every 6 months if on tenofovir disoproxil fumarate/tenofovir alafenamide
Thyroid-stimulating hormone	If symptomatic	
Ophthalmologic examination	See comments	Comprehensive examination once at age 40, follow-up as recommended until age 60; every 1–2 y after age 60; annual dilated retinal examination if diabetes
Hearing screen	If symptomatic	Consider regular symptom assessment
Dental examination	Every 3–12 mo	
Abdominal ultrasound examination	Once, men aged 65–75 with smoking history	
Sleep quality	Annually	
Cancer screening		
Colonoscopy	Starting at age 50[c]	Consider alternative screening if colonoscopy not available
Prostate-specific antigen	Starting at age 50[c]	Screening based on shared decision making
Digital rectal examination	Annually	For rectal cancer (any age) and prostate cancer ($\geq$50 y)
Anal pap smear	Consider annually, if high-resolution anoscopy available	Pending randomized, clinical trial results
BRCA gene screening	If family history	

(continued on next page)

Table 1
(continued)

Screening/Prevention	Frequency	Comments
Mammography	Every 1–2 y beginning at age 50 (or 40)[c]	Screening initiation and frequency varies on guidelines, risk, and patient preference
Cervical pap smear	Every 1–3 y	Annually for 3 y, then every 3 y if 3 consecutive tests are negative; if HPV cotesting available; see footnote for further details[d]
Low-dose chest computed tomography scan	Annually, starting at age 55 if risk (see comment)	Adults ages 55–80 y with a 30 pack-year smoking history, who currently smoke or have quit ≤15 y
Hepatocellular carcinoma screening	If cirrhosis or HBV/HCV with additional risk	
Skin cancer screening	Periodic skin examination if high risk	
Additional considerations for geriatric/aging issues		
Loneliness Elder mistreatment Safety in home Driving safety Financial support Social support Activities of daily living IADLs Gait and balance Cognition Bowel/bladder function Sexual function	Consider at least annually[a]	
Polypharmacy and drug-drug interactions	Every visit	
Goals of care	Regularly	
Advanced directives	Annually[b]	
Falls	Every visit	
Fall prevention interventions	Exercise interventions, especially if high risk	
Serum testosterone	If symptoms	

Abbreviations: A1c, hemoglobin A1c; ACIP, Advisory Committee on Immunization Practices; DXA, dual energy x-ray absorptiometry; FDA, US Food and Drug Administration; GC, gonococcus; HBV, hepatitis B virus; HCV, hepatitis C virus; IADLs, instrumental activities of daily living; MenACQY, meningitis subtypes A, C, Q, and Y; MMR, measles mumps rubella; OI, opportunistic infection; PCV, pneumococcal conjugate vaccine; PPSV, pneumococcal polysaccharide vaccine; Tdap, tetanus diphtheria acellular pertussis; USPSTF, US Preventive Services Task Force.

[a] In the opinion of the authors.
[b] More frequently, depending on risk.
[c] Earlier screening may be indicated depending on family history.
[d] If cotests are both negative, repeat every 3 years; If human papilloma virus (HPV)16 or HPV16/18 are detected, refer for colposcopy. If negative pap but positive cotest for other HPV types, repeat in 1 y and refer for colposcopy of either cotest positive. If ASC-US pap, repeat if HPV cotest is negative, refer to colposcopy of HPV is positive. If low-grade squamous intraepithelial lesion or greater, refer for colposcopy. Recommendations based on references.[37,45,67–73]

people with HIV reported at least 1 fall in the prior year and 18% were recurrent fallers; poor balance was the strongest contributing factor to falls.[91] The identification of mobility impairments as falls risk factors can guide development of more effective fall interventions.[94–96]

Medications are particularly relevant in the care of older adults with HIV. The American Geriatrics Society developed the Beers criteria to assist clinicians in identifying potentially inappropriate medications for older adults, supported by research that demonstrate a high risk-over-benefit profile.[97] This list contains commonly used medications among older adults with HIV, including antidepressants, antipsychotics, benzodiazepines, hypnotics, and testosterone, among many others. Polypharmacy (ie, ≥ 5 medications) is also very common in older adults with HIV, and contributes to drug–drug interactions, poorer adherence, and increased mortality in both people with HIV and uninfected controls.[98–100] Among 248 older adults with HIV in 1 clinic, the average number of non-ART medications was 11.6, with 35% receiving 16 or more medications and 63% receiving inappropriate medication by the Beers Criteria.

Polypharmacy is one of the challenges born from the multicomplexity of older adults with HIV and is a potential consequence of aggressive screening and management of this population. Managing multiple conditions can often result in a prescribing cascade, where the side effects of a medication are misdiagnosed as a new condition.[101,102] For example, a 70-year-old man with HIV, peripheral neuropathy, chronic kidney disease, and heart failure who is taking ritonavir-boosted darunavir, emtricitabine, tenofovir alafenamide, gabapentin, and lisinopril is prescribed amlodipine for improved blood pressure control; subsequent edema is treated with furosemide rather than cessation of amlodipine, and the subsequent nocturnal urinary frequency with furosemide is treated with prazosin and zolpidem. Ultimately, he experiences confusion and falls. Approaching multicomplexity by taking a step back to see the whole person rather than a collection of conditions is useful in avoiding such clinical care pitfalls. Multicomplexity also embraces the evaluation and management of persons within their socioeconomic situation. Encouraging HIV case management and social work to develop a better understanding of the resources available for older adults may enhance the team care of older adults with HIV.

Last, geriatricians actively incorporate what "matters most": patients' personal goals and priorities into medical decision making and risk/benefit counseling. This approach allows management prioritization within the context of multicomplexity and is likely to improve patient adherence to recommendations. Considering what matters most may also allow smooth transitions to discussions regarding advanced care planning and overall goals of care.

INTRODUCING THE SIXTH M FOR OLDER ADULTS WITH HUMAN IMMUNODEFICIENCY VIRUS: MODIFIABLE

HIV-associated chronic inflammation, direct HIV-1 effects, ART-related toxicities on aging-related biologic pathways, and higher rates of cooccurring psychosocial conditions are thought to contribute to the aging phenotype observed in older adults with HIV.[103–106] Although we cannot change the historic impact that more toxic ART and immune suppression have had on the aging process of older adults with HIV, we can and should focus on the contributing factors that are modifiable. Arguably one of the most important targets of the screening and management of older adults with HIV with multimorbidity are lifestyle factors that maximize health span and decrease medication burden. Lifestyle management is often not addressed in the clinical setting,[42] although studies suggest that adherence is improved with

Table 2
A new approach to prioritizing key care components for the older adult with HIV: The six Ms

		Components	Interventions
[a]Modifiable: Prioritization of interventions that target the most modifiable risk factors (physical activity, obesity, nutrition, substance use) that impact multiple bio/psycho/social systems	Mind	Cognition, depression, mood	Evaluate and treat mood disorders Evaluate and treat comorbidities and polypharmacy that may contribute to cognitive decline Physical activity and mentally stimulating activities across the lifespan to maintain cognitive function Ensure safety (ie, consideration of driving safety, social support at home, medication administration)
	Mobility	Gait, balance, falls	Fall intervention programs Physical activity Physical/occupational therapy Home safety assessments
	Medications	Polypharmacy and drug–drug interactions	Reduce polypharmacy Prescribe treatments specific for older person's needs Identify medication adverse effects
	Multicomplexity	Consideration of comorbidities within complex social circumstances and limitations	Consideration of the highest priority screening and treatment guidelines, without contributing to polypharmacy. Assess living conditions and competing priorities Help older adults manage a variety of health conditions
	Matters most to me	An individual's own health outcome goals and care preferences	Coordinate advance care planning Manage goals of care Risk/benefit discussions when considering priorities and goals of care

[a] Added to the Geriatric 5 Ms Model.

provider-recommended lifestyle changes in the context of a clinic visit.[107–111] The US Preventative Services Task Force recognizes the importance of behavior change interventions through an evidence level B recommendation for intensive behavioral counseling interventions for physical activity and diet among adults with obesity or additional cardiovascular risk.[112] Multiple organizations, including the American Heart Association, have emphasized the importance of physical activity in comorbidity management, with a call for routine identification of physical inactivity as a vital sign and better incorporation of physical activity counseling throughout multiple levels of care. As in the general population, the importance of addressing these lifestyle factors across the lifespan of people with HIV cannot be emphasized enough. Improvement of lifestyle factors such as smoking cessation and other substance use counseling, routine physical activity, and a healthy diet can improve comorbidity burden, mood, inflammation and the immune system, and life expectancy among people with HIV.[113] Recommendations on smoking cessation among older adults with HIV exist,[38] and recent publications provide practical guidelines for obesity management[68] and physical activity.[113] Both the US HIV ART[67] and primary care guidelines[37] provide essentially no emphasis on screening or management of these modifiable factors. Because the magnitude of these lifestyle effects increases with increasing lifespan, behavioral counseling and therapy should become standard metrics of excellence assessed by US Health Resources and Services Administration and Ryan White, and treatment guidelines should emphasize the importance of these factors in the long-term care of all people with HIV.

SUMMARY

The health care of older adults with HIV can be highly complex, resource intensive, with a high administrative burden. Thus, improving the health span and wellness of older adults with HIV will likely require changes to the current model of HIV care. Unfortunately, research guiding the clinical management of older adults with HIV remains in a nascent stage with many unanswered questions. For example, should HIV providers consider an annual Medicare wellness visit to focus on comorbidity screening and management? Should primary care physicians be integrated into HIV specialty clinics? Should we be performing comprehensive geriatric assessments for all older adults with HIV or providing regular screening for cognitive impairment, frailty, and physical function? Do we pursue the integration of providers dual-trained in geriatrics and HIV management[114,115]? Do we broadly implement these interventions across all older adults with HIV, or stratify based on measures such as the Veterans Aging Cohort Study Index? When do we stop screening and aggressively managing comorbidities?

Growing data from aging longitudinal HIV cohorts and feedback from the HIV community suggest that the current model is not meeting the needs of older adults with HIV. In this review, we introduce the 6 Ms approach as a starting point to addressing the non–HIV-specific health issues that increasingly impact older adults with HIV. This approach acknowledges the multicomplexity of older adults with HIV, simplifies geriatric principles for non–geriatrics-trained providers, and minimizes extensive training and specialized screening tests or tools that may add to administrative burden.

Unfortunately, owing to dissatisfaction with salary/reimbursement and substantial administrative burden,[116] the projected workforce growth in HIV providers is unlikely to support the demand of a growing and complex population of older adults with HIV. Ultimately, we expect that caring for older adults with HIV will result in more frequent outpatient visits and depend on participation from other specialties, in-clinic pharmacists, case managers, social workers, and strong collaborations with community groups and advocates. Successful and sustainable implementation of novel approaches to care will also require support at both the local and national levels of health care administrators and health insurance providers and will likely depend on changes to the standards of care used to measure the quality of HIV clinics by the US Health Resources and Services Administration and Ryan White.

REFERENCES

1. Centers for Disease Control and Prevention. HIV among people aged 50 and older. 2018. Available at: https://www.cdc.gov/hiv/group/age/olderamericans/index.html. Accessed November 27, 2018.
2. Smit M, Brinkman K, Geerlings S, et al. Future challenges for clinical care of an ageing population infected with HIV: a modelling study. Lancet Infect Dis 2015; 15(7):810–8.
3. Buchacz K, Battalora L, Armon C, et al. Hospitalizations with AIDS and chronic end-organ conditions in HIV outpatient study. Presented at Conference on Retroviruses and Opportunistic Infections, Boston, MA, February 22–25, 2016. Abstract #708.
4. Smith C. Data Collection on Adverse events of Anti-HIV Drugs (D:A:D) Study. Association between modifiable and nonmodifiable risk factors and specific causes of death in the HAART Era: the data collection on adverse events of anti-HIV drugs study [abstract 145]. Paper presented at: program and abstracts of the 16th Conference on Retroviruses and Opportunistic Infections. Montreal, Canada, February 8–11, 2009.
5. Patterson S, Jose S, Samji H, et al. A tale of two countries: all-cause mortality among people living with HIV and receiving combination antiretroviral therapy in the UK and Canada. HIV Med 2017;18(9):655–66.
6. GBD 2015 Eastern Mediterranean Region HIV/AIDS Collaborators. Trends in HIV/AIDS morbidity and mortality in Eastern Mediterranean countries, 1990–2015: findings from the Global Burden of Disease 2015 study. Int J Public Health 2017;63(Suppl 1):123–36.
7. Reniers G, Blom S, Calvert C, et al. Trends in the burden of HIV mortality after roll-out of antiretroviral therapy in KwaZulu-Natal, South Africa: an observational community cohort study. Lancet HIV 2017;4(3):e113–21.
8. Maciel RA, Klück HM, Durand M, et al. Comorbidity is more common and occurs earlier in persons living with HIV than in HIV-uninfected matched controls, aged 50 years and older: a cross-sectional study. Int J Infect Dis 2018;70:30–5.
9. Pathai S, Bajillan H, Landay AL, et al. Is HIV a model of accelerated or accentuated aging? J Gerontol A Biol Sci Med Sci 2014;69(7):833–42.
10. Deeks SG. Immune dysfunction, inflammation, and accelerated aging in patients on antiretroviral therapy. Top HIV Med 2009;17(4):118–23.
11. Deeks SG. HIV infection, inflammation, immunosenescence, and aging. Annu Rev Med 2011;62:141–55.
12. Guaraldi G, Orlando G, Zona S, et al. Premature age-related comorbidities among HIV-infected persons compared with the general population. Clin Infect Dis 2011;53(11):1120–6.
13. Erlandson KM, Schrack JA, Jankowski CM, et al. Functional impairment, disability, and frailty in adults aging with HIV-infection. Curr HIV/AIDS Rep 2014;11(3):279–90.
14. Mayer KH, Loo S, Crawford PM, et al. Excess clinical comorbidity among HIV-infected patients accessing primary care in US community health centers. Public Health Rep 2018;133(1):109–18.
15. Schouten J, Wit FW, Stolte IG, et al. Cross-sectional comparison of the prevalence of age-associated comorbidities and their risk factors between HIV-

infected and uninfected individuals: the AGEhIV cohort study. Clin Infect Dis 2014;59(12):1787–97.

16. Koram N, Vannappargari V, Sampson T. Comorbidity prevalence and its influence on non-ARV comedication burden among HIV positive patients. IDWeek 2013;2013:2–6 [abstract: 323].

17. Allavena C, Hanf M, Rey D, et al. Antiretroviral exposure and comorbidities in an aging HIV-infected population: The challenge of geriatric patients. PLoS One 2018;13(9):e0203895.

18. Greene M, Covinsky KE, Valcour V, et al. Geriatric syndromes in older HIV-infected adults. J Acquir Immune Defic Syndr 2015;69(2):161.

19. Kilbourne A, Justice A, Rabeneck L, et al. General medical and psychiatric comorbidity among HIV-infected veterans in the post-HAART era. J Clin Epidemiol 2001;54(12):S22–8.

20. Balderson BH, Grothaus L, Harrison RG, et al. Chronic illness burden and quality of life in an aging HIV population. AIDS Care 2013;25(4):451–8.

21. Oursler KK, Goulet JL, Crystal S, et al. Association of age and comorbidity with physical function in HIV-infected and uninfected patients: results from the Veterans Aging Cohort Study. AIDS Patient Care STDS 2011;25(1):13–20.

22. Rodriguez-Penney AT, Iudicello JE, Riggs PK, et al. Co-morbidities in persons infected with HIV: increased burden with older age and negative effects on health-related quality of life. AIDS Patient Care STDS 2013;27(1):5–16.

23. Zingmond DS, Arfer KB, Gildner JL, et al. The cost of comorbidities in treatment for HIV/AIDS in California. PLoS One 2017;12(12):e0189392.

24. Grov C, Golub SA, Parsons JT, et al. Loneliness and HIV-related stigma explain depression among older HIV-positive adults. AIDS Care 2010;22(5):630–9.

25. Fekete EM, Williams SL, Skinta MD. Internalised HIV-stigma, loneliness, depressive symptoms and sleep quality in people living with HIV. Psychol Health 2018; 33(3):398–415.

26. Greene M, Hessol NA, Perissinotto C, et al. Loneliness in older adults living with HIV. AIDS Behav 2018;22(5):1475–84.

27. Fang X, Vincent W, Calabrese SK, et al. Resilience, stress, and life quality in older adults living with HIV/AIDS. Aging Ment Health 2015;19(11):1015–21.

28. Halkitis PN. The AIDS generation: stories of survival and resilience. New York: Oxford University Press; 2013.

29. Emlet CA. An examination of the social networks and social isolation in older and younger adults living with HIV/AIDS. Health Soc work 2006;31(4):299–308.

30. Poindexter C, Shippy RA. Networks of older New Yorkers with HIV: fragility, resilience, and transformation. AIDS Patient Care STDS 2008;22(9):723–33.

31. Emlet CA. "You're awfully old to have this disease": experiences of stigma and ageism in adults 50 years and older living with HIV/AIDS. Gerontologist 2006; 46(6):781–90.

32. Johnson MJ, Jackson NC, Arnette JK, et al. Gay and lesbian perceptions of discrimination in retirement care facilities. J Homosex 2005;49(2):83–102.

33. Shippy RA, Karpiak SE. Perceptions of support among older adults with HIV. Res Aging 2005;27(3):290–306.

34. Baker S. Social networks and community resources among older, African American caregivers of people living with HIV/AIDS. J Cult Divers 1999;6(4):124.

35. Fairchild SK, Carrino GE, Ramirez M. Social workers' perceptions of staff attitudes toward resident sexuality in a random sample of New York State nursing homes: a pilot study. J Gerontol Soc Work 1996;26(1–2):153–69.

36. Stein GL, Bonuck KA. Physician–patient relationships among the lesbian and gay community. J Gay Lesbian Med Assoc 2001;5(3):87–93.

37. Aberg JA, Gallant JE, Ghanem KG, et al. Primary care guidelines for the management of persons infected with HIV: 2013 update by the HIV Medicine Association of the Infectious Diseases Society of America. Clin Infect Dis 2014; 58(1):1–10.

38. Abrass CK, Applebaum JS, Boyd CM, et al. The HIV and aging consensus project: recommended treatment strategies for clinicians managing older patients with HIV 2014. Available at: www.hiv-ageorg/wp-content/uploads2013/11/HIVandAgingConsensusProject051815pdf. Accessed November 28, 2018.

39. Lichtenstein KA, Armon C, Buchacz K, et al. Provider compliance with guidelines for management of cardiovascular risk in HIV-infected patients. Prev Chronic Dis 2013;10:E10.

40. Molloy A, Curtis H, Burns F, et al. Routine monitoring and assessment of adults living with HIV: results of the British HIV Association (BHIVA) national audit 2015. BMC Infect Dis 2017;17(1):619.

41. Landovitz RJ, Desmond KA, Gildner JL, et al. Quality of Care for HIV/AIDS and for Primary Prevention by HIV Specialists and Nonspecialists. AIDS Patient Care STDS 2016;30(9):395–408.

42. Ladapo JA, Richards AK, DeWitt CM, et al. Disparities in the quality of cardiovascular care between HIV-infected versus HIV-uninfected adults in the United States: a cross-sectional study. J Am Heart Assoc 2017;6(11) [pii:e007107].

43. Burkholder GA, Tamhane AR, Salinas JL, et al. Underutilization of aspirin for primary prevention of cardiovascular disease among HIV-infected patients. Clin Infect Dis 2012;55(11):1550–7.

44. McComsey GA, Tebas P, Shane E, et al. Bone disease in HIV infection: a practical review and recommendations for HIV care providers. Clin Infect Dis 2010; 51(8):937–46.

45. Brown TT, Hoy J, Borderi M, et al. Recommendations for evaluation and management of bone disease in HIV. Clin Infect Dis 2015;60(8):1242–51.

46. Alvarez E, Belloso WH, Boyd MA, et al. Which HIV patients should be screened for osteoporosis: an international perspective. Curr Opin HIV AIDS 2016;11(3): 268–76.

47. Jackson T. Does Medicare cover bone density tests?. 2018. Available at: https://medicare.com/coverage/does-medicare-cover-bone-density-tests/. Accessed November 15, 2018.

48. Battalora L, Buchacz K, Armon C, et al. Low bone mineral density and risk of incident fracture in HIV-infected adults. Antivir Ther 2016;21(1):45–54.

49. Stephens KI, Rubinsztain L, Payan J, et al. Dual-energy X-ray absorptiometry and calculated FRAX risk scores may underestimate osteoporotic fracture risk in vitamin D-deficient veterans with HIV infection. Endocr Pract 2016;22(4):440–6.

50. Yang J, Sharma A, Shi Q, et al. Improved fracture prediction using different fracture risk assessment tool adjustments in HIV-infected women. AIDS 2018; 32(12):1699–706.

51. Yin MT, Shiau S, Rimland D, et al. Fracture prediction with modified-FRAX in older HIV-infected and uninfected men. J Acquir Immune Defic Syndr 2016; 72(5):513–20.

52. Yin MT, Falutz J. How to predict the risk of fracture in HIV? Curr Opin HIV AIDS 2016;11(3):261–7.

53. Centers for Disease Control and Prevention. Vaccine recommendations and guidelines of the ACIP. Zoster (shingles) ACIP vaccine recommendations

2018. Available at: https://www.cdc.gov/vaccines/hcp/acip-recs/vacc-specific/shingles.html. Accessed November 27, 2018.

54. Hawkins KL, Gordon KS, Levin MJ, et al. Herpes zoster and herpes zoster vaccine rates among adults living with and without HIV in the Veterans Aging Cohort Study. J Acquir Immune Defic Syndr 2018;79(4):527–33.

55. Erlandson KM, Streifel A, Novin AR, et al. Low rates of vaccination for herpes zoster in older people living with HIV. AIDS Res Hum Retroviruses 2018;34(7):603–6.

56. Benson CA, Andersen JW, Macatangay BJC, et al. Safety and immunogenicity of zoster vaccine live in human immunodeficiency virus-infected adults with CD4+ cell counts >200 Cells/mL virologically suppressed on antiretroviral therapy. Clin Infect Dis 2018;67(11):1712–9.

57. Shafran SD. Live attenuated herpes zoster vaccine for HIV-infected adults. HIV Med 2016;17(4):305–10.

58. Berkowitz EM, Moyle G, Stellbrink HJ, et al. Safety and immunogenicity of an adjuvanted herpes zoster subunit candidate vaccine in HIV-infected adults: a phase 1/2a randomized, placebo-controlled study. J Infect Dis 2015;211(8):1279–87.

59. Rubin LG, Levin MJ, Ljungman P, et al. 2013 IDSA clinical practice guideline for vaccination of the immunocompromised host. Clin Infect Dis 2014;58(3):e44–100.

60. Mahale P, Engels EA, Coghill AE, et al. Cancer risk in older persons living with human immunodeficiency virus infection in the United States. Clin Infect Dis 2018;67(1):50–7.

61. Colon-Lopez V, Shiels MS, Machin M, et al. Anal Cancer Risk Among People With HIV Infection in the United States. J Clin Oncol 2018;36(1):68–75.

62. Coghill AE, Engels EA, Schymura MJ, et al. Risk of breast, prostate, and colorectal cancer diagnoses among HIV-infected individuals in the United States. J Natl Cancer Inst 2018;110(9):959–66.

63. Shiels MS, Islam JY, Rosenberg PS, et al. Projected cancer incidence rates and burden of incident cancer cases in HIV-infected adults in the United States through 2030. Ann Intern Med 2018;168(12):866–73.

64. Engels EA, Yanik EL, Wheeler W, et al. Cancer-attributable mortality among people with treated human immunodeficiency virus infection in North America. Clin Infect Dis 2017;65(4):636–43.

65. Coghill AE, Pfeiffer RM, Shiels MS, et al. Excess mortality among HIV-infected individuals with cancer in the United States. Cancer Epidemiol Biomarkers Prev 2017;26(7):1027–33.

66. Calkins K, Geentanjali C, Joshu C, et al. Cancer stage, treatment, and survival comparing HIV clinic enrollees and SEER. Paper presented at: Conference on Retrovirals and Opportunistic Infections 2018. Boston, MA.

67. U.S. Department of Health and Human Services. Guidelines for the use of antiretroviral agents in adults and adolescents living with HIV 2018. Available at: https://aidsinfo.nih.gov/guidelines/html/1/adult-and-adolescent-arv/0. Accessed November 29, 2018.

68. Lake JE, Stanley TL, Apovian CM, et al. Practical review of recognition and management of obesity and lipohypertrophy in human immunodeficiency virus infection. Clin Infect Dis 2017;64(10):1422–9.

69. Kennel KA, Drake MT, Hurley DL. Vitamin D deficiency in adults: when to test and how to treat. Mayo Clin Proc 2010;85(8):752–7 [quiz: 757–8].

70. U.S. Preventive Services Task Force. Recommendations for primary care Practice 2018. Available at: https://www.uspreventiveservicestaskforce.org/Page/Name/recommendations. Accessed November 28, 2018.

71. Sokol HN. Preventive care in adults: recommendations 2018. Available at: www.uptodate.com/contents/preventive-care-in-adults-recommendations. Accessed November 12, 2018.

72. Wintemute GJ, Betz ME, Ranney ML. Yes, you can: physicians, patients, and firearms. Ann Intern Med 2016;165(3):205–13.

73. Rubenstein LZ, Wieland D. Comprehensive geriatric assessment. Annu Rev Gerontol Geriatr 1989;9:145–92.

74. Starrels JL, Peyser D, Haughton L, et al. When human immunodeficiency virus (HIV) treatment goals conflict with guideline-based opioid prescribing: a qualitative study of HIV treatment providers. Subst Abus 2016;37(1):148–53.

75. Tinetti ME, Fried T. The end of the disease era. Am J Med 2004;116(3):179–85.

76. Bradley EH, Bogardus ST Jr, Tinetti ME, et al. Goal-setting in clinical medicine. Soc Sci Med 1999;49(2):267–78.

77. Tinetti ME, McAvay GJ, Fried TR, et al. Health outcome priorities among competing cardiovascular, fall injury, and medication-related symptom outcomes. J Am Geriatr Soc 2008;56(8):1409–16.

78. Moore A, Patterson C, Nair K, et al. Minding the gap: prioritization of care issues among nurse practitioners, family physicians and geriatricians when caring for the elderly. J Interprof Care 2015;29(4):401–3.

79. Tinetti M, Huang A, Molnar F. The Geriatrics 5M's: a new way of communicating what we do. J Am Geriatr Soc 2017;65(9):2115.

80. Alisky JM. The coming problem of HIV-associated Alzheimer's disease. Med Hypotheses 2007;69(5):1140–3.

81. Justice AC, McGinnis KA, Atkinson JH, et al. Psychiatric and neurocognitive disorders among HIV-positive and negative veterans in care: veterans aging cohort five-site study. AIDS 2004;18:49–59.

82. Kalichman SC, Heckman T, Kochman A, et al. Depression and thoughts of suicide among middle-aged and older persons living with HIV-AIDS. Psychiatr Serv 2000;51(7):903–7.

83. Tate D, Paul RH, Flanigan TP, et al. The impact of apathy and depression on quality of life in patients infected with HIV. AIDS Patient Care STDs 2003; 17(3):115–20.

84. Jia H, Uphold CR, Wu S, et al. Health-related quality of life among men with HIV infection: effects of social support, coping, and depression. AIDS Patient Care STDS 2004;18(10):594–603.

85. Bierman AS. Functional status: the six vital sign. J Gen Intern Med 2001;16(11):785–6.

86. Erlandson KM, Wu K, Koletar SL, et al. Association between frailty and components of the frailty phenotype with modifiable risk factors and antiretroviral therapy. J Infect Dis 2017;215(6):933–7.

87. Schrack JA, Althoff KN, Jacobson LP, et al. Accelerated longitudinal gait speed decline in HIV-infected older men. J Acquir Immune Defic Syndr 2015;70(4):370–6.

88. Althoff KN, Jacobson LP, Cranston RD, et al. Age, comorbidities, and AIDS predict a frailty phenotype in men who have sex with men. J Gerontol A Biol Sci Med Sci 2013;69(2):189–98.

89. Onen NF, Patel P, Baker J, et al. Frailty and pre-frailty in a contemporary cohort of HIV-infected adults. J Frailty Aging 2014;3(3):158–65.

90. Petit N, Enel P, Ravaux I, et al. Frail and pre-frail phenotype is associated with pain in older HIV-infected patients. Medicine (Baltimore) 2018;97(6):e9852.

91. Erlandson KM, Allshouse AA, Jankowski CM, et al. Risk factors for falls in HIV-infected persons. J Acquir Immune Defic Syndr 2012;61(4):484–9.

92. Sharma A, Hoover DR, Shi Q, et al. Falls among middle-aged women in the Women's Interagency HIV Study. Antivir Ther 2016;21(8):697–706.

93. Erlandson KM, Plankey MW, Springer G, et al. Fall frequency and associated factors among men and women with or at risk for HIV infection. HIV Med 2016;17(10):740–8.

94. Xue Q-L. The frailty syndrome: definition and natural history. Clin Geriatr Med 2011;27(1):1–15.

95. Cadore EL, Rodríguez-Mañas L, Sinclair A, et al. Effects of different exercise interventions on risk of falls, gait ability, and balance in physically frail older adults: a systematic review. Rejuvenation Res 2013;16(2):105–14.

96. Sihvonen S, Kulmala J, Kallinen M, et al. Postural balance and self-reported balance confidence in older adults with a hip fracture history. Gerontology 2009; 55(6):630–6.

97. By the American Geriatrics Society Beers Criteria Update Expert Panel. American Geriatrics Society 2015 updated beers criteria for potentially inappropriate medication use in Older Adults. J Am Geriatr Soc 2015;63(11):2227–46.

98. Justice AC, Gordon KS, Skanderson M, et al. Nonantiretroviral polypharmacy and adverse health outcomes among HIV-infected and uninfected individuals. AIDS 2018;32(6):739–49.

99. Siefried KJ, Mao L, Cysique LA, et al. Concomitant medication polypharmacy, interactions and imperfect adherence are common in Australian adults on suppressive antiretroviral therapy. AIDS 2018;32(1):35–48.

100. Greene M, Steinman MA, McNicholl IR, et al. Polypharmacy, drug–drug interactions, and potentially inappropriate medications in older adults with human immunodeficiency virus infection. J Am Geriatr Soc 2014;62(3):447–53.

101. Rochon PA, Gurwitz JH. Optimising drug treatment for elderly people: the prescribing cascade. BMJ 1997;315(7115):1096–9.

102. Caughey GE, Roughead EE, Pratt N, et al. Increased risk of hip fracture in the elderly associated with prochlorperazine: is a prescribing cascade contributing? Pharmacoepidemiol Drug Saf 2010;19(9):977–82.

103. Cahill S, Valadéz R. Growing older with HIV/AIDS: new public health challenges. Am J Public Health 2013;103(3):e7–15.

104. Cohen J, Torres C. HIV-associated cellular senescence: a contributor to accelerated aging. Ageing Res Rev 2017;36:117–24.

105. Nasi M, Pinti M, De Biasi S, et al. Aging with HIV infection: a journey to the center of inflammAIDS, immunosenescence and neuroHIV. Immunol Lett 2014;162(1): 329–33.

106. Patel P, Hanson DL, Sullivan PS, et al. Incidence of types of cancer among HIV-infected persons compared with the general population in the United States, 1992–2003. Ann Intern Med 2008;148(10):728–36.

107. Neff HA, Kellar-Guenther Y, Jankowski CM, et al. Turning disability into ability: barriers and facilitators to initiating and maintaining exercise among older men living with HIV. AIDS Care 2018;1–5 [Epub ahead of print].

108. Petrella RJ, Lattanzio CN, Overend TJ. Physical activity counseling and prescription among Canadian primary care physicians. Arch Intern Med 2007; 167(16):1774–81.

109. Elley CR, Kerse N, Arroll B, et al. Effectiveness of counselling patients on physical activity in general practice: cluster randomised controlled trial. BMJ 2003; 326(7393):793.

110. Stead LF, Buitrago D, Preciado N, et al. Physician advice for smoking cessation. Cochrane Database Syst Rev 2013;(5):CD000165.

111. Rodriguez MM, Castillo JM, Sanchez JA, et al. Associations among physician advice, physical activity, and socio-demographic groups in older Spanish adults. Can J Aging 2012;31(3):349–56.

112. LeFevre ML, U.S. Preventive Services Task Force. Behavioral counseling to promote a healthful diet and physical activity for cardiovascular disease prevention in adults with cardiovascular risk factors: U.S. Preventive Services Task Force Recommendation statement. Ann Intern Med 2014;161(8):587–93.

113. Montoya JL, Jankowski CM, O'Brien KK, et al. Evidence-informed practical recommendations for increasing physical activity among persons living with HIV. AIDS 2019;33(6):931–9.

114. Siegler EL, Brennan-Ing M. Adapting systems of care for people aging with HIV. J Assoc Nurses AIDS Care 2017;28(5):698–707.

115. Siegler EL, Burchett CO, Glesby MJ. Older people with HIV are an essential part of the continuum of HIV care. J Int AIDS Soc 2018;21(10):e25188.

116. Weiser J, Beer L, West BT, et al. Qualifications, demographics, satisfaction, and future capacity of the HIV care provider workforce in the United States, 2013–2014. Clin Infect Dis 2016;63(7):966–75.

Key Principles of Antiretroviral Pharmacology

Brandon Dionne, PharmD[a,b,*]

KEYWORDS

- HIV • Antiretroviral • Pharmacology • Pharmacokinetics • Drug interactions

KEY POINTS

- Nearly every major step in the human immunodeficiency virus (HIV) life cycle is targeted by at least 1 class of antiretrovirals, but not all classes of antiretrovirals are commonly used.
- Combination antiretroviral therapy is very effective but can also come with adverse effects and complex drug interactions that need to be managed carefully.
- Differences in pill burden, tolerability, and barrier to resistance may help determine the choice of agent for an individual patient.
- Long-acting agents may play a role in improving adherence and eliminating the need for daily medications for both treatment and prevention of HIV.

Antiretroviral pharmacology has progressed significantly since the Food and Drug Administration's (FDA) approval of the first antiretroviral, the nucleoside reverse transcriptase inhibitor zidovudine, in 1987; classes of antiretrovirals have been developed with mechanisms of action that target nearly every major step in the human immunodeficiency virus (HIV) life cycle (**Fig. 1**).[1] Combination antiretroviral therapy (ART) that includes agents from at least 2 different classes is effective at suppressing viral replication, restoring immune status, and ultimately improving patient survival. The benefits are so widespread that essentially everyone with HIV is on treatment. Because multiple medications are required to prevent the development of resistance, clinicians need to understand the off-target effects of antiretrovirals, their metabolic pathways, and the important range of potential drug interactions (**Table 1**).

Before initiating or changing ART, or when starting any new medications in a patient currently on ART, providers should consult authoritative resources for potential drug interactions. Commonly used sites include the Department of Health and Human Services' AIDSinfo guidelines[1] and The University of Liverpool's drug interaction web site (hiv-druginteractions.org) or app (HIV iChart). The latter, in particular, is updated

Disclosure Statement: Nothing to disclose.
[a] Department of Pharmacy and Health System Sciences, Northeastern University, 360 Huntington Avenue, R218TF, Boston, MA 02115, USA; [b] Infectious Diseases, Pharmacy Department, Brigham and Women's Hospital, Boston, MA, USA
* 360 Huntington Avenue, R218TF, Boston, MA 02115.
E-mail address: b.dionne@northeastern.edu

Infect Dis Clin N Am 33 (2019) 787–805
https://doi.org/10.1016/j.idc.2019.05.006
0891-5520/19/© 2019 Elsevier Inc. All rights reserved.

id.theclinics.com

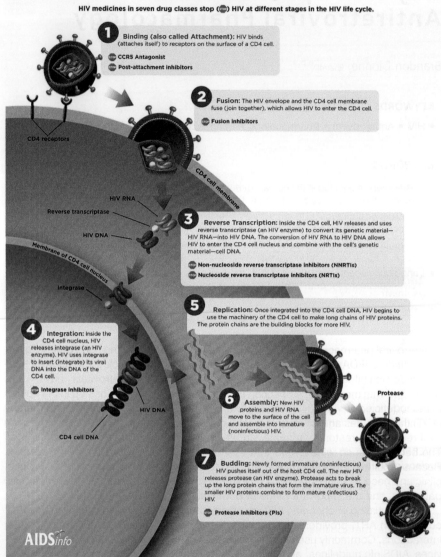

Fig. 1. The HIV life cycle and antiretroviral targets. (*From* Panel on Antiretroviral Guidelines for Adults and Adolescents. Guidelines for the Use of Antiretroviral Agents in Adults and Adolescents Living with HIV. Department of Health and Human Services. Available at: https://aidsinfo.nih.gov/contentfiles/lvguidelines/adultandadolescentgl.pdf. Published 2018. Accessed.)

frequently and often identifies potentially significant interactions that other resources do not.[2] Adherence and management of drug interactions are very important for maintaining trough concentrations of antiretrovirals above the minimum effective concentration to prevent viral replication (**Fig. 2**). The remainder of this article focuses on the individual drug classes, agents, and dosing used primarily in adults.

Table 1
Pharmacokinetic effects and metabolism of antiretrovirals on select enzymes

Antiretroviral	CYP3A4	CYP2D6	CYP2B6	CYP2C9	CYP2C19	P-gp	UGT	OCT2/ MATE1	OATP
EIs									
Maraviroc	S					S			
NRTIs									
Tenofovir						S			S
NNRTIs									
Efavirenz	S/↑/↓		S/↑		↑				
Rilpivirine	S								
Doravirine	S								
INSTIs									
Raltegravir							S		
Elvitegravir	S		↑				S		
Dolutegravir	S (minor)					S	S	↓	
Bictegravir	S					S	S	↓	
PIs									
Atazanavir	S/↓							↓	↓
Darunavir	S/↓			↑					↓
Boosters									
Ritonavir	S/↓	S/↓	↑	↑	↑	S/↓	↑		
Cobicistat	S/↓	↓					↓		

Abbreviations: ↑, inducer; ↓, inhibitor; EI, entry inhibitor; OATP, organic anion-transporting polypeptide; S, substrate.

Adapted from Panel on Antiretroviral Guidelines for Adults and Adolescents. Guidelines for the Use of Antiretroviral Agents in Adults and Adolescents Living with HIV. Department of Health and Human Services. Available at: https://aidsinfo.nih.gov/contentfiles/lvguidelines/adultandadolescentgl.pdf. Published 2018. Accessed.

REVERSE TRANSCRIPTASE INHIBITORS
Nucleoside Reverse Transcriptase Inhibitors

Nucleoside and nucleotide reverse transcriptase inhibitors (NRTIs) are the oldest class of antiretrovirals and are still commonly used as a "backbone" of therapy. They undergo phosphorylation intracellularly to their active diphosphate or triphosphate metabolites with different NRTIs acting as analogues of different deoxyribonucleotide triphosphates (dNTPs). They are incorporated into the viral DNA in place of their analogues by reverse transcriptase and lack a 3'-hydroxyl group, which prevents binding of the next dNTP, resulting in chain termination. HIV can develop resistance to NRTIs through discrimination, which is when reverse transcriptase is able to differentiate an NRTI from its analogue (eg, M184V or K65R point mutations), or phosphorolytic removal of NRTIs after incorporation into viral DNA (eg, T215Y point mutation), also known as thymidine analogue mutations. NRTIs are not metabolized by cytochrome P450 (CYP) enzymes, which results in fewer drug interactions with NRTIs than with other antiretrovirals. Class side effects can include lactic acidosis and hepatic steatosis, although these were more common with the older NRTIs (stavudine and didanosine) and are rare with the commonly used agents today. **Table 2** summarizes their characteristics.

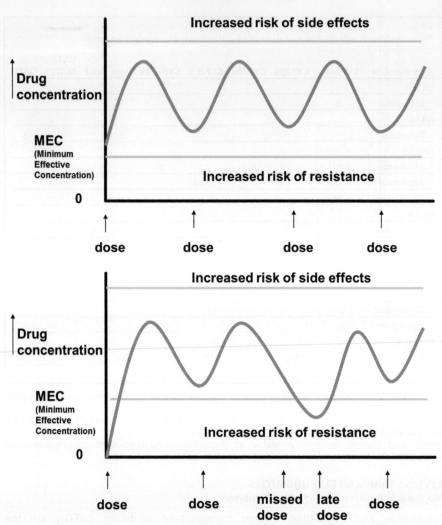

Fig. 2. Consequences of adherence on effective drug concentrations.

Abacavir

Abacavir (Ziagen) is an analogue of guanine. It is absorbed readily and completely, and although it was originally approved at a dose of 300 mg twice daily, it is now typically given as 600 mg once daily, generally in a combination tablet with lamivudine (Epzicom) or a fixed-dose single-tablet regimen with lamivudine and dolutegravir (Triumeq). Abacavir can cause a life-threatening hypersensitivity reaction and is contraindicated in patients who have HLA-B*5701, so testing for this allele must be conducted before initiating any regimen containing abacavir.[3] Abacavir has been associated with increased risk of myocardial infarction in some studies,[4] although this has not been consistently demonstrated[5]; one plausible mechanism is increased platelet activation through interference in nitric oxide–mediated inhibition of platelet aggregation.[6] Abacavir has also been associated with discordance between hemoglobin A1C and serum glucose, although the mechanism of this is unclear.[7]

Table 2
Characteristics of nucleoside reverse transcriptase inhibitors

	Abacavir (Ziagen)	Tenofovir Disoproxil (Viread)	Tenofovir Alafenamide	Emtricitabine (Emtriva)	Lamivudine (Epivir)	Zidovudine (Retrovir)
Usual adult dose	600 mg po daily or 300 mg po twice daily	300 mg po daily	25 mg po daily; 10 mg po daily with cobicistat	200 mg po daily	300 mg po daily	300 mg po twice daily
Dose adjusted in renal insufficiency?	No	Yes; Adjust or avoid when CrCl <50 mL/min	No; Avoid in CrCl <15 mL/min and not on hemodialysis	Yes; Avoid when CrCl <30 mL/min if coformulated; adjust when CrCl <50 mL/min when given separately	Yes; Adjust when CrCl <50 mL/min	Yes; Adjust for CrCl <15 mL/min
Fixed-dose combinations	Epzicom (w/ lamivudine) Triumeq (w/ lamivudine and dolutegravir) Trizivir (w/ lamivudine and zidovudine)	Truvada (w/emtricitabine) Cimduo/Temixys (w/ lamivudine) Atripla (w/emtricitabine and efavirenz) Symfi/Symfi Lo (w/ lamivudine and efavirenz) Complera (w/emtricitabine and rilpivirine) Stribild (w/emtricitabine, elvitegravir, and cobicistat)	Descovy (w/ emtricitabine) Odefsey (w/ emtricitabine and rilpivirine) Genvoya (w/ emtricitabine, elvitegravir, and cobicistat) Biktarvy (w/ emtricitabine and bictegravir) Symtuza (w/ emtricitabine, darunavir, and cobicistat)	Truvada (w/tenofovir disoproxil) Atripla (w/tenofovir disoproxil and efavirenz) Complera (w/tenofovir disoproxil and rilpivirine) Stribild (w/tenofovir disoproxil, elvitegravir, and cobicistat) Descovy (w/tenofovir alafenamide) Odefsey (w/tenofovir alafenamide and rilpivirine) Genvoya (w/tenofovir alafenamide, elvitegravir, and cobicistat) Biktarvy (w/tenofovir alafenamide and bictegravir) Symtuza (w/tenofovir alafenamide, darunavir, and cobicistat)	Combivir (w/ zidovudine) Cimduo/Temixys (w/tenofovir disoproxil) Symfi/Symfi Lo (w/tenofovir disoproxil and efavirenz) Epzicom (w/ abacavir) Triumeq (w/abacavir and dolutegravir)	Combivir (w/ lamivudine) Trizivir (w/ lamivudine and abacavir)

(continued on next page)

Table 2 (*continued*)

	Abacavir (Ziagen)	Tenofovir Disoproxil (Viread)	Tenofovir Alafenamide	Emtricitabine (Emtriva)	Lamivudine (Epivir)	Zidovudine (Retrovir)
Dosage forms	Tablets: 300 mg Solution: 20 mg/mL	Tablets: 150 mg, 200 mg, 250 mg, 300 mg Powder: 40 mg/g	Not available separately for HIV (25 mg tablet for hepatitis B treatment)	Tablets: 200 mg Solution: 10 mg/mL	Tablets: 100 mg, 150 mg, 300 mg Solution: 10 mg/L	Tablets: 300 mg Capsules: 100 mg Syrup: 50 mg/5 mL IV solution: 10 mg/mL
Number of daily tablets	1–2	1	1	1	1	2
Major drug interactions	None	P-gp inducers and inhibitors	Avoid with strong P-gp inducers	None	None	Inhibitors/inducers of glucuronidation
Common/ significant adverse effects	Rash Possible increased risk of cardiovascular events	Nephrotoxicity (including Fanconi syndrome) Bone mineral density loss	Less likely than tenofovir disoproxil: Nephrotoxicity (including Fanconi syndrome) Bone mineral density loss	Generally well tolerated	Generally well tolerated	Bone marrow suppression (macrocytic anemia, neutropenia) Rash Headache
Other notes	HLA-B*5701 allele must be tested for before starting abacavir because it is contraindicated if present	HBV symptoms can flare upon starting or stopping tenofovir in coinfection	HBV symptoms can flare upon starting or stopping tenofovir in coinfection	HBV symptoms can flare upon starting or stopping emtricitabine in coinfection	HBV symptoms can flare upon starting or stopping lamivudine in coinfection	Used in pregnancy during delivery to prevent maternal-fetal transmission when mother's HIV viral load is >1000 copies/mL

Lamivudine and emtricitabine

Lamivudine (Epivir) and emtricitabine (Emtriva) are analogues of cytosine. Because they have nearly the same structure, except for the addition of a fluorine on emtricitabine, they are essentially interchangeable and should never be used together. Emtricitabine is typically combined with tenofovir disoproxil or tenofovir alafenamide in a combination tablet (Truvada or Descovy, respectively) or in multiple fixed-dose single-tablet regimens with third agents. Lamivudine is often combined with abacavir (Epzicom), but recently branded generic combinations with tenofovir disoproxil (Cimduo, Temyxis) have been approved. Both drugs have activity against hepatitis B virus (HBV) and may be used with tenofovir in a patient with HIV-HBV coinfection; acute exacerbations of HBV can occur when starting or stopping ART containing these medications. Lamivudine and emtricitabine are primarily renally eliminated and require renal dose adjustment, generally when creatinine clearance (CrCl) is less than 50 mL/min; however, emtricitabine may be used at full dose in fixed-dose combination tablets when CrCl is $\geq$30 mL/min.[8-10] In end-stage renal disease (ESRD) on hemodialysis, the recommended lamivudine dose is 25 mg, but doses up to 150 mg have been used in this population without toxicity to avoid splitting tablets or using the liquid formulation.[11]

Tenofovir

Tenofovir is an analogue of adenine. It is available as 2 different prodrugs, tenofovir disoproxil (Viread, TDF) and tenofovir alafenamide (TAF), which are converted to tenofovir diphosphate intracellularly. Tenofovir alafenamide and tenofovir disoproxil are both available coformulated with emtricitabine (Descovy and Truvada, respectively) and in multiple fixed-dose single-tablet regimens. Tenofovir alafenamide achieves higher intracellular tenofovir concentrations, whereas more tenofovir disoproxil remains in serum.[12] The higher serum concentration of TDF likely leads to higher rates of nephrotoxicity and bone mineral density reduction as compared with TAF, although this may be less pronounced when TDF is given without a booster.[13] Concentrations of tenofovir are generally lower in the female genital tract than in the gastrointestinal (GI) tract, suggesting that adherence is crucial for efficacy of pre-exposure prophylaxis (PrEP) in women.[14]

Tenofovir prodrugs rely on P-glycoprotein (P-gp) for absorption; TAF is contraindicated with P-gp inducers, whereas TDF may be used with careful monitoring. Tenofovir exposure is increased with P-gp inhibitors (eg, ritonavir and cobicistat), which is why a lower dose of TAF 10 mg is used in fixed-dose single-tablet regimens containing cobicistat (ie, Genvoya and Symtuza). Tenofovir is primarily eliminated renally through both glomerular filtration and tubular secretion, so concentrations can be increased by drugs that undergo active tubular secretion due to competitive inhibition (eg, acyclovir). Urinalysis to look for proteinuria is used to screen for tenofovir-induced nephrotoxicity, and a low urine albumin to protein ratio is suggestive of tubular injury due to tenofovir. Tenofovir disoproxil is dose adjusted when CrCl is less than 50 mL/min, whereas tenofovir alafenamide can be used safely at full dose when CrCl $\geq$15 mL/min or ESRD on hemodialysis[15] but is generally avoided when CrCl is less than 30 mL/min because it is coformulated with emtricitabine.[16]

Zidovudine

Zidovudine (Retrovir) is an analogue of thymidine. It is the only NRTI available in an intravenous formulation and is also available as a tablet or suspension. Zidovudine is available in a combination tablet with lamivudine (Combivir). Zidovudine is rarely used today because of numerous subjective side effects (headache, nausea, fatigue), and the risk of bone marrow suppression, particularly macrocytic anemia and neutropenia. The most common use in adults is as a continuous intravenous infusion during delivery in pregnant women with HIV viral loads greater than 1000 copies/mL to prevent maternal-to-fetal transmission. It is still occasionally used in pediatric patients, particularly neonates, because other antiretrovirals are not as well studied in this population.[17]

Nonnucleoside Reverse Transcriptase Inhibitors

Nonnucleoside reverse transcriptase inhibitors (NNRTIs) bind to reverse transcriptase at the same allosteric site, causing a conformational change in HIV-1 reverse transcriptase, which reduces its ability to bind to dNTPs.[18] The second-generation NNRTIs were developed to retain activity in the presence of certain high-level resistance mutations to the first-generation NNRTIs (ie, K103N). Some cross-resistance may occur between doravirine and rilpivirine, but etravirine may retain activity depending on the specific mutations. Most NNRTIs can cause rash, which often can be rechallenged, although the older NNRTI nevirapine had a higher risk of Stevens-Johnson syndrome. **Table 3** summarizes their characteristics.

Table 3
Characteristic of nonnucleoside reverse transcriptase inhibitors

	Efavirenz (Sustiva)	Rilpivirine (Edurant)	Doravirine (Pifeltro)
Usual adult dose	600 mg po daily 800 mg po daily with strong 3A4 inducers 300 mg po daily with strong inhibitors	25 mg po daily 25 mg po twice daily with moderate CYP3A4 inducer	100 mg po daily; 100 mg po twice daily with moderate CYP3A4 inducer
Dose adjusted in renal insufficiency?	No	No	No
Fixed-dose combinations	Atripla (w/emtricitabine and tenofovir disoproxil) Symfi/Symfi Lo (w/lamivudine and tenofovir disoproxil)	Complera (w/emtricitabine and tenofovir disoproxil) Odefsey (w/emtricitabine and tenofovir alafenamide)	Delstrigo (w/lamivudine and tenofovir disoproxil)
Dosage forms	Tablets: 600 mg Capsule: 50 mg, 200 mg	Tablets: 25 mg	Tablets: 100 mg
Number of daily tablets	1–3	1–2	1–2
Major drug interactions	CYP3A4 and CYP2B6 substrates, inducers, and inhibitors CYP2C19 substrates	CYP3A4 inducers and inhibitors, acid suppressants	CYP3A4 inducers and inhibitors
Common/ significant adverse effects	CNS effects (insomnia, depression, vivid dreams) Rash	CNS effects (insomnia, depression), less than efavirenz	CNS effects (insomnia, depression), less than efavirenz
Other notes	Should be taken on an empty stomach to minimize adverse effects	Should be taken with food to increase absorption	Can be taken without food

Efavirenz

Efavirenz (Sustiva) is available as both a tablet and a capsule as a 600-mg dose given once daily, but it is most commonly included as a component of the first fixed-dose single-tablet regimen with emtricitabine and tenofovir disoproxil (Atripla). It is also part of the first branded generic single-tablet regimens with tenofovir disoproxil and lamivudine (Symfi and Symfi Lo). The dose of efavirenz in Symfi Lo is 400 mg, which is adequate to maintain viral suppression in treatment-naïve patients with potentially fewer side effects.[19] Efavirenz is an inducer of CYP2B6, an inhibitor of CYP2C9, CYP2C19, and both an inducer and an inhibitor of CYP3A4, so it can have complex effects on substrates of these enzymes. Because it is primarily metabolized by CYP3A4 and CYP2B6, it autoinduces its own metabolism. Adverse effects include new or worsened psychiatric symptoms, central nervous system (CNS) effects such as vivid dreams, and elevations in lipids. Absorption is increased when taken with a meal, which can lead to increased adverse events, so it is recommended to be given on an empty stomach, typically before bed.[20]

Rilpivirine

Rilpivirine (Edurant) is a second-generation NNRTI available as a 25-mg tablet and in fixed-dose single-tablet regimens with emtricitabine and TDF (Complera), emtricitabine and TAF (Odefsey), and dolutegravir (Juluca). Because of an excess risk of virologic failure, rilpivirine should not be used when a patient's CD4 count is less than 200 cells/mm^3 or HIV viral load is greater than 100,000 copies/mL. It is primarily metabolized by CYP3A4, so strong inducers are contraindicated, whereas an increased dose of 25 mg twice daily may be necessary when given with moderate inducers (eg, rifabutin). It can cause minimal QT prolongation of approximately 2 milliseconds. Because rilpivirine requires an acidic pH for absorption, concomitant proton pump inhibitor (PPI) use is contraindicated; it should be given at the same time or 12 hours after histamine 2 receptor antagonists (H2RAs) and 4 hours before or 2 hours after antacids. It should be taken with food to increase absorption.[21]

Doravirine

Doravirine (Pifeltro) is the newest second-generation NNRTI. It is given as a 100-mg tablet once daily and is also part of a fixed-dose single-tablet regimen with lamivudine and tenofovir disoproxil (Delstrigo). It is metabolized primarily through CYP3A4, so it should not be coadministered with strong inducers of this enzyme and should be given twice daily with moderate inducers such as rifabutin. It can be given without food.[22]

INTEGRASE INHIBITORS

The integrase strand transfer inhibitors (INSTIs) bind to a magnesium moiety on the integrase enzyme, preventing insertion of the viral DNA (provirus) into the cellular DNA. The site that binds magnesium can be chelated by polyvalent cations (eg, calcium, aluminum, zinc, iron), which reduces absorption, so integrase inhibitors should generally be given 2 hours before or 6 hours after medicines containing polyvalent cations (eg, antacids, supplements). This chelation may be reduced when both are taken with food, however.[23] The first-generation INSTIs have a low barrier to resistance, but the second-generation INSTIs are considered to have a relatively high barrier to resistance, requiring several point mutations to confer resistance. Although resistance is uncommon, cross-resistance between the INSTIs is a concern. Integrase inhibitors have also been associated with increased weight gain compared with other antiretrovirals.[24,25] **Table 4** summarizes their characteristics.

Table 4
Characteristics of integrase inhibitors

	Raltegravir (Isentress)	Elvitegravir	Dolutegravir (Tivicay)	Bictegravir
Usual adult dose	1200 mg po daily 400 mg po twice daily	150 mg po daily	50 mg po daily 50 mg po twice daily with certain resistance mutations	200 mg po daily
Dose adjusted in renal insufficiency?	No	No; however it should not be started if CrCl <70 mL/min when coformulated with tenofovir disoproxil or <30 mL/min when coformulated with tenofovir alafenamide	No	No; however it is avoided when CrCl <30 mL/min because it is only available coformulated with emtricitabine and tenofovir alafenamide
Fixed-dose combinations	No	Stribild (w/emtricitabine, tenofovir disoproxil, and cobicistat) Genvoya (w/emtricitabine, tenofovir alafenamide, and cobicistat)	Triumeq (w/lamivudine and abacavir)	Biktarvy (w/emtricitabine and bictegravir)
Dosage forms	Tablets: 400 mg, 600 mg Chewable tablets: 25 mg, 100 mg Powder: 100 mg/packet	Not available separately	Tablets: 10 mg, 25 mg, 50 mg	Not available separately
Number of daily tablets	2	1	1–2	1
Major drug interactions	UGT inducers Polyvalent cations	CYP3A4 inducers Polyvalent cations	CYP3A4 and UGT inducers Polyvalent cations	CYP3A4 and UGT inducers Polyvalent cations
Common/significant adverse effects	Creatine kinase elevations	GI upset	Headache, insomnia	Headache GI upset
Other notes	May cause weight gain	Should be taken with food to increase absorption May cause weight gain	May cause weight gain Can cause benign elevations in serum creatinine	May cause weight gain Can cause benign elevations in serum creatinine

Raltegravir

Raltegravir was the first INSTI approved by the FDA. It is available as a 400-mg tablet (Isentress), which is given as 1 tablet twice daily, and a 600-mg tablet (Isentress HD), which is given as 2 tablets once daily. It is not metabolized by CYP enzymes but instead undergoes glucuronidation by uridine diphosphate glucuronosyltransferase (UGT)1A1, so a higher dose of 800 mg twice daily may be necessary with strong inducers of this enzyme (eg, rifampin). It can cause increased creatine kinase levels, but myopathy and rhabdomyolysis are rare.[26] Raltegravir has become less commonly used because of the lower barrier to resistance and higher pill burden (at least 3 tablets for a complete regimen) compared with other antiretroviral regimens. It remains a first-line option in the US Department of Health and Human Services (DHHS) guidelines, particularly in women who are pregnant or want to become pregnant, because of its favorable tolerability and lack of reported adverse effects on pregnancy outcomes.[1]

Elvitegravir

Elvitegravir is a first-generation INSTI that is only available in fixed-dose combinations with cobicistat, emtricitabine, and tenofovir disoproxil (Stribild) or with cobicistat, emtricitabine, and tenofovir alafenamide (Genvoya). It is primarily metabolized through CYP3A4 and requires boosting to achieve adequate serum levels for once-daily dosing. Because it must be boosted, it has many significant drug interactions and cannot be given with any strong inducers. It was used frequently when it was the only single-tablet regimen containing an integrase inhibitor with a tenofovir-based backbone, but its role has largely been supplanted by bictegravir. The most common adverse effects are GI (nausea, vomiting, and diarrhea).[27]

Dolutegravir

Dolutegravir (Tivicay) is a second-generation INSTI available in a 50-mg tablet for adults and 10- and 25-mg tablets for pediatric patients as well as in fixed-dose single-tablet regimens with abacavir and lamivudine (Triumeq), rilpivirine (Juluca), or lamivudine (Dovato). Dolutegravir is metabolized primarily by glucuronidation through UGT1A1 and partially by CYP3A4. It may need to be dosed twice daily with strong inducers of these enzymes (eg, rifampin, carbamazepine). Dolutegravir is an inhibitor of the organic cation transporter 2 (OCT2) and multidrug and toxin extrusion transporter 1 (MATE1), which leads to inhibition of tubular secretion of creatinine, which causes benign increases in serum creatinine. Inhibition of OCT2 and MATE1 also can increase concentrations of drugs eliminated via these pathways (eg, metformin), which may require dose reductions of the affected drugs. Dolutegravir has been associated with headaches and insomnia, which may lessen over time.[28] A recent study of dolutegravir in pregnant women in Botswana suggested a possible increased risk of neural tube defects when dolutegravir was used at the time of conception, so the DHHS guidelines currently recommend avoiding dolutegravir in women in the first trimester of pregnancy and in those of childbearing age who are planning to become pregnant or not using effective contraception.[1] However, it is still safe and effective in women in the second or third trimester, and it will be important to follow up on the final results of this study to determine whether this is a true effect. It is also important to note that this warning does not yet apply to other INSTIs, reflecting a lack of comprehensive data on their safety.

Bictegravir

Bictegravir is a second-generation INSTI and is currently only available in a fixed-dose single-tablet regimen with emtricitabine and tenofovir alafenamide (Biktarvy). Like dolutegravir, it is primarily metabolized through UGT1A1 and partially through CYP3A4 and inhibits both OCT2 and MATE1, so it also causes a benign increase in serum creatinine. Given the similar metabolism and inhibition, the drug interactions with bictegravir are very similar to those of dolutegravir. Two notable differences are the interactions of the 2 INSTIs with metformin and the rifamycins. Metformin does not require empiric dose adjustments when given with bictegravir because concentrations are increased to a lesser extent than by dolutegravir; conversely, rifampin and rifabutin metabolize bictegravir to a greater degree, leading to the recommendation that coadministration should be avoided. It can be taken without respect to food and has one of the smallest tablet sizes of all full-regimen ART options. Bictegravir's high barrier to resistance, availability as a single-tablet regimen with the most effective backbone (TAF and emtricitabine), and limited drug interactions have made it a commonly chosen option for first-line therapy.[10]

Cabotegravir

Cabotegravir is an investigational drug currently in phase 3 trials with an oral lead in with a 2-NRTI backbone followed by transition after viral suppression to an intramuscular (IM) injection of cabotegravir and rilpivirine every 4 weeks.[29] It is also being studied in treatment-experienced patients who are virally suppressed with 4-week oral cabotegravir and rilpivirine lead in followed by a transition to the IM injection every 4 weeks. The IM injection acts as a depot, slowly releasing the drug over the month to maintain adequate serum levels. Because of its long-acting activity, IM cabotegravir is also being evaluated for use in PrEP.[30] Cabotegravir is primarily metabolized by glucuronidation through UGT1A1 and UGT1A9 and is an inhibitor of organic anion transporter 1 (OAT1) and OAT3.[31,32] It is a promising alternative to daily oral antiretrovirals because it reduces concerns for nonadherence, although 1 limitation is that it would require monthly visits for injection, and mild to moderate injection site reactions were common.

PROTEASE INHIBITORS

Protease inhibitors (PIs) bind to protease and prevent cleavage of Gag-Pol polyproteins in infected cells, which prevents maturation of viral particles.[33] The PIs have more metabolic effects than other antiretrovirals, with the older PIs causing insulin resistance and hyperlipidemia, although these side effects are less common or less severe with the newer agents. GI side effects are also very common with the PIs, resulting in more discontinuation than with other agents. **Table 5** summarizes their characteristics.

Atazanavir

Atazanavir (Reyataz) is available as a 300-mg capsule, which is used with ritonavir and as a tablet coformulated with cobicistat (Evotaz). Atazanavir also has an FDA-approved unboosted dose of 400 mg, but this is not recommended by the DHHS guidelines for most patients because treatment failure with resistance may occur. Tenofovir disoproxil can decrease atazanavir concentrations, but it is not clear that this same effect occurs with tenofovir alafenamide. Atazanavir increases tenofovir concentrations, which may increase nephrotoxicity; in addition, atazanavir can crystallize in the urine, which may lead to nephrolithiasis and interstitial nephritis. The incidence of renal impairment increases with duration of use of atazanavir.[34] Like rilpivirine, atazanavir requires an acidic environment for absorption, so it should be coadministered or given 12 hours after H2RAs with a maximum dose equivalent to famotidine 40 mg twice daily in treatment-naïve patients or 20 mg twice daily in

Table 5 Characteristics of protease inhibitors		
	Atazanavir (Reyataz)	Darunavir (Prezista)
Usual adult dose	300 mg po daily with booster 400 mg po daily unboosted	800 mg po daily with booster 600 mg po twice daily with booster with certain resistance mutations or in pregnancy
Dose adjusted in renal insufficiency?	No	No
Fixed-dose combinations	Evotaz (w/cobicistat)	Prezcobix (w/cobicistat) Symtuza (w/emtricitabine, tenofovir alafenamide, and cobicistat)
Dosage forms	Capsules: 150 mg, 200 mg, 300 mg Powder: 50 mg/packet	Tablets: 150 mg, 200 mg, 250 mg, 300 mg Powder: 40 mg/g
Number of daily tablets	1	1–2
Major drug interactions	CYP3A4 inducers	CYP3A4 inducers
Common/significant adverse effects	GI upset Hyperbilirubinemia (indirect, asymptomatic) Dyslipidemia Nephrolithiasis	GI upset Rash Dyslipidemia
Other notes	Hyperbilirubinemia may be cardioprotective, but may also cause discontinuation for cosmetic reasons (jaundice)	Has very high barrier to resistance and is often active in the presence of multiple PI mutations

treatment-experienced patients and should also be separated from antacids by 2 hours before or 1 hour after. Atazanavir should only be used with PPIs in treatment-naïve patients at a maximum of omeprazole 20 mg or equivalent per day, and PPIs should be avoided in treatment-experienced patients. Atazanavir is an inhibitor of CYP3A4 and UGT1A1 and a weak inhibitor of CYP2C8. It can increase indirect bilirubin levels through inhibition of UGT, leading to hyperbilirubinemia and, in some cases, jaundice. Although this may be disturbing cosmetically to some patients, bilirubin functions as an antioxidant and may account for the observation that this PI does not appear to increase cardiovascular risk.[33,35]

Darunavir

Darunavir (Prezista) is the most recently approved PI and is available as an 800-mg tablet given once daily with ritonavir or a 600-mg tablet given twice daily with ritonavir when certain PI resistance mutations are present. It is also coformulated with cobicistat (Prezcobix) or in a fixed-dose single-tablet regimen with cobicistat, emtricitabine, and tenofovir alafenamide (Symtuza) for once-daily use. Darunavir has a sulfonamide moiety so should be used with caution in patients with sulfa allergies; however, the incidence and severity of rash were similar between those with and without an allergy in the clinical trials, so practically, patients may receive darunavir with a history of a sulfa allergy if the adverse reaction was not life threatening. Darunavir is an inhibitor of CYP3A4, CYP2D6, and P-gp and is a substrate of CYP3A4 and P-gp. It should generally be given with food to increase absorption and minimize GI side effects. Darunavir has a high barrier to resistance, requiring multiple point mutations to select for resistance; in addition, it retains activity against many viral isolates with extensive PI resistance.[36]

BOOSTERS

The pharmacokinetic boosters are used to increase concentrations of elvitegravir and the PIs because of their inhibition of CYP3A4. They also increase concentrations of tenofovir because of inhibition of P-gp, so lower doses of TAF are used in fixed-dose single-tablet regimens containing cobicistat. **Table 6** summarizes their characteristics.

Ritonavir

Ritonavir (Norvir) was originally developed as a PI, but because of adverse effects (primarily GI) when given at therapeutic doses, it is no longer used as an antiretroviral. Because of its inhibition of CYP3A4 at lower doses (100–200 mg/daily), it was used as a booster for other PIs. In addition to CYP3A4, it also inhibits CYP2D6 and induces CYP1A2, CYP2C9, CYP2C19, CYP2B6, and UGT. Because of the mixed inhibition and induction, ritonavir has multiple complex drug interactions. Ritonavir is difficult to coformulate with other antiretrovirals because of its size, so it is generally given separately as a 100-mg tablet.[37]

Cobicistat

Cobicistat was developed specifically to be used as a pharmacokinetic booster with no antiretroviral activity. It is available as a 150-mg tablet (Tybost) and is also

Table 6
Characteristics of pharmacokinetic boosters

	Ritonavir (Norvir)	Cobicistat (Tybost)
Usual adult dose	100 mg po daily 100 mg po twice daily when used with twice-daily darunavir	150 mg po daily
Dose adjusted in renal insufficiency?	No	No
Fixed-dose combinations	Kaletra (w/lopinavir)	Evotaz (w/atazanavir) Prezcobix (w/darunavir) Stribild (w/emtricitabine, tenofovir disoproxil, and elvitegravir) Genvoya (w/emtricitabine, tenofovir alafenamide, and elvitegravir) Symtuza (w/emtricitabine, tenofovir alafenamide, and darunavir)
Dosage forms	Tablets: 100 mg Solution: 80 mg/mL Powder: 100 mg/packet	Tablets: 150 mg
Number of daily tablets/injections	1–2	1
Major drug interactions	Multiple CYP substrates	CYP3A4 and CYP2D6 substrates
Common/significant adverse effects	GI upset	Benign increase in serum creatinine
Other notes	Should be taken with food to improve tolerability	Not interchangeable with ritonavir when higher exposures needed (pregnancy, twice-daily darunavir)

coformulated with atazanavir (Evotaz) and darunavir (Prezcobix) as well as in fixed-dose single-tablet regimens with elvitegravir (Stribild and Genvoya) or darunavir (Symtuza). Cobicistat does not increase levels of darunavir or atazanavir as much as ritonavir does, so it is not interchangeable and should not be used when higher doses are needed (eg, in pregnancy or when twice-daily darunavir is used for resistance mutations). It inhibits CYP3A4, CYP2D6, P-gp, BCRP, OATP1B1, and OATP1B3, so it can significantly increase concentrations of drugs that are substrates of these enzymes. It also inhibits tubular secretion of serum creatinine, so it can cause benign increases without actually affecting the glomerular filtration rate.[38]

ENTRY INHIBITORS

The entry inhibitors are more of a group than a class because the 3 agents each have different mechanisms of action. They are often reserved for patients with multiple drug resistance mutations to other classes because of lower efficacy or administration challenges (eg, higher pill burden or parenteral formulation). **Table 7** summarizes their characteristics.

Postattachment Inhibitors

The only postattachment inhibitor currently approved by the FDA is ibalizumab (Trogarzo). It is a humanized monoclonal antibody that binds to domain 2 of CD4, which blocks HIV from fusing with the host cell without impairing CD4-mediated immune function. Ibalizumab is administered intravenously as a loading dose of 2000 mg

Table 7
Characteristics of entry inhibitors

	Ibalizumab (Trogarzo)	Maraviroc (Selzentry)	Enfuvirtide (Fuzeon)
Usual adult dose	2000 mg intravenously loading dose followed by 800 mg intravenously every 2 wk	300 mg po twice daily; 150 mg po twice daily with strong CYP3A4 inhibitor; 600 mg po twice daily with strong CYP3A4 inducer	90 mg subcutaneously twice daily
Dose adjusted in renal insufficiency?	No	Only if orthostatic hypotension	No
Dosage forms	150 mg/mL (200 mg per vial)	Tablets: 25 mg, 75 mg, 150 mg, 300 mg Solution: 20 mg/mL	90 mg/vial
Number of daily tablets/injections	1 every other week	2–4	2
Major drug interactions	None	CYP3A4 inhibitors and inducers	None
Common/significant adverse effects	Possible hypersensitivity reactions	Orthostatic hypotension (renal insufficiency)	Injection site reactions
Other notes	Must be diluted in 250 mL of normal saline Restart loading dose if more than 3 d late for maintenance dose	Viral tropism test must be done before starting: can only be used with CCR5-tropic virus	May be given intravenously

followed by 800 mg every 2 weeks, which achieves steady state after the first 800-mg maintenance dose (see **Table 2**). Ibalizumab must be diluted in 250 mL of normal saline and is only stable for 4 hours at room temperature and 24 hours refrigerated and therefore should be administered at a medical office or infusion clinic. As with other monoclonal antibodies, there is a chance for infusion-related reactions; for this reason, the loading dose should be administered over at least 30 minutes, and patients should be observed for at least 1 hour after the initial dose. If no reactions occur, future maintenance doses can be shortened to a 15-minute infusion followed by a 15-minute observation period. However, if the maintenance dose is delayed by 3 or more days, a loading dose of 2000 mg should be administered as soon as possible before returning to maintenance dosing. Because of the challenges of administration and timing and less clinical experience with ibalizumab than with other classes of medications, it is reserved for patients with multidrug-resistant HIV who have failed other regimens. One advantage, however, is that the mechanism and target of ibalizumab mean that it is not expected to have any significant drug-drug interactions. In addition, it should be used in combination with other antiretrovirals to prevent the emergence of drug resistance.[39]

CCR5 Antagonists

Maraviroc (Selzentry) is the only CCR5 antagonist FDA approved for treatment of HIV. It binds to the chemokine coreceptor CCR5 on the surface of $CD4^+$ cells, preventing the HIV surface protein gp120 from interacting with the coreceptor. HIV can use CCR5, CXCR4, or both (dual-tropic) as coreceptors, so tropism testing of the patient's virus must be done before initiation of maraviroc because it is not effective for CXCR4- or dual-tropic virus. Maraviroc has high bioavailability, with full absorption occurring within 4 hours, and is typically given as 300-mg twice-daily dosing to maintain adequate trough concentrations to fully suppress viral replication. In 1 study of maraviroc, patients with higher trough concentrations were more likely to have viral suppression at 48 weeks with 57% suppressed in the lowest quartile versus 84% in the highest quartile. Of those in the lowest quartile, 24% had undetectable concentrations for at least 1 measurement, whereas only 1 patient in the highest quartile had at least 1 undetectable level. This association between trough concentrations and viral suppression demonstrates the importance of adherence and significant effect that missed doses can have on efficacy.[40]

Maraviroc is primarily eliminated hepatically by CYP3A4 to an inactive metabolite, and therefore, a higher dose of 600 mg twice daily is used when taken with strong inducers (eg, rifampin), whereas a reduced dose of 150 mg twice daily is used when taken with strong inhibitors (eg, ritonavir) of this isoenzyme. Approximately 20% of maraviroc is eliminated renally, which results in higher exposures in patients with severe renal dysfunction (CrCl <30 mL/min) or ESRD. Despite this higher exposure, no dose adjustment is needed unless patients with CrCl less than 30 mL/min experience postural hypotension on 300 mg twice daily (ie, not taking any strong CYP3A4 inducers or inhibitors), in which case the dose should be lowered to 150 mg twice daily.[40]

Fusion Inhibitors

The only fusion inhibitor currently approved by the FDA for treatment of HIV is enfuvirtide (Fuzeon), which works by binding to the gp41 subunit of the HIV-1 viral envelope protein to prevent conformational changes, which inhibits fusion of the viral and CD4 cell membranes. Enfuvirtide is administered as a subcutaneous injection of 90 mg twice daily, which commonly results in injection site reactions, which can be painful and occasionally result in induration or nodules.[41] For patients unable to tolerate the injection site reactions, intravenous infusion of enfuvirtide may be an option.[42] The drug has also been associated with an increased risk of bacterial pneumonia, although the mechanism of this is unclear. Enfuvirtide is not a substrate, inducer, or inhibitor of CYP enzymes and does not have any significant drug-drug interactions. As a peptide, it is expected to be metabolized to its component amino acids, so it does not require any dose adjustments for renal or hepatic function.[41]

SUMMARY

Antiretrovirals have dramatically improved survival and the quality of life of people with HIV. Current antiretroviral therapies are generally well tolerated with manageable adverse effects and low pill burdens. Understanding the dosage forms, adverse effects, and drug interactions of antiretrovirals allows clinicians to choose the most appropriate regimen for their patient.

REFERENCES

1. Panel on Antiretroviral Guidelines for Adults and Adolescents. Guidelines for the use of antiretroviral agents in adults and adolescents living with HIV. Department of Health and Human Services; 2018. Available at: https://aidsinfo.nih.gov/contentfiles/lvguidelines/adultandadolescentgl.pdf.
2. University of Liverpool. HIV drug interactions. 2019. Available at: https://hiv-druginteractions.org/. Accessed March 29, 2019.
3. Food and Drug Administration. Ziagen (product label). 2018. Available at: https://www.accessdata.fda.gov/drugsatfda_docs/label/2018/020977s033s034,020978s036s037lbl.pdf. Accessed March 29, 2019.
4. Elion RA, Althoff KN, Zhang J, et al. Recent Abacavir use increases risk of type 1 and type 2 myocardial infarctions among adults with HIV. J Acquir Immune Defic Syndr 2018;78(1):62–72.
5. Nan C, Shaefer M, Urbaityte R, et al. Abacavir use and risk for myocardial infarction and cardiovascular events: pooled analysis of data from clinical trials. Open Forum Infect Dis 2018;5(5):ofy086.
6. Taylor KA, Smyth E, Rauzi F, et al. Pharmacological impact of antiretroviral therapy on platelet function to investigate human immunodeficiency virus-associated cardiovascular risk. Br J Pharmacol 2019;176(7):879–89.
7. Kim PS, Woods C, Georgoff P, et al. A1C underestimates glycemia in HIV infection. Diabetes Care 2009;32(9):1591–3.
8. Food and Drug Administration. Emtriva (product label). 2018. Available at: https://www.accessdata.fda.gov/drugsatfda_docs/label/2018/021500s029lbl.pdf. Accessed March 29, 2019.
9. Food and Drug Administration. Epivir (product label). 2018. Available at: https://www.accessdata.fda.gov/drugsatfda_docs/label/2018/020564s038,020596s037lbl.pdf. Accessed March 29, 2019.
10. Food and Drug Administration. Biktarvy (product label). 2018. Available at: https://www.accessdata.fda.gov/drugsatfda_docs/label/2018/210251s000lbl.pdf. Accessed March 29, 2019.
11. Fischetti B, Shah K, Taft DR, et al. Real-world experience with higher-than-recommended doses of Lamivudine in patients with varying degrees of renal impairment. Open Forum Infect Dis 2018;5(10):ofy225.
12. Podany AT, Bares SH, Havens J, et al. Plasma and intracellular pharmacokinetics of tenofovir in patients switched from tenofovir disoproxil fumarate to tenofovir alafenamide. AIDS 2018;32(6):761–5.

13. Hill A, Hughes SL, Gotham D, et al. Tenofovir alafenamide versus tenofovir disoproxil fumarate: is there a true difference in efficacy and safety? J Virus Erad 2018;4(2):72–9.

14. Cottrell ML, Yang KH, Prince HM, et al. A translational pharmacology approach to predicting outcomes of preexposure prophylaxis against HIV in men and women using tenofovir disoproxil fumarate with or without emtricitabine. J Infect Dis 2016; 214(1):55–64.

15. Food and Drug Administration. Vemlidy (product label). 2019. Available at: https://www.accessdata.fda.gov/drugsatfda_docs/label/2019/208464s007lbl.pdf. Accessed March 29, 2019.

16. Food and Drug Administration. Viread (product label). 2018. Available at: https://www.accessdata.fda.gov/drugsatfda_docs/label/2018/021356s057,022577s013 lbl.pdf. Accessed March 29, 2019.

17. Food and Drug Administration. Retrovir (product label). 2018. Available at: https://www.accessdata.fda.gov/drugsatfda_docs/label/2018/019655s058,019910 s045,019951s036lbl.pdf. Accessed March 29, 2019.

18. Schauer GD, Huber KD, Leuba SH, et al. Mechanism of allosteric inhibition of HIV-1 reverse transcriptase revealed by single-molecule and ensemble fluorescence. Nucleic Acids Res 2014;42(18):11687–96.

19. ENCORE1 Study Group. Efficacy of 400 mg efavirenz versus standard 600 mg dose in HIV-infected, antiretroviral-naive adults (ENCORE1): a randomised, double-blind, placebo-controlled, non-inferiority trial. Lancet 2014;383(9927): 1474–82.

20. Food and Drug Administration. Sustiva (product label). 2017. Available at: https://www.accessdata.fda.gov/drugsatfda_docs/label/2017/021360s044,020972s056 lbl.pdf. Accessed March 29, 2019.

21. Food and Drug Administration. Edurant (product label). 2018. Available at: https://www.accessdata.fda.gov/drugsatfda_docs/label/2018/202022s011lbl.pdf. Accessed March 29, 2019.

22. Food and Drug Administration. Pifeltro (product label). 2018. Available at: https://www.accessdata.fda.gov/drugsatfda_docs/label/2018/210806s000lbl.pdf. Accessed March 29, 2019.

23. Song I, Borland J, Arya N, et al. Pharmacokinetics of dolutegravir when administered with mineral supplements in healthy adult subjects. J Clin Pharmacol 2015; 55(5):490–6.

24. Menard A, Meddeb L, Tissot-Dupont H, et al. Dolutegravir and weight gain: an unexpected bothering side effect? AIDS 2017;31(10):1499–500.

25. Norwood J, Turner M, Bofill C, et al. Brief report: weight gain in persons with HIV switched from Efavirenz-based to integrase strand transfer inhibitor-based regimens. J Acquir Immune Defic Syndr 2017;76(5):527–31.

26. Food and Drug Administration. Isentress (product label). 2018. Available at: https://www.accessdata.fda.gov/drugsatfda_docs/label/2018/022145s038,205 786s007,0203045s015lbl.pdf. Accessed March 29, 2019.

27. Food and Drug Administration. Genvoya (product label). 2019. Available at: https://www.accessdata.fda.gov/drugsatfda_docs/label/2019/207561s023lbl.pdf. Accessed March 29, 2019.

28. Food and Drug Administration. Tivicay (product label). 2018. Available at: https://www.accessdata.fda.gov/drugsatfda_docs/label/2018/204790s016s018lbl.pdf. Accessed March 29, 2019.

29. Margolis DA, Gonzalez-Garcia J, Stellbrink HJ, et al. Long-acting intramuscular cabotegravir and rilpivirine in adults with HIV-1 infection (LATTE-2): 96-week

results of a randomised, open-label, phase 2b, non-inferiority trial. Lancet 2017; 390(10101):1499–510.

30. Markowitz M, Frank I, Grant RM, et al. Safety and tolerability of long-acting cabotegravir injections in HIV-uninfected men (ECLAIR): a multicentre, double-blind, randomised, placebo-controlled, phase 2a trial. Lancet HIV 2017;4(8):e331–40.

31. Bowers GD, Culp A, Reese MJ, et al. Disposition and metabolism of cabotegravir: a comparison of biotransformation and excretion between different species and routes of administration in humans. Xenobiotica 2016;46(2):147–62.

32. Reese MJ, Bowers GD, Humphreys JE, et al. Drug interaction profile of the HIV integrase inhibitor cabotegravir: assessment from in vitro studies and a clinical investigation with midazolam. Xenobiotica 2016;46(5):445–56.

33. Food and Drug Administration. Reyataz (product label). 2018. Available at: https://www.accessdata.fda.gov/drugsatfda_docs/label/2018/021567s042,206 352s007lbl.pdf. Accessed March 29, 2019.

34. Mocroft A, Lundgren JD, Ross M, et al. Cumulative and current exposure to potentially nephrotoxic antiretrovirals and development of chronic kidney disease in HIV-positive individuals with a normal baseline estimated glomerular filtration rate: a prospective international cohort study. Lancet HIV 2016;3(1):e23–32.

35. Dekker D, Dorresteijn MJ, Pijnenburg M, et al. The bilirubin-increasing drug atazanavir improves endothelial function in patients with type 2 diabetes mellitus. Arterioscler Thromb Vasc Biol 2011;31(2):458–63.

36. Food and Drug Administration. Prezista (product label). 2019. Available at: https://www.accessdata.fda.gov/drugsatfda_docs/label/2019/021976s053,202 895s024lbl.pdf. Accessed March 29, 2019.

37. Food and Drug Administration. Norvir (product label). 2018. Available at: https://www.accessdata.fda.gov/drugsatfda_docs/label/2018/022417s021lbl.pdf. Accessed March 29, 2019.

38. Food and Drug Administration. Tybost (product label). 2018. Available at: https://www.accessdata.fda.gov/drugsatfda_docs/label/2018/203094s012lbl.pdf. Accessed March 29, 2019.

39. Food and Drug Administration. Trogarzo (product label). 2018. Available at: https://www.accessdata.fda.gov/drugsatfda_docs/label/2018/761065lbl.pdf. Accessed March 29, 2019.

40. Food and Drug Administration. Selzentry (product label). 2018. Available at: https://www.accessdata.fda.gov/drugsatfda_docs/label/2018/022128s018,208 984s001lbl.pdf. Accessed March 29, 2019.

41. Food and Drug Administration. Fuzeon (product label). 2018. Available at: https://www.accessdata.fda.gov/drugsatfda_docs/label/2018/021481s032lbl.pdf. Accessed March 29, 2019.

42. Neijzen RW, Van Maarseveen EM, Hoepelman AI, et al. Continuous intravenous infusion of enfuvirtide in a patient with a multidrug-resistant HIV strain. Int J Clin Pharm 2016;38(4):749–51.

How Big Data Science Can Improve Linkage and Retention in Care

Aadia I. Rana, MD*, Michael J. Mugavero, MD

KEYWORDS

• HIV • AIDS • Prevention • Treatment • Continuum • Data • Surveillance

KEY POINTS

- "Ending the HIV Epidemic: A Plan for America" is predicated on using data to inform prevention, treatment, and care at the local level aligned with strategies to diagnose, treat, protect, and respond.
- Big data science holds potential to advance utilization of existing data systems and novel data platforms to address gaps in the understanding of human immunodeficiency virus (HIV) transmission risks, social networks, and progress across a status-neutral HIV prevention and care continuum.
- Current gaps in big data system infrastructure and qualified personnel as well as ethical considerations must be addressed to maximize the potential of big data approaches toward actionable HIV testing, prevention, and treatment initiatives.

INTRODUCTION

With the "Ending the HIV Epidemic: A Plan for America" (EtHE), the US Department of Health and Human Services (DHHS) proposes ambitious goals for reductions in new human immunodeficiency virus (HIV) infections by 75% in 5 years and at least a 90% reduction by 2030. The initiative calls for unparalleled coordination across DHHS agencies, with a targeting of resources to the 48 highest burden counties; Washington, DC; San Juan, Puerto Rico; and the 7 states with substantial rural HIV burden.[1] The plan is centered on 3 major areas of action, among them the use of data to inform prevention, care, and treatment at the local level, aligned with 4 key strategies—diagnose, treat, protect, and respond—and a commitment to establish local teams, referred to as the HIV HealthForce, committed to the success of the

Disclosure Statement: Dr. Rana was supported to complete this work though a career developmental grant from the National Institute of Mental Health (K23MH100955).
Department of Medicine, Division of Infectious Diseases, University of Alabama at Birmingham School of Medicine, 845 19th Street South BBRB 206, Birmingham, AL 35205, USA
* Corresponding author.
E-mail address: airana@uabmc.edu

Infect Dis Clin N Am 33 (2019) 807–815
https://doi.org/10.1016/j.idc.2019.05.009
0891-5520/19/© 2019 Elsevier Inc. All rights reserved.

initiative. A status-neutral continuum of HIV prevention and care provides an over-arching framework on which to situate the EtHE strategies, with HIV testing (diagnose) as the gateway for the treat, protect, and respond components of the initiative (**Fig. 1**).[2] Beyond tracking and monitoring the success of the EtHE initiative, data per-taining to all 4 strategies are imperative to inform programs and clinical, community, and public health action in providing testing, prevention, treatment, and care services. To this end, there are opportunities to utilize data already captured via existing sys-tems in new ways as well as the potential to harness novel sources of big data toward achieving the ambitious EtHE goals.

Advancements in biomedical research for both treatment and prevention of HIV illu-minate a path to the end of the epidemic: well-tolerated, fixed-dose combination ther-apy taken once daily,[3] clinical trials clearly indicating that immediate treatment benefits individuals with HIV[4] and minimizes transmission,[5,6] and the use of pre-exposure prophylaxis (PrEP)—a single pill containing 2 anti-HIV drugs that can reduce an individual's risk of contracting HIV by more than 90%.[7] Yet, among the 1.2 million people estimated to be living with HIV (PLWH) in the United States, almost 15% remain unaware of their diagnosis and barely half achieve viral suppression (VS), the goal necessary to ensure optimal individual and public health outcomes.[8] Additionally, PrEP as a prevention strategy is vastly underutilized. The Centers for Disease Control and Prevention estimate that more than 1.2 million people in the United States are at substantial risk of HIV infection and could benefit from PrEP; however, less than 5% of these people are taking it. Moreover, only one-third of primary care doctors and nurses are unaware of PrEP and its potential health advantages.[9] To target services and funding accordingly, there is a need to identify more precisely who, where, when, and how new HIV infections are being transmitted and to better characterize those PLWH who are not linked to care, engaged in prevention and treatment ser-vices, or virally suppressed.

As large data sets are becoming increasingly available to the research community, new opportunities to analyze and intervene on the health care indicators are emerging.[10–12] Big data science (BDS) specifically refers to research that capitalizes on the increased analytical speed, data storage capacity, and liquidity of large amounts of diverse data from health, genomics, environment, social media, and com-mercial activities. Data sources are characterized by their high volume and variety, and the field is developing approaches to capture, manage, organize, harmonize, and analyze them. BDS technologies, computing, informatics, and analytics may allow

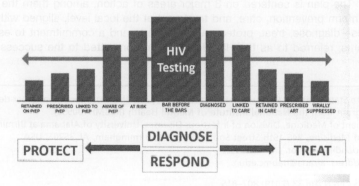

Fig. 1. Status-neutral continuum of HIV prevention and care as a framework to situate the diagnose, treat, protect, and respond strategies articulated in the EtHE.

addressing gaps in the understanding of HIV transmission risks, social networks, and the status-neutral HIV prevention and treatment continuum of care.[13,14] More broadly, BDS, by providing this level of precision, could allow programmatic activities to hone in on a clearly defined subgroup and locality with the most effective interventions until HIV incidence is driven to zero.

   BDS can provide insight into actionable approaches to improve HIV prevention and treatment. Its ability to elucidate associations not seen in less diverse data sets and the potential scalability of BDS compared wih traditional study designs and data sets may promote the discovery of transformative approaches in HIV prevention, treatment, and long-term outcomes. BDS research also may be able to shed light on behaviors that occur outside of venues surveyed by health professionals or the reporting of behaviors that are significantly modified in the presence of others (ie, social desirability bias) and thus are difficult to document. Along with the potential advances with BDS research and discovery, however, there also are ethical considerations. Research that seeks to identify rare, unseen, or perhaps transient events, networks, risks, and health-seeking behaviors as they pertain to HIV will fundamentally improve the quality of the inferences but may risk a loss of privacy or confidentiality. The BDS approach also may increase the potential that the ongoing social, structural, and other challenges faced by people affected by HIV and AIDS, such as stigma, are obscured from view.

PREVENTION

Between 2010 and 2016, HIV incidence in the United States declined 17% among heterosexuals and 30% among injecting drug users; yet, new infections continue to increase in men of color who have sex with men and bisexuals, with the biggest burden in the Southern United States.[15,16] Furthermore, challenging prevention efforts is the reality that HIV infection is concentrated in subpopulations at high risk. Prevention and HIV health care messaging that are directed at the broader demographic group may fail to reach high-risk subgroups, stalling efforts to reduce the rate of HIV transmission in the United States. The gaps in identifying those at greatest risk and vulnerability to HIV point to a need for innovative strategies to improve and tailor HIV prevention efforts. BDS may provide the ability to characterize social, behavioral, and contextual life courses of events and decisions that put individual people at risk for HIV acquisition using the linkage, modeling, and iterative processing of social media,[17,18] pharmaceutical or commercial data, or clinical data, including deidentified laboratory test results.

   Research on analysis of social media big data for HIV epidemiologic monitoring and prevention interventions seems promising. After filtering tweets for HIV risk-related keywords and phrases suggesting the occurrence of present or future HIV risk (eg, sexual behaviors and drug use behaviors), researchers found a high correlation between the geography of county-level HIV-related tweets and actual Centers for Disease Control and Prevention (CDC)-reported HIV cases.[19] Another study utilized Google search data from 2007 to 2014 to develop a model to predict HIV cases using a subset of significant predictor keywords entered into the searches across the United States. Combined with state-level HIV case reports provided by the CDC, this method was able to train a model to predict the number of new HIV diagnoses by state from 2011 to 2014.[18] Social media data have also aided researchers in assessing the utilization of HIV prevention interventions. After analyzing free-text posts from an online community focused on HIV prevention, 1 study found that individuals who posted about HIV prevention and testing, compared with those who posted about other topics, wound up significantly more likely to request an HIV self-testing kit.[20] These types of insights based on social media could be valuable in providing health departments with information on how many tests or prevention products might be needed and determining real-time information on where those health services are about to be requested and perhaps best proactively deployed.

Another developing application of BDS for prevention involves using viral phylogenetics and data characterizing human phenotypes to define HIV transmission networks that can inform the development of approaches to disrupt them.[21–24] Molecular surveillance is an important tool to track HIV transmission in relative real time and implement programs to intervene; nearly 10% of the viral sequence can be obtained via sequencing data from viral genotypes routinely obtained for clinical care. There have been substantial efforts by the CDC to work with state health departments in implementing HIV sequencing for cluster identification to inform public health action, in real time, to interrupt transmission networks. Among the 4 key strategies articulated in EtHE, the "respond" strategy is predicated on ensuring the technology and personnel are in place in designated localities for successful deployment of laboratory and epidemiologic techniques for cluster identification, linked with programmatic assets, resources, and personnel.

ENGAGEMENT WITH CARE AND TREATMENT

The most frequent use of BDS to evaluate HIV care engagement involves analysis of public health surveillance data, often at jurisdiction levels. Surveillance data, through the electronic HIV/AIDS reporting system (eHARS) database contains information from PLWH, including identifiable data, such as name, address, and date of birth, as well as laboratory, pharmacy, and health service utilization information. A deidentified data set is reported by each jurisdiction to the CDC that forms the basis of the nationwide HIV care continuum estimates. A challenging aspect of utilizing public health surveillance data is related to the delay in data reporting. Outcomes often are reported with upward of a 1-year to 2-year delay in final reporting. In addition, surveillance data provide cross-sectional evaluation of the success of the HIV prevention and care system in the United States but provide relatively little insight into the system's success in meeting the needs of persons with recently diagnosed HIV infection. Moreover, the individual-level characteristics ascertained by HIV surveillance data are limited and do not include some key factors informing care engagement, including social determinants of health, history of incarceration, mental illness, substance use, stigma, or community influences.

Utilizing surveillance data to estimate time from initial HIV diagnosis to VS (<200 copies/mL) as a novel public health indicator can capture the collective effectiveness of HIV prevention and treatment activities in a given locale, including testing, clinical, antiretroviral therapy (ART), and supportive services provided by public health and community-based organizations and clinical entities.[25] An analysis of time from HIV diagnosis to the initial report of VS using surveillance data from 19 jurisdictions in 2009 found a median time of 19 months from HIV diagnosis to VS among 17,028 newly diagnosed persons, with linkage to care within 3 months of diagnosis (hazard ratio [HR] 4.84; 95% CI, 4.27, 5.48) and a higher number of HIV care visits (HR 1.51 per additional visit; 95% CI, 1.48, 1.52), associated with more expeditious suppression.[26] An analysis of geographic differences in time from diagnosis to VS across the 11 public health areas (PHAs) in Alabama found that among 1979 persons with HIV infection newly diagnosed from 2012 to 2014, there was considerable geographic variability, with cross-sectional 12-month VS ranging from 41% to 83% and time to VS ranging from 5 months to 13 months across the 11 PHAs.[26] These findings raise critical questions as to the drivers of this heterogeneity within the PHAs of even a single state; answering these questions is essential in the development of population health approaches to achieve more rapid VS and, consequently, to attain optimal HIV individual-level and community-level outcomes and a reduction in transmission. More recently, investigators in New York City identified an improvement in the percentage of persons newly diagnosed with HIV achieving VS within 3 months from 9% in 2007% to 37% in 2016,[27] with calls to make time to VS after diagnosis a metric of HIV care success.[28] Many rapid ART start programs have already adopted time from initial HIV diagnosis to VS as an indicator of programmatic success.[29,30] Beyond relying on existing indicators reported to DHHS agencies, the adoption and uptake of novel measures utilizing existing data systems are imperative both for monitoring success of the EtHE initiative as well as informing resource allocation and HIV testing, prevention, and treatment service delivery. Time from diagnosis to VS represents 1 such measure that could leverage readily available surveillance data to inform relatively real-time public health action.

Data to Care (D2C) is a public health strategy that uses HIV surveillance and other data to support the HIV care continuum, by identifying persons with HIV who are in need of HIV medical care or other services and facilitating linkage to those services.[31] It is a collaborative effort between the health department, HIV medical providers/clinics, and essential support service providers. D2C approaches may vary and range in scope and design. Some examples of D2C activities include using HIV surveillance data routinely collected by state and local health departments to identify persons who are not in care and then link or re-engage them in care. D2C also has been used to identify persons who are in care but are not virally suppressed and to work with the clients and their providers to support attaining VS. When implemented as part of a comprehensive strategy, D2C programs have the ability to result in improved surveillance data quality, successful linkage to or re-engagement in care for persons with HIV, and improved partner notification to offer testing and other prevention services, including PrEP. Data from D2C programs in early adopting and implementing jurisdictions and states, however, have called into question the potential population-level impact of this approach.

A limitation of the D2C approach is its reliance on accurate HIV surveillance data to identify out-of-care persons. Differentiating persons who have moved out of the area from persons who are out of HIV care is a major time-consuming challenge for health departments, and the extent to which migration varies geographically is not known. A novel multiorganization data-sharing approach, termed the *Black Box*, sought to improve the timeliness and quality of HIV surveillance data in 3 jurisdictions where persons often may travel across the borders of the District of Columbia, Maryland, and Virginia. The Black Box uses a deterministic algorithm, including a person-matching system with eHARS variables following a privacy technology approach.[32] No direct access existed between jurisdictions' eHARS servers and the privacy device. Instead, jurisdictions posted information onto a secure file transfer protocol site that then sent information (synthetic test and real eHARS data) to the privacy device. Of 161,343 uploaded eHARS records from the District of Columbia (N = 49,326), Maryland (N = 66,200), and Virginia (N = 45,817), a total of 21,472 persons were matched across jurisdictions over various strengths in a matching process that took 21 minutes and 58 seconds, leaving 139,871 uniquely identified with only 1 jurisdiction. Three separate validation methods were conducted for this study, and they all found greater than or equal to 90% accuracy between records matched by this novel method and traditional matching methods. This study illustrated a BDS approach that may facilitate timelier and better-quality HIV surveillance data for public health action by reducing the effort needed for traditional person-matching reviews, without compromising matching accuracy. Successful scale up of such approaches in other settings is essential to have accurate, actionable data to inform EtHE programmatic activities from a public health action framework, leveraging the eHARS big data surveillance system.

LIMITATIONS AND ETHICAL CONSIDERATIONS

There are both limitations and ethical considerations in using BDS, particularly for those at risk for or with HIV. There are usability issues with big data approaches because many government agencies, local organizations, and even academic public health departments currently lack the infrastructure to handle big data.[33,34] Traditional statistical infrastructure is not powerful enough to address the complexity of big data and unstructured data. Instead, collaborations between public health researchers and computer scientists trained in machine learning/data mining are necessary and perhaps essential to provide the necessary infrastructure for storing and analyzing big data. In addition, quality and timeliness of surveillance data are critical and must be prioritized and updated frequently in order to better develop methods of using big data to monitor HIV cases to inform service delivery.

Ethical issues also must be taken into consideration. Foremost, privacy and confidentiality concerns of PLWH relate to the risk of unintentional disclosure as a result of BDS approaches, whether through compromised computer systems or as a result of BDS analyses itself.[34,35] There also is an issue of consent, because some data in BDS methods are collected or combined in ways unanticipated by the community initially sharing the data.[36,37] Advancing an ethical framework to evaluate BDS methods in the constantly changing environment of available digital data will be critical.[36,37] Such dialogues have been initiated[38] and likely will be brought to the fore by the EtHE initiative and need for innovative approaches to the utilization of existing and untapped big data systems toward achieving the ambitious goal of a 90% reduction in new HIV cases in the next decade.

SUMMARY

The National Institutes of Health established the Big Data to Knowledge and Data Science programs to promote research and develop biomedical computing and informatics focused on important biomedical and behavioral problems, including the HIV epidemic. Data are currently insufficient in some areas of the country to fully describe the landscape of epidemiologic patterns in HIV transmission and engagement in preventive and treatment care. Furthermore, data are not as timely as is necessary to describe the rapidly changing landscape of transmission. Current surveillance systems operate on a slower basis, resulting in delays at the national level. These current systems do not provide the level of granularity necessary to target the existing tools necessary to end the HIV epidemic in the most vulnerable and at risk populations. The advent of rapid ART strategies, increases in the use of PrEP, changes in health care access, and fluctuations in substance abuse have an impact on transmission risk on a relatively rapid time course. BDS methods that can measure these fluctuations much closer to real time can appropriately guide public health responses and improve understanding of HIV risk, health-seeking behaviors, and the complex contextual environment in which they occur. Moreover, utilizing data already captured by big data systems in new ways, such as the population-level estimate of time from initial HIV diagnosis to VS at a jurisdiction level utilizing eHARS surveillance, for programmatic action represents opportunities to leverage existing resources via taking such novel indicators to scale nationally. More research is needed to refine the methods of using big data in HIV as well as in other areas of public health, providing an important and necessary opportunity for HIV and public health researchers. Accelerating the pace of this research and implementation of proved and promising BDS approaches are imperative to achieving the ambitious goals of the EtHE initiative, toward the optimization of individual and population health HIV prevention and treatment outcomes.

REFERENCES

1. Fauci AS, Redfield RR, Sigounas G, et al. Ending the HIV epidemic: a plan for the United States. JAMA 2019;321(9):844–5.
2. Myers JE, Braunstein SL, Xia Q, et al. Redefining prevention and care: a status-neutral approach to HIV. Open Forum Infect Dis 2018;5(6):1–4.
3. Panel on antiretroviral guidelines for adults and adolescents. Guidelines for the use of antiretroviral agents in adults and adolescents with HIV. Department of Health and Human Services. Available at http://aidsinfo.nih.gov/contentfiles/lvguidelines/AdultandAdolescentGL.pdf. Section F1-F5, Accessed March 1, 2019.
4. Group ISS, Lundgren JD, Babiker AG, et al. Initiation of antiretroviral therapy in early asymptomatic HIV infection. N Engl J Med 2015;373(9):795–807.
5. Montaner JS, Lima VD, Barrios R, et al. Association of highly active antiretroviral therapy coverage, population viral load, and yearly new HIV diagnoses in British Columbia, Canada: a population-based study. Lancet 2010;376(9740):532–9.
6. Cohen MS, Chen YQ, McCauley M, et al. Prevention of HIV-1 infection with early antiretroviral therapy. N Engl J Med 2011;365(6):493–505.
7. Grant RM, Lama JR, Anderson PL, et al. Preexposure chemoprophylaxis for HIV prevention in men who have sex with men. N Engl J Med 2010;363(27):2587–99.
8. Centers for Disease Control and Prevention. Selected national HIV prevention and care outcomes in the United States. 2018. Available at: https://www.cdc.gov/hiv/pdf/library/factsheets/cdc-hiv-national-hiv-care-outcomes.pdf. Accessed February 5, 2019.
9. Smith DK, Van Handel M, Wolitski RJ, et al. Vital signs: estimated percentages and numbers of adults with indications for preexposure prophylaxis to prevent HIV acquisition–United States, 2015. MMWR Morb Mortal Wkly Rep 2015;64(46):1291–5.
10. Mervis J. U.S. science policy. Agencies rally to tackle big data. Science 2012;336(6077):22.
11. Ohno-Machado L. Big science, big data, and a big role for biomedical informatics. J Am Med Inform Assoc 2012;19(e1):e1.
12. Wang W, Krishnan E. Big data and clinicians: a review on the state of the science. JMIR Med Inform 2014;2(1):e1.
13. Bushman FD, Barton S, Bailey A, et al. Bringing it all together: big data and HIV research. AIDS 2013;27(5):835–8.
14. Young SD. A "big data" approach to HIV epidemiology and prevention. Prev Med 2015;70:17–8.
15. Centers for Disease Control and Prevention. Estimated HIV incidence and prevalence in the United States, 2010–2016. HIV Surveillance Supplemental Report 2019;24(No.1). Available at: http://www.cdc.gov/hiv/library/reports/hiv-surveillance.html. Accessed March 13, 2019.
16. CDC. HIV in The United States by geography. November 2017 2017. Available at: https://www.cdc.gov/hiv/pdf/statistics/cdc-hiv-geographic-distribution.pdf.

17. Jena AB, Karaca-Mandic P, Weaver L, et al. Predicting new diagnoses of HIV infection using internet search engine data. Clin Infect Dis 2013;56(9):1352–3.

18. Young SD, Zhang Q. Using search engine big data for predicting new HIV diagnoses. PLoS One 2018;13(7):e0199527.

19. Young SD, Rivers C, Lewis B. Methods of using real-time social media technologies for detection and remote monitoring of HIV outcomes. Prev Med 2014;63:112–5.

20. Young SD, Jaganath D. Online social networking for HIV education and prevention: a mixed-methods analysis. Sex Transm Dis 2013;40(2):162–7.

21. Kostaki EG, Nikolopoulos GK, Pavlitina E, et al. Molecular analysis of human immunodeficiency virus type 1 (HIV-1)-Infected individuals in a network-based intervention (transmission reduction intervention project): phylogenetics identify HIV-1-infected individuals with social links. J Infect Dis 2018;218(5):707–15.

22. Kusejko K, Kadelka C, Marzel A, et al. Inferring the age difference in HIV transmission pairs by applying phylogenetic methods on the HIV transmission network of the Swiss HIV Cohort Study. Virus Evol 2018;4(2):vey024.

23. Lubelchek RJ, Hoehnen SC, Hotton AL, et al. Transmission clustering among newly diagnosed HIV patients in Chicago, 2008 to 2011: using phylogenetics to expand knowledge of regional HIV transmission patterns. J Acquir Immune Defic Syndr 2015;68(1):46–54.

24. Pasquale DK, Doherty IA, Sampson LA, et al. Leveraging phylogenetics to understand HIV transmission and partner notification networks. J Acquir Immune Defic Syndr 2018;78(4):367–75.

25. Hall HI, Tang T, Westfall AO, et al. HIV care visits and time to viral suppression, 19 U.S. jurisdictions, and implications for treatment, prevention and the national HIV/AIDS strategy. PLoS One 2013;8(12):e84318.

26. Rogers R, Tang T, Batey DS, et al. Geographic variability in time from HIV diagnosis to viral suppression in Alabama. Abstract #185. Paper presented at: 12th International Conference on HIV Treatment and Prevention Adherence, June 4–6, 2017; Miami, Florida.

27. Xia Q, Coeytaux K, Braunstein SL, et al. Proposing a new indicator for the national human immunodeficiency virus/AIDS strategy: percentage of newly diagnosed persons achieving viral suppression within 3 months of diagnosis. J Infect Dis 2018;219(6):851–5.

28. Dombrowski JC, Baeten JM. It's time to make the time to viral suppression after hiv diagnosis a metric of hiv care success. The Journal of Infectious Diseases 2019;219(6):845–7.

29. Pilcher CD, Ospina-Norvell C, Dasgupta A, et al. The effect of same-day observed initiation of antiretroviral therapy on HIV viral load and treatment outcomes in a US Public health setting. J Acquir Immune Defic Syndr 2017;74(1):44–51.

30. Colasanti J, JS, Mehta C, et al. A rapid Entry program in the South: Improving access to care and viral suppression. Abstract#1109. Paper presented at: Conference on Retroviruses and Opportunistic Infection March 4–7, 2018; Boston, MA.

31. CDC. Effective interventions data to care. Available at: https://effectiveinterventions. cdc.gov/data-to-care/group-1/data-to-care. Accessed March 15, 2019.

32. Ocampo JMF, Smart JC, Allston A, et al. Improving HIV surveillance data for public health action in Washington, DC: a novel multiorganizational data-sharing method. JMIR Public Health Surveill 2016;2(1):e3.

33. Coffron M, Opelka F. Big promise and big challenges for big heath care data. Bull Am Coll Surg 2015;100(4):10–6.

34. Craven M, Page CD. Big data in healthcare: opportunities and challenges. Big Data 2015;3(4):209–10.

35. Zhang X, Perez-Stable EJ, Bourne PE, et al. Big data science: opportunities and challenges to address minority health and health disparities in the 21st century. Ethn Dis 2017;27(2):95–106.
36. Bourne PE. Confronting the ethical challenges of big data in public health. PLoS Comput Biol 2015;11(2):e1004073.
37. Vayena E, Salathe M, Madoff LC, et al. Ethical challenges of big data in public health. PLoS Comput Biol 2015;11(2):e1003904.
38. Sweeney P, Gardner LI, Buchacz K, et al. Shifting the paradigm: using HIV surveillance data as a foundation for improving HIV care and preventing HIV infection. Milbank Q 2013;91(3):558–603.

The Reproductive Years of Women with Perinatally Acquired HIV

From Gynecologic Care to Obstetric Outcomes

Saba Berhie, MD[a],*, Lynn Yee, MD, MPH[a], Jennifer Jao, MD, MPH[b]

KEYWORDS

- Perinatal HIV • HIV • Reproductive health • Pregnancy • Pregnancy outcomes

KEY POINTS

- Women with perinatally acquired HIV (PHIV) have unique medical and psychosocial issues compared with their counterparts with nonperinatally acquired HIV (NPHIV) as they have been exposed to multiple HIV regimens, grapple with antiretroviral therapy (ART) resistance, and engage with the health care system from a young age.
- Women with PHIV are less likely to have appropriate cervical cancer screening and are more likely to have higher rates of sexually transmitted infections (STIs) and unintended pregnancies than peers with NPHIV or without HIV.
- There may be increased risk of mother-to-child transmission of HIV for infants of pregnant women with PHIV.
- Emerging data suggest that infants of women with PHIV may have increased morbidity compared with infants of women with NPHIV, with higher rates of low birth weight and non–HIV-related infections requiring hospitalizations within the first year of life.

INTRODUCTION

Advances in HIV care and antiretroviral therapy (ART) have led to more young men and women with perinatally acquired HIV (PHIV) surviving to adulthood. In 2011, the World Health Organization estimated that 4500 children 15 years or younger in the United States were with PHIV.[1] As these children transition into young adulthood, they may face distinctive challenges due to living with a chronic disease, including stigma and more complex HIV care, compared with those with nonperinatally acquired HIV

Disclosure Statement: The authors have no conflicts of interest to disclose.
[a] Department of Obstetrics and Gynecology, Division of Maternal Fetal Medicine, Northwestern University Feinberg School of Medicine, 250 E Superior Street, Suite 5-2149, Chicago, IL 60611, USA; [b] Ann & Robert H. Lurie Children's Hospital of Chicago, Box 20, 225 E Chicago Avenue, Chicago, IL 60611, USA
* Corresponding author.
E-mail address: saba.berhie@northwestern.edu

Infect Dis Clin N Am 33 (2019) 817–833
https://doi.org/10.1016/j.idc.2019.04.004
0891-5520/19/© 2019 Elsevier Inc. All rights reserved.

id.theclinics.com

(NPHIV). Substantial work has focused on potential biological differences between children and young adults with PHIV compared with those with NPHIV. For example, individuals with PHIV may have differential risks due to immune system alterations in the setting of lifelong immunosuppression and may incur metabolic complications of lifelong ART such as insulin resistance and dyslipidemia.[2–4] Such differences enhance the complexity of medical care for individuals with PHIV.

For young women with PHIV transitioning into adulthood, unique concerns include reproductive health and outcomes. The first case report of a successful pregnancy by an adolescent with PHIV was described in 1998[5]; although over 20 years have passed since that report, the concerns raised then remain relevant today, including issues of contraception, strategies to prevent mother-to-child transmission (MTCT) of HIV, and potential adverse maternal or neonatal outcomes. Comprehensive health care for this population centers around maintaining a healthy and productive life for women with PHIV and also shepherding women through their reproductive years with appropriate gynecologic care and—if desired–safe and successful childbearing. Although the gynecologic and obstetric care of young women with PHIV is understudied compared with other medical and psychosocial issues experienced by individuals with PHIV, these issues are nonetheless of critical importance to achieving these goals. This article reviews the existing evidence regarding the gynecologic and obstetric issues unique to reproductive age women with PHIV.

REPRODUCTIVE HEALTH
Cervical Cancer Prevention

The foundation of gynecologic care for young women generally begins with family planning counseling, access to contraception when desired, sexually transmitted infection (STI) screening, and cervical cancer screening and prevention. Women with HIV (WLHIV) are at disproportionate risk for cervical dysplasia and cancer.[6] Per the NIH and American College of Obstetricians and Gynecologists (ACOG), cervical cancer screening for all WLHIV should begin with cervical cytology within a year of onset of sexual activity or at age 21, whichever occurs earliest.[7,8] This recommendation differs from recommendations for women without chronic immunosuppression, who begin screening no earlier than age 21 regardless of potentially earlier onset of sexual activity. Furthermore, in contrast to women without HIV, WLHIV are recommended to have annual cervical cancer screening, which can be reduced to every 3 years once there are 3 annual normal results. Finally, cervical cancer screening should continue throughout the lifetime of women with PHIV and not stop at 65 years of age given chronic immunosuppression.

Some data suggest that women with PHIV are not undergoing appropriate cervical dysplasia screening compared with their NPHIV counterparts. Setse and colleagues[9] found that 34% of women with PHIV received appropriate screening compared with 62% of women with NPHIV. When screened, the risk of abnormal findings is also high; abnormal cervical cytology has been reported at 30% in a cohort of female adolescents with PHIV and 54% among all young female adolescents with HIV.[9,10] Reassuringly, in the Longitudinal Epidemiologic Study to Gain Insight into HIV/AIDS in Children and Youth (LEGACY) cohort, only 2% of adolescents had high-grade lesions and there were no cases of invasive cervical cancer.[9] However, this finding is likely due to the indolent natural history of human papillomavirus (HPV) and the young age of the women in this study, because HPV infections are known to be more persistent in WLHIV. When appropriate screening and treatment are not performed, WLHIV are 2 to 8 times more likely to develop cervical cancer than women without HIV.[6,11]

The only known strategy to prevent HPV acquisition and progression to cervical cancer is HPV vaccination. There are no data on the rates of HPV vaccine counseling or uptake in WLHIV or specifically among women with PHIV. The quadrivalent HPV vaccine should be offered to all adolescent and reproductive age women, including women with PHIV; notably, the Food and Drug Administration recently expanded approval of the vaccine to age 45 years (from a previous maximum of 26) based on data showing efficacy beyond the age of 26 years.[12] There are data that HPV vaccination is effective in WLHIV and can prevent high-risk HPV acquisition.[13] As in women without HIV, HPV vaccination is most effective when given before onset of sexual activity and exposure to HPV, and thus is recommended in early adolescence. Greater work is needed to understand rates of implementation of HPV vaccination for young women with PHIV and the potential altered efficacy of such vaccination in this high-risk population.

Sexual Health and Sexually Transmitted Infections

Though young women with PHIV are less likely to be sexually active and to have an STI compared with their counterparts with NPHIV,[14,15] sexual activity among women with PHIV is associated with poor HIV control due to behavioral and social factors that lead to poorer adherence to the ART regimen. Sexually active adolescent women with PHIV are more likely to have a higher viremia and lower CD4 counts than nonsexually active women with PHIV.[10] Furthermore, sexually active young women with PHIV are less likely to be on ART.[10] Importantly, sexually active adolescents with PHIV may not be aware of their HIV status; in the LEGACY study, 19% of sexually active adolescents with PHIV were unaware of their HIV status because of guardian nondisclosure.[14]

HPV is the most common STI diagnosed among adolescents with HIV.[9] Reported ranges of other STIs vary in the PHIV and NPHIV populations. From the Pediatric AIDS Clinical Trials Group 219 (PACTG 219), there was a 9% rate of trichomoniasis and chlamydia seen in adolescent women with PHIV, whereas the Reaching for Excellence in Adolescent Care and Health cohort—which also included adolescent women with NPHIV—report rates of trichomoniasis of 12.6% and 22.4% for chlamydia.[10,16] By comparison, the rate of trichomoniasis among women without HIV in the United States is 3.1%, whereas rates of chlamydial infection in sexually active women 14 to 24 years old was most recently reported at 4.7%.[17,18] The higher incidence of STIs among adolescents with PHIV further emphasizes the need for attention to the US Preventive Services Task Force recommendations, which include annual gonorrhea and chlamydia screening in sexually active women 24 years or younger and a consideration for trichomoniasis screening as well.[19]

Contraception and Preconception Counseling

Half of all pregnancies in the United States are unintended.[20] In a case series of 30 pregnant women with PHIV, 81% reported that their pregnancies were unplanned.[21] For women with PHIV, unintended pregnancy may have even greater consequences, because of the impact of pregnancy on maternal health as well as the risk of MTCT, which is directly associated with maternal viral control.[22] In a US survey of young WLHIV, women with PHIV were less likely to discuss contraception with a health care provider compared with women with NPHIV, although women with NPHIV were more likely to have been pregnant.[23] One driving hypothesis for this difference in discussion of contraception with providers may be that women with PHIV have been connected to the health care system for their entire lives and may believe they have more knowledge of contraception owing to this interaction with the system, resulting in decreased discussion with their provider regarding contraception.

Notably, however, baseline knowledge of contraception among WLHIV has been found to be high but translation of that knowledge to uptake of long-acting reversible forms of contraception has been low.[24]

Data on abortion rates, access, and complications among women with PHIV are limited. In 1 small cohort study of women with PHIV in India, 13% underwent abortions in the setting of undesired pregnancy, whereas in a case series of women with PHIV in the United Kingdom and Ireland, 36% had abortions.[21,25] These data on abortion frequency are likely to be underreported due to the complexity of ascertaining accurate abortion data. Moreover, no data on abortion among US women with PHIV exist, and data on early pregnancy loss among women with PHIV are also lacking.

Although preconception counseling is recommended for all women contemplating pregnancy, there are some salient differences in the recommendations for WLHIV.[26] Preconception counseling topics must include safer conception if a serodiscordant relationship is present, future fetal concerns, and maternal health concerns, including routine preconception issues as well as specific ART recommendations. Preexposure prophylaxis may be an effective tool that should be discussed in the preconception period when a serodiscordant relationship is present and pregnancy is desired.[27] In addition, as with any woman contemplating pregnancy, optimal control of comorbidities that can affect pregnancy such as obesity, hypertension, and diabetes, is essential to maternal and fetal health. Unique to WLHIV is that the preconception period is a critical opportunity to minimize risk of MTCT by emphasizing ART adherence and virologic suppression as well as optimizing the ART regimen. **Table 1** summarizes key studies that evaluate the reproductive health of women with PHIV.

OBSTETRIC CARE
Antenatal Care

The framework of obstetric care for women with NPHIV and PHIV follows the same general structure for all pregnant women.[28] We recommend closely referencing the Department of Health and Human Services Recommendations for the Use of Antiretroviral Drugs in Pregnant Women with HIV Infection and Interventions to Reduce Perinatal HIV Transmission in the United States (referred to as the "US Perinatal Guidelines") when caring for pregnant and postpartum WLHIV. Data regarding obstetric care and outcomes relevant to women with PHIV are discussed here.[29] Although most aspects of prenatal care, such as nutrition counseling, prenatal laboratories, and fetal surveillance are similar to women without HIV, there are several unique concerns for pregnant WLHIV, including that of invasive diagnostic genetic testing.

Genetic screening is offered to all pregnant women. During the first trimester and early second trimester there are many available noninvasive screening tests available including serum marker screening and cell-free DNA. If screening tests demonstrate increased risk for aneuploidy, then an invasive diagnostic test should be offered to the patient in the form of a chorionic villus sampling or amniocentesis depending on gestational age.[30] These procedures require needle sampling through the maternal abdomen or cervix to access the placenta or amniotic fluid. The sample can be analyzed by way of karyotype and/or microarray analysis.[31] WLHIV may be at increased risk of vertical transmission if viremic at the time of invasive diagnostic procedures such as amniocentesis or chorionic villus sampling, and thus counseling about genetic screening and testing must include shared decision making about the risks and benefits of testing. In 1 multicenter case series, WLHIV on ART who underwent invasive diagnostic testing had similar rates of MTCT as women who did not undergo invasive testing.[32] Furthermore, an undetectable viral load (VL) is preferable as a

Table 1
Key articles describing gynecologic and reproductive health outcomes of women with perinatally acquired HIV

Authors	Study Population	Setting	Study Design	Sample Size	Outcomes Measured	Results
Koenig et al,[15] 2010	Adolescents with HIV (LEGACY Study)	US	Cohort	N = 56 PHIV N = 88 NPHIV	Demographics, sexual behavior, psychosocial characteristics	• Unprotected sex more common among those with NPHIV (OR = 4.5 1.46–13.9; $P = .009$) • NPHIV adolescents more likely to have been sexually abused than PHIV (48% vs 18%; $P = .001$) • NPHIV adolescents more likely to be sexually active (82% vs 56%; $P = .008$)
Setse et al,[14] 2011	Adolescents with HIV (LEGACY Study)	US	Cohort	N = 116 PHIV N = 181 NPHIV	Sexual behavior, STI, awareness of HIV diagnosis	• 34% of PHIV and 90% PHIV participants were sexually active • No difference in rates of condom use between the 2 groups • NPHIV adolescents more likely to have an STI (32% vs 10%, $P<.01$) • HPV most common STI in both groups • 22% (120) PHIV participants unaware of HIV diagnosis • 19% (34) of PHIV participants who did not know HIV status were sexually active
Setse et al,[9] 2012	Adolescents with HIV (LEGACY Study)	US	Cohort	N = 107 PHIV N = 124 NPHIV	Cervical Pap screening	• PHIV vs NPHIV adolescents less likely to undergo appropriate Pap screening (APR 0.66; 95% CI, 0.45–0.96) • 43% (48) had normal cervical test results • 2% (2) had high-grade lesions (HSIL/CINIII) • No women had invasive cervical cancer)

(continued on next page)

Table 1
(continued)

Authors	Study Population	Setting	Study Design	Sample Size	Outcomes Measured	Results
Brogly et al,[10] 2007	Women with PHIV from PACTG 219	US	Cohort	N = 638 PHIV	Sexual behavior, STI exposure, Pap screening, pregnancy rates	• 174 (27%) sexually active • 30 (30%) abnormal cytology at first Pap • Sexually active adolescents: more likely to be Hispanic (36% vs 26%), live on their own (23% vs 1%), have higher VL (44% > 1000 vs 32% vs 1%) • 17% of women experienced first pregnancy by age 19
Echenique et al,[23] 2017	Young women with HIV (16–29 y)	US	Survey	N = 21 PHIV N = 13 NPHIV	Contraception knowledge, patient behavior, depression	• PHIV women less likely to discuss pregnancy prevention with health care provider compared with NPHIV (71% vs 100% P = .04) • PHIV women more likely to be prescribed ART (100% vs 62%, P = .005) • NPHIV women more likely to have moderate to severe depression (69% vs 33%, P = .042) • NPHIV women more likely to have been pregnant compared with PHIV (92% vs 48% P = .01)
Jones et al,[24] 2017	Young women with HIV (16–29 y)	US	RCT	N = 21 PHIV N = 13 NPHIV	Preconception counseling intervention, contraceptive and pregnancy knowledge	• Contraceptive use and pregnancy planning knowledge similar between women with PHIV and NPHIV

Abbreviations: APR, adjusted prevalence ratio; ART, antiretroviral therapy; HPV, human papilloma virus; LEGACY, longitudinal epidemiologic study to gain insight into HIV/AIDS in children and youth; NPHIV, nonperinatally acquired HIV; OR, odds ratio; PACTG, Pediatric AIDS Clinical Trials Group; PHIV, perinatally acquired HIV; RCT, randomized controlled trial; STI, sexually transmitted infection; VL, viral load.

prerequisite to invasive testing to lessen the risk of MTCT.[33] There are no data specifically on these issues of genetic counseling among women with PHIV, although it should be noted that the risk of aneuploidy is not thought to be higher for women with PHIV compared with other age-matched women. There are also no data on rates of congenital anomalies among PHIV women.

ART adherence and viral suppression are the backbone of prevention of MTCT of HIV. Reassuringly, women with PHIV are more likely to be on ART at the first prenatal visit compared with women with NPHIV.[34] Despite great strides in the reduction of MTCT to approximately less than 1% in high-income countries such as the United States, continued counseling of women with PHIV includes discussion of the risks of MTCT, recommendations for reducing this risk, and the importance of ART adherence.[35,36]

Antiretroviral Therapy Initiation and Adherence

The US Perinatal Guidelines provide direction on ART choice for pregnant WLHIV. Recommendations are the same for both women with PHIV and NPHIV.[37] If a woman has an elevated VL entering pregnancy, antiretroviral drug resistance studies should be obtained. Because women with PHIV have been exposed to multiple ART throughout their lives they enter pregnancy with higher rates of ART resistance than their NPHIV counterparts and have higher rates of multiclass resistance.[34,38,39] A small Spanish cohort reported 71% of the women with PHIV had been on 6 or more ART regimens throughout her lifetime, while a small Brazilian cohort reported 41% of women with PHIV on third-line ART.[40,41]

In addition to recommendations regarding early initiation of ART and performing resistance studies, the guidelines also advise on drug choice. The ART regimen choice for women with PHIV is generally separated into 2 categories: (1) pregnant women already on ART at conception or (2) those who previously received ART but did not conceive on ART, thus requiring initiation of ART during pregnancy. Women with PHIV will typically have had exposure to multiple previous regimens, which must be carefully considered when determining optimal ART regimens for pregnancy. Women who conceive on a regimen and are already doing well on that regimen are generally counseled to continue it during pregnancy, particularly if it is a preferred or alternative regimen, whereas women who are on nonpreferred regimens require a discussion about the risks and benefits of continuing the regimen versus changing during early pregnancy. For those women who have been on ART in the past, but are not currently on medications, their provider should investigate the past history of ART regimens, previous resistance data, overall VL trajectory, and any previous adherence challenges.

One unique issue is regarding the use of dolutegravir (DTG) at the time of conception. At the time of this writing, the US Perinatal Guidelines were recently updated and addressed controversy around early data from Botswana in 2018, which reported a higher prevalence of neural tube defects among fetuses of women receiving DTG during the first trimester (0.95% rate among infants exposed to in utero DTG vs 0.12% among those exposed to non–DTG-containing ART).[42] Current recommendations from the US Perinatal Guidelines recommend DTG not be initiated during the first trimester of pregnancy or in women attempting conception. Further data from this study are expected in 2019.

Intrapartum and Postpartum Care

Similar to women with NPHIV, decision making about mode of delivery for women with PHIV hinges on VL near the time of anticipated delivery. ACOG and the US Perinatal

Guidelines both recommend a scheduled cesarean delivery at 38 weeks gestation for WLHIV with VL greater than 1000 copies/mL to avoid labor or rupture of membranes.[29,43] Intravenous zidovudine should be administered before cesarean delivery. Given the maternal morbidity of cesarean delivery, counseling throughout pregnancy about ART adherence to avoid requiring this intervention is of utmost importance. For women with a VL ≤1000 copies/mL, delivery timing and route should be based on other comorbidities and usual obstetric indications for delivery.[29,43] In the 5 cohort studies comparing mode of delivery between women with NPHIV versus PHIV, 3 show women with PHIV experience cesarean delivery at greater frequency than women with NPHIV due to greater likelihood of viremia.[38,44,45] In addition, cesarean delivery increases the risk of maternal and neonatal morbidity and mortality in subsequent pregnancies due to the risk of uterine rupture, placenta previa, and placenta accreta. Thus cesarean delivery places women at greater risk of morbidity and mortality; women undergoing cesarean delivery have higher rates of postpartum infection, hemorrhage requiring transfusion or hysterectomy, and venous thromboembolism compared with women who deliver vaginally.[46] The potentially higher frequency of cesarean delivery among women with PHIV may have greater long-term implications for women with PHIV due to their young age, lesser use of effective contraception, and potentially longer period of reproductive capacity.

After delivery, the postpartum period—also known as the "fourth trimester"—can be a time of joy and challenge for women and their families. ACOG recommends close postpartum follow-up for all women, including a comprehensive assessment of maternal well-being, attention to chronic health conditions, and support for transition to primary care or specialist care.[47] Women with PHIV have the additional strain of maintaining an ART regimen during this transitional time and needing to coordinate infectious disease follow-up in addition to routine postpartum care. Women with PHIV also may be more likely to require administration of a multidrug neonatal prophylaxis regimen, because they are more likely to be viremic at delivery, which may be an added postpartum stressor.

Moreover, once the motivations of pregnancy have ended, some have hypothesized that women with PHIV may have reduced adherence to HIV care; for example, in 1 study, women with PHIV had lower postpartum CD4 counts and higher VLs compared with their NPHIV counterparts.[45] In a small cohort study of US WLHIV, the rare maternal deaths occurred solely among women with PHIV; in 3 of the 4 cases, it was noted that these women stopped their ART and were severely immunocompromised with CD4 less than 50 cells/mm³.[44]

Few data exist regarding best practices to promote retention in care for postpartum women with PHIV. However, 1 study reported case management during pregnancy and up to 1 year postpartum to be effective for WLHIV; at 1 year postpartum, more women with case management remained in infectious disease care (53% vs 34%, P<.0001).[48] Although viral suppression remained suboptimal among women with PHIV and NPHIV, case management or similar approaches may be an important area worthy of further investigation for women with PHIV.

Maternal Outcomes

Limited data exist examining maternal health and obstetric complications in women with PHIV compared with NPHIV. In 1 single-site US cohort there were no differences in rates of preeclampsia, gestational hypertension, or gestational diabetes between women with PHIV versus NPHIV.[38] Perinatal depression, defined as depression or depressive symptoms anytime during pregnancy and up to a year postpartum, is another important maternal outcome.[49,50] In the largest study to date on perinatal depression and WLHIV, women with PHIV were more likely to experience perinatal depression compared with women without HIV.[51] However, perinatal depression rates were similar between PHIV and NPHIV women.[52] Although data on perinatal depression in the PHIV population are limited, depression screening should be standardized and routine in prenatal and postpartum care for all women.[49,50] Women with PHIV may face unique psychosocial morbidities such as stigma or disclosure issues that amplify their risk for perinatal depression.

Findings regarding HIV-related maternal outcomes suggest potentially greater morbidity for women with PHIV. Although women with PHIV are more likely to conceive on an ART regimen, multiple studies have reported that they enter pregnancy with lower CD4 counts and higher VLs compared with NPHIV counterparts.[53–55] Women with PHIV are also less likely to have a suppressed VL at delivery but are more likely to have had a previous or current history of opportunistic infections.[34,38,52]

Neonatal Outcomes

A primary concern for any child born to a mother with HIV is MTCT of HIV. The baseline rate of MTCT for infants of women with PHIV ranges from 0.45% to 2%, similar to or slightly higher than rates reported for infants of women with NPHIV.[55,56] In contrast, the largest study of pregnant women with PHIV is from the Surveillance Monitoring of ART Toxicities Study (SMARTT) of the Pediatric HIV/AIDS Cohort Study (PHACS), which demonstrated MTCT among women with PHIV as almost 3 times that among women with NPHIV (1.1% among women with PHIV vs 0.4% among women with NPHIV).[56] However, it is reassuring that rates of MTCT among women with PHIV are still similar to those with NPHIV currently in the United States.[36]

In addition, women with PHIV may be at greater risk of other fetal and neonatal complications due to greater comorbidities, inflammation, and immunosuppression. There are reports of lower birth weight for infants of women with PHIV compared with women with NPHIV; however, there are no data on intrauterine growth restriction.[44,45,54] In 1 study of birth outcomes in the Bronx, NY, 66% of infants born to women with NPHIV weighed more than 3000 g, while 12.5% of the infants of women with PHIV weighed more than 3000 g.[45] An updated report 2 years later from the same group noted 62.5% of infants of NPHIV women weighed more than 3000 g, while 32.4% of infants of PHIV women weighed more than 3000 g.[44] However, there were no differences in the numbers of low-birth-weight (LBW) infants between groups. Another study in New York reported that infants born to women with PHIV had an increased odds of small for gestational age (SGA) status with an adjusted odds ratio of 5.67 (95% CI, 1.03–31.61) compared with infants of women with NPHIV.[52] However, data from a large combined analysis of PHACS SMARTT and the International Maternal Pediatric Adolescent AIDS Clinical Trials P1025 did not show an association between maternal PHIV status and LBW or SGA outcomes, although in subgroup analyses, women with PHIV in the oldest age category (23–30 years of age) were at increased risk for having LBW infants compared with women with NPHIV of the same age.[54] Given the long-term morbidity associated with LBW and SGA status, these conflicting data, as well as the specific relationship between maternal PHIV status and LBW among older pregnant women with PHIV, warrant future research.[57]

Preterm birth is a major contributor to short-term and long-term child morbidity and mortality worldwide. The rate of preterm births among WLHIV is higher than the general population for a multitude of theorized reasons, and data on preterm birth specifically among women with PHIV are sparse. For reference, the preterm birth rate in the United States is approximately 9.8%, and reported rates globally for WLHIV range

Table 2
Key articles describing maternal, obstetric, and HIV transmission outcomes in women with perinatally acquired HIV

Authors	Study Setting	Study Design	Sample Size	Results
Maternal Outcomes				
Cruz et al,[41] 2016	Brazil	Cohort	N = 22 PHIV	• 7 (41%) on third-line ART • 11 (69%) with mutations consistent with ARV resistance • 7 (41%) had VL <50 at time of delivery
Angrand et al,[51] 2018	US	Cohort	N = 23 PHIV N = 98 NPHIV N = 124 HIV-U	• PHIV women at increased risk of perinatal depression than HIV-U women (aOR = 15.9, 95% CI, 1.8–143.8) • PHIV women not more likely to have perinatal depression than NPHIV women (aOR = 1.9, 95% CI, 0.5–7.6)
Badell et al,[38] 2013	US	Cohort	N = 20 PHIV N = 80 NPHIV	• PHIV women with higher rates of ARV resistance (40% vs 12.5, $P \leq .01$) • PHIV women more likely to have detectable VL (65% vs 37% $P \leq .01$) • PHIV women with higher rates of CD due to HIV (64% vs 22% $P \leq .5$) • No differences in frequency of preeclampsia, gestational hypertension, GDM, preterm birth, chorioamnionitis
Byrne et al,[53] 2017	UK and Ireland	Cohort	N = 45 PHIV N = 118 NPHIV	• PHIV women more likely to conceive on cART (65% vs 39%; $P<.01$) • Baseline CD4 count lower for PHIV women (21% PHIV <200 vs 6% NPHIV; $P<.01$) • PHIV women with higher rates of pregnancy termination (13% vs 3% $P = .02$) • No difference in mode of delivery • PHIV women more likely to have detectable VL at delivery aOR = 3.22 (1.22–8.48, $P = .02$)
Calitr et al,[39] 2014	Italy	Registry	N = 23 PHIV	• Median number of ARV regimens pregnant women had been exposed to before pregnancy: 4
Jao et al,[52] 2012	US	Cohort	N = 14 PHIV N = 60 NPHIV	• PHIV women more likely to have OI ($P = .008$), nadir CD4 count $\leq$200 ($P = .01$), and receive second-line ART in pregnancy ($P<.001$)
Jao et al,[54] 2017	US, multicenter	Cohort	N = 235 PHIV N = 2035 NPHIV	• PHIV women more likely to have CD4 <200 (19% vs 11%, $P<.01$) and delivery VL $\geq$400 (28% vs 17%, $P<.01$) • PHIV women more likely to be on ART regimen with $\geq$ 3-class ARV (23% vs 2%, $P<.01$)
Kenny et al,[21] 201	UK and Ireland	Case series	N = 30 PHIV	• Eight (19%) pregnancies were planned, 15 (36%) pregnancies were electively terminated, 6 (14%) first trimester miscarriages

Reference	Country	Study Type	N	Findings
Lazenby et al,[34] 2016	Canada and US, multicenter	Cohort	N = 41 PHIV, N = 41 NPHIV	• PHIV women more likely to be taking ARVs at first prenatal visit (68% vs 23% P<.0001) and to have VL >1000 at first prenatal visit (46% vs 0, P = .01) • PHIV women exclusively had multiclass ARV resistance (16% vs 0%, P = .030) • PHIV women with higher rates of psychiatric illness (50% vs 27%, P = .03) • Only PHIV women had prior history of OIs • Similar rates of pregnancy complications, mode of delivery for PHIV vs NPHIV women
Munjal et al,[44] 2013	US	Cohort	N = 30 PHIV, N = 35 NPHIV	• PHIV women more likely to have CD due to high VL (P = .03) • Four deaths of PHIV women postpartum and no deaths in the NPHIV women (3 of these women had CD4 <50 at 1 y after delivery and stopped taking ARVs after delivery)
Phillips et al,[45] 2011	US	Cohort	N = 11 PHIV, N = 27 NPHIV	• Third trimester CD4 (P=.003) lower and VL higher (P = .02) for PHIV women • 6-mo postpartum CD4 (P = .0006) lower and VL higher (P = .001) for PHIV women • 88% NPHIV women with undetectable VL at delivery vs 60% PHIV women (P = .03) • 80% PHIV women delivered by CD vs 39% NPHIV (P = .009)
Prieto et al,[40] 2017	Spain	Cohort	N = 22 PHIV	• 71% had been on 6 or more ARV regimens • VL at conception ≤50 for 50% and ≥10,000 for 29%
Lundberg et al,[55] 2018	Brazil	Cohort	N = 32 PHIV, N = 595 NPHIV	• PHIV women younger than NPHIV (19 y/o vs 22 y/o P = .01) • PHIV women more likely to be on cART in the first trimester OR = 12.5 (95% CI, 5.7–27.3; P<.01) • No difference in mode of delivery
Goodenough et al,[56] 2018	US, multicenter	Cohort	N = 232 PHIV, N = 1646 NPHIV	• PHIV women more likely to have final VL during pregnancy >1000 (19% vs 9%, P<.001) and final CD4 <200 (19% vs 8%, P<.001)

Obstetric Outcomes

Reference	Country	Study Type	N	Findings
Chibber,[25] 2005	India	Cohort	N = 30 primiparous PHIV	• 13% had TABs • PTB: 1 (3.3%) • Mean birth weight: 3072 ± 450 g • 3.3% LBW <2500 g
Munjal et al,[44] 2013	US	Cohort	N = 30 PHIV, N = 35 NPHIV	PHIV newborn lower mean birth weight (2834 ± 545 g vs 3093 ± 528 g, P = .03) then newborns to NPHIV women
Phillips et al,[45] 2011	US	Cohort	N = 11 PHIV, N = 27 NPHIV	PHIV newborn lower mean birth weight than NPHIV newborns (2688 vs 3117 g, P = .003)

(continued on next page)

Table 2
(continued)

Authors	Study Setting	Study Design	Sample Size	Results
Prieto et al,[40] 2017	Spain	Cohort	N = 22 PHIV	30% neonates SGA
Lundberg et al,[55] 2018	Brazil	Cohort	N = 32 PHIV N = 595 NPHIV	No difference in infant birth weight between groups
Cruz et al,[41] 2016	Brazil	Cohort	N = 22 PHIV	4 (18%) PTB
Byrne et al,[53] 2017	UK and Ireland	Cohort	N = 45 PHIV N = 118 NPHIV	No difference in PTB between groups
Calitri et al,[39] 2014	Italy	Registry	N = 23 PHIV	8/23 (35%) PTB
Jao et al,[52] 2012	US	Cohort	N = 17 PHIV, n = 70 NPHIV	• Similar rates of PTB between groups • PHIV neonates: more likely to be born SGA. aOR = 5.67 (95% CI, 103–31.61)
Jao et al,[54] 2017	US	Prospective	N = 235 PHIV N = 2035 NPHIV	• Mean BWZ lower in infants of PHIV women vs NPHIV (−0.45 vs −0.33, P = .03) • PHIV women (23–30 y) with higher proportions of LBW infants (aRR = 1.74, 95% CI, 1.18–2.58, P<.01) • No differences in rates of PTB between PHIV vs NPHIV women
Mother-to-child transmission of HIV				
Lazenby et al,[34] 2016	Canada and US, multicenter	Cohort	N = 41 PHIV N = 41 NPHIV	2 (5%) MTCT NPHIV, 0 PHIV
Lundberg et al,[55] 2013	Brazil	Cohort	N = 32 PHIV N = 595 NPHIV	29 (2%) MTCT NPHIV, 0 PHIV
Byrne et al,[53] 2017	UK and Ireland	Cohort	N = 45 PHIV N = 118 NPHIV	1 (3%) MTCT PHIV, 0 NPHIV
Goodenough et al,[56] 2018	US	Cohort	N = 232 PHIV N = 1646 NPHIV	9 (0.5%) PHIV, 0 NPHIV

Abbreviations: aOR, adjusted odds ratio; aRR, adjusted relative risk; ART, antiretroviral therapy; ARV, antiretroviral; BWZ, birth weight Z score; cART, combination antiretroviral therapy; CD, cesarean delivery; CI, confidence interval; GA, gestational age; GDM, gestational diabetes mellitus; HIV-U, HIV uninfected; LBW, low birth weight; MTCT, mother-to-child transmission; NPHIV, nonperinatally acquired HIV; OI, opportunistic infections; PHIV, perinatally acquired HIV; PTB, preterm birth; SGA, small for gestational age; TAB, termination abortion; VL, viral load.

from 16% to 30%.[53,58,59] In 2 cohorts of women with PHIV in the United States, United Kingdom, and Ireland, rates of preterm birth were comparable with women with NPHIV.[53,54] **Table 2** summarizes major studies that assess maternal, obstetric, and neonatal outcomes of women with PHIV.

Finally, another outcome of interest is the long-term health of the HIV-exposed uninfected (HEU) infant born to a woman with PHIV. A recent US-based study found increased hospitalizations related to infectious causes in the first year of life for this population of infants compared with HEU infants born to a mother with NPHIV.[60] Another postnatal study revealed that HEU infants of women with PHIV also showed decreased weight and length for their age throughout the first year of life.[61] The long-term potential comorbidities are uncertain but investigating targeted interventions to potentially mitigate these complications may be an area for future work.

SUMMARY AND FUTURE DIRECTIONS

The gynecologic and obstetric care of women with PHIV is complex and multifaceted. Women with PHIV have the unique experience of managing and with HIV as a lifelong disease and are more exposed to the health care industrial complex than other women in their peer group. Beyond the medical care of women with PHIV, there are added psychosocial determinants of health and health inequities that should also be evaluated and addressed, each of which may affect their obstetric and gynecologic health. We note multiple areas in need of future research, including understanding HPV vaccination uptake and efficacy, improving contraception use and counseling, and elucidating the pathways underlying the elevated rates of preterm birth among women with PHIV. Other areas of work include the potentially altered maternal-fetal interface and placentation in the setting of chronic immunosuppression and heightened inflammation and understanding the long-term health of HEU children born to women with PHIV. As young women with PHIV age worldwide in areas of low resource, the concerns brought up in this review need to be prioritized and addressed by collaborative efforts between the pediatric, obstetric, gynecologic, infectious disease, and public health communities.

REFERENCES

1. WHO, UNAIDS, UNICEF. Global HIV/AIDS response: epidemic update and health sector progress towards universal access, 2011 progress report. Geneva (Switzerland): World Health Organization; 2011.
2. Deeks SG. HIV infection, inflammation, immunosenescence, and aging. Annu Rev Med 2011;62:141–55.
3. Roider JM, Muenchhoff M, Goulder PJ. Immune activation and paediatric HIV-1 disease outcome. Curr Opin HIV AIDS 2016;11(2):146–55.
4. Barlow-Mosha L, Eckard AR, McComsey GA, et al. Metabolic complications and treatment of perinatally HIV-infected children and adolescents. J Int AIDS Soc 2013;16:18600.
5. Crane S, Sullivan M, Feingold M, et al. Successful pregnancy in an adolescent with perinatally acquired human immunodeficiency virus. Obstet Gynecol 1998;92(4 Pt 2):711.
6. Ghebre RG, Grover S, Xu MJ, et al. Cervical cancer control in HIV-infected women: past, present and future. Gynecol Oncol Rep 2017;21:101–8.
7. American College of Obstetricians and Gynecologists. Practice Bulletin No. 167: gynecologic care for women and adolescents with human immunodeficiency virus. Obstet Gynecol 2016;128(4):e89–110.

8. Masur H, Brooks JT, Benson CA, et al. Prevention and treatment of opportunistic infections in HIV-infected adults and adolescents: updated guidelines from the centers for disease control and prevention, National Institutes of Health, and HIV Medicine Association of the Infectious Diseases Society of America. Clin Infect Dis 2014;58(9):1308–11.

9. Setse R, Siberry GK, Moss WJ, et al. Cervical pap screening cytological abnormalities among HIV-infected adolescents in the LEGACY cohort. J Pediatr Adolesc Gynecol 2012;25(1):27–34.

10. Brogly SB, Watts DH, Ylitalo N, et al. Reproductive health of adolescent girls perinatally infected with HIV. Am J Public Health 2007;97(6):1047–52. Available at: https://www.ncbi.nlm.nih.gov/pmc/articles/PMC1874205/.

11. Abraham AG, Strickler HD, D'Souza G. Invasive cervical cancer risk among HIV-infected women is a function of CD4 count and screening. J Acquir Immune Defic Syndr 2013;63(5):e163.

12. Wheeler CM, Skinner SR, Del Rosario-Raymundo MR, et al. Efficacy, safety, and immunogenicity of the human papillomavirus 16/18 AS04-adjuvanted vaccine in women older than 25 years: 7-year follow-up of the phase 3, double-blind, randomised controlled VIVIANE study. Lancet Infect Dis 2016;16(10):1154–68.

13. Kojic EM, Rana AI, Cu-Uvin S. Human papillomavirus vaccination in HIV-infected women: need for increased coverage. Expert Rev Vaccines 2016;15(1):105–17.

14. Setse RW, Siberry GK, Gravitt PE, et al. Correlates of sexual activity and sexually transmitted infections among human immunodeficiency virus-infected youth in the LEGACY cohort, United States, 2006. Pediatr Infect Dis J 2011;30(11):967–73.

15. Koenig LJ, Pals SL, Chandwani S, et al. Sexual transmission risk behavior of adolescents with HIV acquired perinatally or through risky behaviors. J Acquir Immune Defic Syndr 2010;55(3):380–90.

16. Vermund SH, Wilson CM, Rogers AS, et al. Sexually transmitted infections among HIV infected and HIV uninfected high-risk youth in the REACH study. Reaching for excellence in adolescent care and health. J Adolesc Health 2001;29(3 Suppl):49–56.

17. Sutton M, Sternberg M, Koumans EH, et al. The prevalence of *Trichomonas vaginalis* infection among reproductive-age women in the United States, 2001–2004. Clin Infect Dis 2007;45(10):1319–26.

18. Torrone E, Papp J, Weinstock H, Centers for Disease Control and Prevention (CDC). Prevalence of *Chlamydia trachomatis* genital infection among persons aged 14–39 years—United States, 2007–2012. MMWR Morb Mortal Wkly Rep 2014;63(38):834–8.

19. LeFevre ML, U.S. Preventive Services Task Force. Screening for chlamydia and gonorrhea: U.S. Preventive Services Task Force recommendation statement. Ann Intern Med 2014;161(12):902–10.

20. Finer LB, Zolna MR. Shifts in intended and unintended pregnancies in the United States, 2001-2008. Am J Public Health 2014;104(Suppl 1):S43–8.

21. Kenny J, Williams B, Prime K, et al. Pregnancy outcomes in adolescents in the UK and Ireland growing up with HIV. HIV Med 2012;13(5):304–8.

22. Garcia PM, Kalish LA, Pitt J, et al. Maternal levels of plasma human immunodeficiency virus type 1 RNA and the risk of perinatal transmission. Women and Infants Transmission Study Group. N Engl J Med 1999;341(6):394–402. Available at: https://www.nejm.org/doi/full/10.1056/NEJM199908053410602.

23. Echenique M, Rodriguez VJ, LaCabe RP, et al. Behaviorally and perinatally HIV-infected young women: targets for preconception counseling. AIDS Care 2017; 29(3):372–7.

24. Jones DL, Echenique M, Potter J, et al. Adolescent girls and young women living with HIV: preconception counseling strategies. Int J Womens Health 2017;9: 657–63.

25. Chibber R, Khurranna A. Birth outcomes in perinatally HIV-infected adolescents and young adults in Manipur, India: a new frontier. Arch Gynecol Obstet 2005; 271(2):127–31.

26. American College of Obstetricians and Gynecologists. ACOG Committee Opinion number 313, September 2005. The importance of preconception care in the continuum of women's health care. Obstet Gynecol 2005;106(3):665–6.

27. Heffron R, Pintye J, Matthews LT, et al. PrEP as peri-conception HIV prevention for women and men. Curr HIV/AIDS Rep 2016;13(3):131–9.

28. Gregory KD, Johnson CT, Johnson TR, et al. The content of prenatal care. Update 2005. Womens Health Issues 2006;16(4):198–215.

29. Panel on treatment of pregnant women with HIV infection and prevention of perinatal transmission. Recommendations for use of antiretroviral drugs in transmission in the United States. Available at: http://aidsinfo.nih.gov/contentfiles/lvguidelines/PerinatalGL.pdf. Accessed November 21, 2018.

30. American College of Obstetricians and Gynecologists. ACOG Committee Opinion #296: first-trimester screening for fetal aneuploidy. Obstet Gynecol 2004;104(1):215–7.

31. American College of Obstetricians and Gynecologists. Practice Bulletin No. 162: prenatal diagnostic testing for genetic disorders. Obstet Gynecol 2016;127(5): e108–22.

32. Somigliana E, Bucceri AM, Tibaldi C, et al. Early invasive diagnostic techniques in pregnant women who are infected with the HIV: a multicenter case series. Am J Obstet Gynecol 2005;193(2):437–42.

33. Watts DH. Management of human immunodeficiency virus infection in pregnancy. N Engl J Med 2002;346(24):1879–91.

34. Lazenby GB, Mmeje O, Fisher BM, et al. Antiretroviral resistance and pregnancy characteristics of women with perinatal and nonperinatal HIV infection. Infect Dis Obstet Gynecol 2016;2016:4897501. Available at: https://www.ncbi.nlm.nih.gov/pmc/articles/PMC4930810/.

35. Paintsil E, Andiman WA. Update on successes and challenges regarding mother-to-child transmission of HIV. Curr Opin Pediatr 2009;21(1):94–101.

36. Centers for Disease Control and Prevention. HIV among pregnant women, infants, and children 2018. https://www.cdc.gov/hiv/group/gender/pregnantwomen/index.html. Accessed December 27, 2018.

37. Panel on treatment of HIV-infected pregnant women and prevention of perinatal transmission. Recommendations for use of antiretroviral drugs in pregnant HIV-1-infected women for maternal health and interventions to reduce perinatal HIV transmission in the United States. Available at: http://aidsinfo.nih.gov/contentfiles/lvguidelines/pediatricguidelines.pdf. Accessed October 20, 2018.

38. Badell ML, Kachikis A, Haddad LB, et al. Comparison of pregnancies between perinatally and sexually HIV-infected women: an observational study at an urban hospital. Infect Dis Obstet Gynecol 2013;2013:301763.

39. Calitri C, Gabiano C, Galli L, et al. The second generation of HIV-1 vertically exposed infants: a case series from the Italian Register for paediatric HIV infection. BMC Infect Dis 2014;14:277.

40. Prieto LM, Fernandez McPhee C, Rojas P, et al. Pregnancy outcomes in perinatally HIV-infected young women in Madrid, Spain: 2000–2015. PLoS One 2017; 12(8):e0183558.

41. Cruz ML, Santos E, Benamor Teixeira Mde L, et al. Viral suppression and resistance in a cohort of perinatally-HIV infected (PHIV+) pregnant women. Int J Environ Res Public Health 2016;13(6) [pii:E568].

42. Zash R, Makhema J, Shapiro RL. Neural-tube defects with dolutegravir treatment from the time of conception. N Engl J Med 2018;379(10):979–81.

43. American College of Obstetricians and Gynecologists. ACOG Committee Opinion No. 751: labor and delivery management of women with human immunodeficiency virus infection. Obstet Gynecol 2018;132(3):e131–7. Available at: https://www.ncbi.nlm.nih.gov/pubmed/30134427.

44. Munjal I, Dobroszycki J, Fakioglu E, et al. Impact of HIV-1 infection and pregnancy on maternal health: comparison between perinatally and behaviorally infected young women. Adolesc Health Med Ther 2013;4:51–8.

45. Phillips UK, Rosenberg MG, Dobroszycki J, et al. Pregnancy in women with perinatally acquired HIV-infection: outcomes and challenges. AIDS Care 2011;23(9): 1076–82.

46. Liu S, Liston RM, Joseph KS, et al. Maternal mortality and severe morbidity associated with low-risk planned cesarean delivery versus planned vaginal delivery at term. CMAJ 2007;176(4):455–60.

47. American College of Obstetricians and Gynecologists. ACOG Committee Opinion No. 736 summary: optimizing postpartum care. Obstet Gynecol 2018; 131(5):949–51.

48. Anderson EA, Momplaisir FM, Corson C, et al. Assessing the impact of perinatal HIV case management on outcomes along the HIV care continuum for pregnant and postpartum women living with HIV, Philadelphia 2005–2013. AIDS Behav 2017;21(9):2670–81.

49. American College of Obstetricians and Gynecologists. Committee Opinion no. 630. Screening for perinatal depression. Obstet Gynecol 2015;125(5):1268–71.

50. Gavin NI, Gaynes BN, Lohr KN, et al. Perinatal depression: a systematic review of prevalence and incidence. Obstet Gynecol 2005;106(5 Pt 1):1071–83.

51. Angrand RC, Sperling R, Roccobono K, et al. Depression in perinatally HIV-infected pregnant women compared to non-perinatally HIV-infected and HIV-uninfected pregnant women. AIDS Care 2018;30(9):1168–72. Available at: https://www.ncbi.nlm.nih.gov/pubmed/29776314.

52. Jao J, Sigel KM, Chen KT, et al. Small for gestational age birth outcomes in pregnant women with perinatally acquired HIV. AIDS 2012;26(7):855–9.

53. Byrne L, Sconza R, Foster C, et al. Pregnancy incidence and outcomes in women with perinatal HIV infection. AIDS 2017;31(12):1745–54.

54. Jao J, Kacanek D, Williams PL, et al. Birth weight and preterm delivery outcomes of perinatally vs nonperinatally human immunodeficiency virus-infected pregnant women in the United States: results from the PHACS SMARTT Study and IMPAACT P1025 Protocol. Clin Infect Dis 2017;65(6):982–9. Available at: https://www.ncbi.nlm.nih.gov/pmc/articles/PMC5849107/.

55. Lundberg P, Andersson R, Machado ES, et al. Pregnancy outcomes in young mothers with perinatally and behaviorally acquired HIV Infections in Rio de Janeiro. Braz J Infect Dis 2018;22(5):412–7.

56. Goodenough CJ, Patel K, Van Dyke RB, Pediatric HIV/AIDS Cohort Study (PHACS). Is there a higher risk of mother-to-child transmission of HIV among

pregnant women with perinatal HIV infection? Pediatr Infect Dis J 2018;37(12): 1267–70. Available at: https://www.ncbi.nlm.nih.gov/pubmed/29742647.

57. Hack M, Klein NK, Taylor HG. Long-term developmental outcomes of low birth weight infants. Future Child 1995;5(1):176–96.

58. Martin JA, Hamilton BE, Osterman MJK, et al. Births: final data for 2016. Natl Vital Stat Rep 2018;67(1):1–55.

59. Cruz ML, Cardoso CA, Joao EC, et al. Pregnancy in HIV vertically infected adolescents and young women: a new generation of HIV-exposed infants. AIDS 2010;24(17):2727–31.

60. Powis KM, Slogrove AL, Okorafor I, et al. Maternal perinatal HIV infection is associated with increased infectious morbidity in HIV-exposed uninfected infants. Pediatr Infect Dis J 2019;38(5):500–2.

61. Jao J, Agwu A, Mhango G, et al. Growth patterns in the first year of life differ in infants born to perinatally vs. nonperinatally HIV-infected women. AIDS 2015;29(1): 111–6. Available at: https://www.ncbi.nlm.nih.gov/pmc/articles/PMC4326225/.

HIV and Substance Use Disorder: Role of the HIV Physician

Christopher M. Bositis, MD, AAHIVS[a],*,
Joshua St. Louis, MD, MPH, AAHIVS[b]

KEYWORDS

- Syndemic • Persons who inject drugs (PWID) • Persons with HIV
- Injection drug use (IDU) • Substance use disorder (SUD)
- Pre-exposure prophylaxis (PrEP) • Syringe service programs (SSPs)
- Supervised injection facilities (SIFs)

KEY POINTS

- People with human immunodeficiency virus experience disproportionate substance use–related morbidity and mortality.
- Substance use disorders have a negative impact on human immunodeficiency virus–related outcomes including retention in care and viral load suppression.
- Evidence-based treatment for substance use disorders by human immunodeficiency virus clinicians is necessary to mitigate the worsened morbidity and mortality these patients experience.
- Adjuvant evidence-based interventions for human immunodeficiency virus–infected and at-risk persons with substance use disorder include naloxone, preexposure prophylaxis, syringe service programs, and supervised injection facilities.
- Physicians may need to serve as advocates to enact an effective national response to the human immunodeficiency virus and substance use disorder syndemic.

INTRODUCTION

Substance use disorders (SUDs) are formally defined in the *Diagnostic and Statistical Manual of Mental Disorders,* 5th edition, as maladaptive patterns of use with social, legal, and occupational consequences.[1] The relationship between human immunodeficiency virus (HIV) infection and SUDs is complex. HIV-infected individuals are more likely than their uninfected peers to suffer from SUD,[2,3] and some SUDs (opioid use disorder [OUD], stimulant use disorder) are risk factors for HIV acquisition, either because of associated intravenous injection, sexual practices, or both.[4,5]

Disclosure Statement: Neither author has any relevant financial disclosures to make.
[a] Greater Lawrence Family Health Center, 34 Haverhill Street, Lawrence, MA 01841, USA;
[b] Lawrence Family Medicine Residency, 34 Haverhill Street, Lawrence, MA 01841, USA
* Corresponding author.
E-mail address: cbositis@glfhc.org

Infect Dis Clin N Am 33 (2019) 835–855
https://doi.org/10.1016/j.idc.2019.04.006
0891-5520/19/© 2019 Elsevier Inc. All rights reserved.

id.theclinics.com

HIV-infected individuals with SUD have been found to have poorer outcomes across all aspects of the HIV care cascade.[2] Although the proportion of new HIV infections attributable to injection drug use (IDU) has decreased over time, the ongoing opioid epidemic poses a major threat to those gains as demonstrated by recent outbreaks in Indiana, Massachusetts, and West Virginia.[6–8] Given their key role at the intersection of these overlapping syndemics,[9] HIV physicians are uniquely situated to mitigate their impact at both the individual and public health levels, and thus should be well versed in the screening, diagnosis and treatment of SUD in HIV-infected and at-risk persons.

Although alcohol use disorder and tobacco use disorder may impact clinical outcomes of patients with HIV, this article focuses on disordered use of other substances, with a particular emphasis on OUD given its dramatic increase in the United States over the last decade.

HISTORY

A causative relationship between illicit use of amyl nitrate inhalants (poppers) and the immunodeficiency syndrome then referred to as gay-related immune deficiency (GRID) was posited early in the AIDS epidemic.[10,11] Although this association proved to be only correlative,[11] the association between HIV and SUD ultimately did prove to be important. The demographics of substance use in people with HIV has changed significantly over time, with heroin declining in popularity during the crack epidemic of the late 1980s[12] and returning to prominence more recently after the debut of extended-release oxycodone in 1996. Amyl nitrate inhalants fell out of favor in the gay male community in the 1990s and were rapidly replaced by methamphetamine, which remains an important risk factor for HIV.[12]

EPIDEMIOLOGY

The disordered use of virtually all substances (alcohol, stimulant, cannabis, opioid, and tobacco) is more prevalent in people with HIV than in the general population.[2] Of particular interest is the epidemiology of IDU and its impact on incident HIV infections. After decreasing steadily from 2008 to 2014 (48%, from 6604 to 3461), new HIV diagnoses attributable to IDU have stabilized.[13] Previous progress on this issue threatens to be reversed, fueled largely by the introduction of synthetic opioids such as fentanyl (**Fig. 1**). Several HIV outbreaks monitored by the Centers for Disease Control and Prevention have been tied to worsening prevalence of OUD, including the 2015 outbreak in Scott County, Indiana,[6] and similar recent outbreaks in Massachusetts[7] and West Virginia.[8]

IMPACT OF SUBSTANCE USE ON ENGAGEMENT, RETENTION, AND VIRAL SUPPRESSION

Studies of the effects of substance use on the HIV care cascade are limited; those that do exist focus primarily on people with HIV who inject drugs.[2] A systematic review demonstrated that HIV-infected people who inject drugs (PWID) have lower rates of engagement, retention and viral suppression compared with those who do not.[2] Similarly, a 2010 review demonstrated that, in the 5 countries with the largest HIV epidemics among PWID, these patients accounted for only 25% of patients receiving antiretroviral therapy (ART) despite comprising 67% of all total cases of HIV.[14] A more recent study showed that only 57% of people with HIV

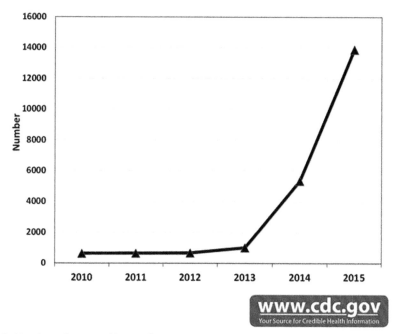

Fig. 1. Number of reported law enforcement encounters testing positive for fentanyl in the United States: 2010 to 2015. (*From* https://www.cdc.gov/drugoverdose/data/fentanyl-le-reports.html. Accessed December 17, 2018.)

and comorbid SUD were retained in care.[15] Finally, it is clear from a number of studies that SUDs (in particular those involving IDU) have a significant negative impact on viral suppression in people with HIV[16] including both OUD[17] and stimulant use disorder (notably methamphetamine).[18] Most of these studies have shown a dose-dependent relationship between lower levels of substance use and higher rates of viral suppression,[19] highlighting that abstinence is not required to improve HIV-related outcomes.

IMPACT OF SUBSTANCE USE DISORDER ON MORBIDITY AND MORTALITY

HIV-infected patients with SUD continue to suffer from disproportionately high all-cause mortality, often from non–HIV-related causes such as overdose, accidents, and suicide.[20–22] This disparity is highlighted by recent data demonstrating that, although the overall risk of death among HIV-infected individuals in the United States decreased by more than 10% from 2011 to 2015, the risk of death from overdose in this population increased by 43% during the same period.[23] Stigma, lack of access to SUD treatment, and comorbid psychiatric problems and infectious diseases perpetuate a vicious cycle of disengagement and worsening illness (**Fig. 2**), which ultimately leads to the excess mortality seen in these patients. A decrease in this mortality is likely to occur only through the expansion of SUD treatment and ART coverage as well as breaking down the complex systemic barriers (eg, criminalization) that contribute to this cycle.[24] Importantly, ART has been found to be just as effective in PWID as in those who do not inject drugs.[16] Moreover, a significant proportion of the excess mortality seen is likely related to untreated chronic hepatitis C virus

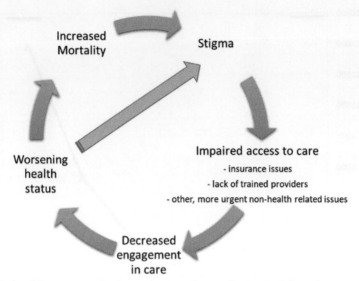

Fig. 2. Cycle of factors contributing to increased mortality in HIV-infected PWID.

(HCV) infection,[25] and given the high cure rates of HCV treatment including among those with SUD[26] there is hope that this cycle can be broken and that mortality rates can improve.

SCREENING FOR SUBSTANCE USE DISORDER

Screening, brief intervention, and referral to treatment is an approach that has been widely implemented based on its efficacy in reducing problem alcohol and tobacco use,[27] although its impact on reducing risky substance use (ie, substance use that puts the patient at risk of developing a SUD[28]) is less clear.[29–31] Nonetheless, the first step to effective treatment of any SUD begins with screening and identification of this problem where it exists. To that end, multiple easy to administer and evidence-based screening tools are available (see **Table 3**). The NM-ASSIST, in particular, is a short, validated screen based on the single question screening test for drug use in primary care (**Box 1**)[32,33] that can be easily integrated into the routine history and provides accompanying resources to help clinicians ensure that patients at risk get appropriate follow-up and treatment.

TREATMENT OF SUBSTANCE USE DISORDER

The treatment of SUD is well within the scope of practice of HIV clinicians.[3] Several, including OUD, may be treated with US Food and Drug Administration (FDA)–

Box 1
Single question screening test for disordered drug use[33]

How many times in the past year have you used an illegal drug or used a prescription medication for nonmedical reasons?

approved medications, although others are treated with behavioral interventions alone. The body of literature supporting the treatments of various SUDs continues to grow, and clinicians are encouraged to attempt treatment even when data are less than robust given the significant benefits of decreased use on HIV-related outcomes. All of the treatments discussed in this article are associated with significant benefit for people with HIV, including improvements in engagement and retention, viral suppression rates, and mortality, and decreased rates of opportunistic infections.[3,17]

Opioid Use Disorder

Although a number of behavioral interventions have been studied in the treatment of OUD (cognitive–behavioral therapy, talk therapy, inpatient detoxification, and group-based abstinence treatment),[34–36] treatment with one of the three FDA-approved medications for treatment of OUD has been shown to be most effective.[28,37] Importantly, methadone and buprenorphine have been shown to significantly improve patient mortality compared with behavioral interventions (in particular inpatient detoxification) or placebo owing largely to a significant decrease in relapse and accidental overdose deaths.[36] Given these compelling data, we recommend prompt initiation of OUD treatment for anyone with HIV and a concomitant OUD who presents to care. There are benefits and drawbacks to each of the 3 medications used, and the decision to initiate one over the others is based on patient preference, severity of OUD, existence of comorbid SUDs, and availability of the 3 options (**Table 1**).

Methadone is a full opioid agonist with extensive data supporting its use. Unlike many illicit and prescription opioids, methadone produces only a minimal high owing to its long half-life. Given its overdose risk, methadone is the most highly regulated of the 3 FDA-approved medications for treatment of OUD and may only be dispensed by federally recognized opioid treatment programs. Patients treated with methadone must follow strict rules (see **Table 1**); failure to do so may incur swift penalties and eventual expulsion from the program.[28] Methadone has the strongest evidence base of the 3 available OUD treatment options. Treatment with methadone improves mortality and is more effective than buprenorphine or naltrexone,[28] in particular showing longer retention in treatment and fewer relapses.

Buprenorphine is a partial opioid agonist that has a large and growing body of evidence to support its use. As a partial agonist, overdose with buprenorphine is extremely unlikely so it is less regulated than methadone. Unlike methadone, buprenorphine may be prescribed by any clinician who has completed the requirements to obtain the Drug Addiction Treatment Act 2000 waiver.[38] Novel delivery forms of buprenorphine include a once monthly subcutaneous injection (Subloclade), implantable subcutaneous rods (Probuphine), and a transdermal patch (Butrans). The latter is not FDA approved for treatment of OUD, and insurance and logistical issues have thus far limited use of the injection and subcutaneous implants in clinical practice.[28,39]

Naltrexone is an opioid antagonist that is approved for the treatment of both OUD and alcohol use disorder. As a once monthly injection (Vivitrol), extended-release naltrexone has no overdose potential and thus is the least regulated of the 3 OUD treatment options. Initiation of extended-release naltrexone requires a period of abstinence from other opioids (generally 7 days for short-acting opioids, 10 days for buprenorphine, and 14 days for methadone) or it will precipitate withdrawal. The newest of the 3 treatment, extended-release naltrexone has not shown a mortality benefit; however, the number of studies published on it thus far is small.[37]

Table 1
Comparison of medication-assisted treatment options for OUD

	Methadone	Buprenorphine	Naltrexone (As Extended-Release Naltrexone)
Date of approval	1972	2002	2006
Mechanism of action	Full opioid agonist	Partial opioid agonist	Opioid antagonist
Administration	Oral liquid	Sublingual tab or film; SQ injection; SQ implant	Deep IM injection
Treatment setting	Methadone opioid treatment program	No restrictions on setting	No restrictions on setting
Prescribing restrictions	Only may be dispensed by a physician in an opioid treatment program	May be prescribed by any physician who has a Drug Addiction Treatment Act 2000 waiver (8 h training required)	No restrictions on prescribing
Patient requirements	Daily visits for ≥3 mo, maximum take-home allowance is 2 weeks, required counseling	Weekly visits until appropriate urine drug screens ×6, maximum prescription duration is 2 months, may require counseling	Usually monthly visits, but may space clinician visits to less often, may require counseling
Overdose risk	High (in combination with illicit opioids and BZDs, usually in times of relapse)	Minimal (blocks binding of other opioids, some risk with BZDs)	Minimal (blocks binding of other opioids, some risk owing to decreased opioid tolerance with relapse)
Preferred patient characteristics	High opioid tolerance Large daily dose of opioids Concomitant chronic pain History of failing other OUD treatment Pregnancy Desires high degree of structure Desires daily counseling	Low to moderate opioid tolerance Low to moderate daily dose of opioids Desire for flexibility Treatment with EFV Complex medication regimen Pregnancy	Intermittent opioid use Concomitant alcohol use disorder Complex medication regimen Treatment with EFV Desire for flexibility Desire for nonopioid treatment Unable to take daily medicine
Not preferred patient characteristics	Restrictive job/home schedules Concerns about stigma Treatment with EFV (possibly also with DRV, ATV, or RPV) Prolonged QTc interval	History of failing other OUD treatment High opioid tolerance Large daily dose of opioids Chronic BZD use Decompensated cirrhosis	Daily opioid use High opioid tolerance Large daily dose of opioids Desires daily counseling Requires continued opioids Decompensated cirrhosis

Abbreviations: ATV, atazanavir; BZD, benzodiazepine; DRV, darunavir; EFV, efavirenz; IM, intramuscularly; SQ, subcutaneously.
Data from Herron AJ, Brennan TK. The ASAM Essentials of Addiction Medicine. 3rd ed. Philadelphia, PA: Wolters Kluwer; 2020.

Some individuals struggling with addiction may be hesitant to consider OUD treatment owing to concerns about replacing one addiction with another. Although we strive to create a safe space for patients to voice such concerns, we also work with them to clarify the difference between addiction (which does not apply to OUD treatment) and dependence (which does), and highlight the overdose and mortality benefits from these medicines compared with inpatient detoxification and rehabilitation.

Stimulant Use Disorder

Both cocaine and methamphetamine use disorders are particular health hazards for people with HIV; methamphetamine use disorder is the predominant SUD in this population in some parts of the country.[2,5] Psychotherapeutic interventions such as cognitive–behavioral therapy and contingency management are efficacious in the management of stimulant use disorder.[40,41] Unfortunately, few medications have proven so and none have gained FDA approval for this indication.[28] In our practice, we consider a trial of a medication with higher quality evidence (topiramate or long-acting stimulants)[42,43] for the treatment of cocaine use disorder in addition to psychotherapeutic interventions in patients when it seems to be having a negative effect on the management of the patient's HIV or concomitant OUD. With regard to methamphetamine use disorder, we strongly emphasize psychosocial treatments and consider the use of either mirtazapine[44] or bupropion[45] if the patient also meets criteria for a mood disorder.

Notable Drug–Drug Interactions

Important drug–drug interactions between medications for OUD and antiretrovirals are highlighted in **Table 2**.

RESOURCES FOR BEGINNING TREATMENTS FOR SUBSTANCE USE DISORDER IN YOUR PRACTICE

Many clinicians are anxious or ambivalent about treating SUD in their practice, in particular treating OUD with buprenorphine. Reasons for not doing so are varied and include concerns about its complexity and how time consuming it might be, despite the reality that it is simpler than many other common primary care treatments and often highly rewarding.[46] Others may express concerns about diversion; although this concern is real, a recent study showed that buprenorphine is rarely abused when diverted and is usually used by people who are seeking treatment but cannot access it.[47] Still others are concerned that they will become a magnet for these patients, overwhelming their staff and capabilities, owing to the paucity of clinicians available to treat OUD.[48]

Table 3 lists a number of resources to support clinicians starting OUD treatment in their practice. Although getting started may feel overwhelming[48] and full staffing may not always be available to allow for observed buprenorphine inductions, excellent evidence exists that unmonitored self-induction is safe and effective[49]; it is also important to remember that buprenorphine is safe, has a minimal risk of overdose, and has the potential to save the lives of those to whom it is prescribed.

STRATEGIES FOR HARM REDUCTION

Despite its effectiveness, not everyone with a SUD is ready to start treatment, underscoring the importance of a harm reductionist approach for such persons.

Table 2
Notable drug-drug interactions between SUD treatments and HIV medicines

Antiretroviral Medicine	Effect on ART	Effect on SUD Treatment	Management
Elvitegravir/cobicistat	None anticipated with methadone or buprenorphine	Increases in buprenorphine levels	Monitor for signs of opioid toxicity, no adjustment usually needed
Darunavir (boosted)	None anticipated with methadone or buprenorphine	Modest increase in norbuprenorphine levels Decreases in methadone levels	Monitor for signs of opioid toxicity, no adjustment usually needed Monitor for signs of withdrawal and adjust methadone dose as needed
Atazanavir (boosted or unboosted)	Possible decrease in ATV concentration if administered unboosted with buprenorphine	Increases in buprenorphine levels (with boosted ATV) Decreases in methadone levels (with boosted ATV)	Monitor for signs of opioid toxicity, titrate using lowest initial dose Monitor for signs of withdrawal and adjust methadone dose as needed
Efavirenz	None anticipated with methadone or buprenorphine	Potential decreases in buprenorphine levels Decreases in methadone levels	Monitor for signs of withdrawal, no dose adjustment of buprenorphine usually needed Monitor for signs of withdrawal and adjust methadone dose as needed
Etravirine	None anticipated with methadone or buprenorphine	Potential decreases in buprenorphine levels	Monitor for signs of withdrawal, no dose adjustment of buprenorphine usually needed
Rilpivirine	None anticipated with methadone or buprenorphine	Slight decrease in methadone levels	Monitor for signs of withdrawal, no dose adjustment of methadone usually needed

This material was accessed on [9/5/2019] on the HIV Clinical Resource website (www.hivguidelines.org). The HIV Clinical Guidelines Program is a collaborative effort of the New York State Department of Health AIDS Institute and the Johns Hopkins University Division of Infectious Diseases. Copyright © Johns Hopkins University HIV Clinical Guidelines Program 2000–2016.

Table 3
Clinician resources

Resource	Location	Description
American Society of Addiction Medicine Fundamentals of Addiction Medicine 40 Hour CME Course	https://elearning.asam.org/products/the-asam-fundamentals-of-addiction-medicine-40-hour-cme-program-online	Online program aimed at primary care and other clinicians to empower them to identify, treat, and/or refer patients at risk for or with addiction.
National Institute on Drug Abuse Drug Screening and Assessment Resources	https://www.drugabuse.gov/nidamed-medical-health-professionals/tool-resources-your-practice/screening-assessment-drug-testing-resources/chart-evidence-based-screening-tools	Chart of evidence-based screening tools and resources based on substance type, patient age, and how administered, with links to the tools themselves
Clinical Guidelines Program—HIV and Substance Use (New York State Department of Health AIDS Institute)	https://www.hivguidelines.org/substance-use/	Extensive set of state-level guidelines on the management of SUDs in people with HIV
Clinical Guidelines Program—HIV and Substance Use Treatment Drug-Drug Interactions (New York State Department of Health AIDS Institute)	https://www.hivguidelines.org/substance-use/drug-drug-interactions/#tab_7	Exhaustive review of all relevant drug–drug interactions between antiretroviral medicines and medicines used for the treatment of SUDs.
DEA-X Drug Addiction Treatment Act waiver training	https://www.asam.org/education/live-online-cme/waiver-training	Free courses to complete the requirements to be able to prescribe buprenorphine
Fundamentals of Addiction Medicine ECHO Series	https://www.asam.org/education/live-online-cme/fundamentals-program/fame-teleecho	Interactive 16-week video conference series for clinicians that addresses topics in the field of addiction medicine and reviews patient cases
HIV Medicine Association Policy Statements	https://www.hivma.org/policy-advocacy/policy-amp-advocacy/	Database of all policy statements produced by the HIV Medicine Association for advocacy-related activities
Integrating Buprenorphine Treatment for Opioid Use Disorder in Primary Care	http://cahpp.org/wp-content/uploads/2017/06/Buprenorphine-Implementation-Manual-for-Primary-Care-Settings-.pdf	Toolkit developed by a multiuniversity collaborative to provide resources and support for clinicians starting an outpatient buprenorphine treatment program

(continued on next page)

Table 3
(continued)

Resource	Location	Description
National HIV Curriculum (University of Washington and AETC National Coordinating Resource Center)	https://www.hiv.uw.edu/go/basic-primary-care/substance-use-disorders/core-concept/all	Online program aimed at primary care and other clinicians focused on teaching the management of HIV and cooccurring conditions, including SUD
"The Nature of Addiction and HIV" and "How Change Happens: Substance Use Disorders and HIV/AIDS" (University of California Los Angeles, Pacific Southwest ATTC, and AETC Pacific)	http://www.uclaisap.org/slides/psattc/nature-change-paetc.html	Online curricula focused on the management of SUDs in people with HIV
Project SHOUT (Support for Hospital Opioid Use Disorder Treatment)	https://www.projectshout.org/	Guidelines, toolkits, and webinars to support clinicians treating SUDs (in particular OUD) in hospitalized adults
Substance Use Management Clinical Consultation Center (University of California San Francisco)	https://nccc.ucsf.edu/clinician-consultation/substance-use-management/	Free online consultation service with SUD experts at the University of California San Francisco. Consults can be submitted by email or by phone
State Targeted Response Technical Assistance (Substance Abuse and Mental Health Services Administration)	https://www.getstr-ta.org/	Technical assistance consortium funded by Substance Abuse and Mental Health Services Administration to provide support and local expertise to help projects focused on addressing the opioid crisis

---

Box 2
Five key questions to promote harm reduction

- When you use street drugs, what do you use and how (including associated rituals)? How much do you use?
- Where do you get your equipment (syringes, needles, cookers, water, cotton)?
- When did do you last share any of the above?
- Have you ever overdosed in the past? What happened?
- How do you support your drug use?

Although the principles of harm reduction have been recognized as a key part of the response to the HIV epidemic since its earliest days, most providers trained in the traditional medical model remain reluctant partners in implementing these principles into their practice with patients.[50] The harm reduction model begins with fostering open, honest communication between the clinician and the patient; this process can be far more difficult in practice than it would seem at face value. Although the principles and practice of motivational interviewing are beyond the scope of this article, the following video is an example of a respectful, nonjudgmental interaction: https://www.youtube.com/watch?v=TGhj06-sM2Y.

To help clinicians integrate harm reduction principles more seamlessly into their practice, we propose 5 basic questions to ask patients with known SUD, as well as a simple harm reduction package that should be reviewed at each visit (**Boxes 2 and 3**). The remainder of this section discusses the evidence behind these and other key harm reduction interventions; treatment of SUD, likely the most effective such intervention, is discussed in detail elsewhere in this article.

Overdose Prevention

Overdose death, primarily opioid related, is now the leading cause of accidental death in the United States, and in 2017 claimed more than 70,000 lives (**Fig. 3**).[51] Naloxone is an opioid antagonist that can reverse opioid-related overdose and is now available through either third-party or non–patient-specific prescriptions in almost every state (**Table 4**).[52] Moreover, when combined with preexposure prophylaxis (PrEP) and linkage to addiction treatment, naloxone distribution was found to significantly decrease the number of HIV and overdose-related deaths, and increase life expectancy by 3 years, when compared with no additional intervention in one recent modeling study.[53] Practical steps that can be taken to reduce the risk of overdose for persons

---

Box 3
Essential harm reduction package

- Overdose prevention: naloxone; practical ways to reduce risk of overdose ("Getting Off Right" publication; see text)
- Prevention of infectious complications other than HIV: where to get clean needles and equipment (syringe service programs [SSPs] where available); safer injecting practices ("Getting Off Right" publication; see text)
- HIV prevention: SSPs, preexposure prophylaxis, condom use

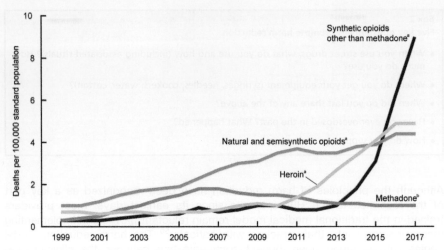

Fig. 3. Age-adjusted drug overdose death rates, by opioid category: United States, 1999 to 2017. [a] Significant increasing trend from 1999 through 2017 with different rates of change over time (P<.05). [b] Significant increasing trend from 1999 through 2006, then decreasing trend from 2006 through 2017 (P<.05). Deaths are classified using the *International Classification of Diseases, 10th Revision*. Drug poisoning (overdose) deaths are identified using underlying cause-of-death codes X40–X44, X60–X64, X85, and Y10–Y14. Drug overdose deaths involving selected drug categories are identified by specific multiple causes of death codes: heroin, T40.1; natural and semisynthetic opioids, T40.2; methadone, T40.3; and synthetic opioids other than methadone, T40.4. Deaths involving more than 1 opioid category (eg, a death involving both methadone and a natural and semisynthetic opioid) are counted in both categories. The percentage of drug overdose deaths that identified the specific drugs involved varied by year, with ranges of 75% to 79% from 1999 through 2013 and 81% to 88% from 2014 through 2017 SOURCE: NCHS, National Vital Statistics System, Mortality. (*From* https://www.cdc.gov/nchs/products/databriefs/db329.htm, Accessed May 29, 2019.)

Table 4
Naloxone prescription variation

Naloxone Prescription Model	What Is It?	Which States Permit the Model?
Traditional	Provider generated prescription to patients at risk of OD	All 50 states and the Washington, DC
Third-party	Prescription issued by a provider to a person not at risk of OD for use on someone else	45 states and Washington, DC Not permitted in DE, MN, KS, MO, VA
Non–patient-specific; includes: Standing orders Collaborative practice agreements Protocol orders	Authorize naloxone distribution to individuals and organizations that meet specific criteria without direct interaction with a provider	49 states and Washington, DC Not permitted in NE

Abbreviation: OD, overdose.
From https://www.samhsa.gov/capt/sites/default/files/resources/naloxone-access-laws-tool.pdf

with SUD include starting with a test dose and using with another, trusted person around.[54]

Preexposure Prophylaxis

PrEP to prevent HIV infection has been found to be effective in PWID. In the Bangkok Tenofovir (TDF) Study, use of TDF reduced incident HIV infections by almost 50% overall, and by 84% in those who were highly adherent.[55,56] Despite its clear benefits, PrEP remains vastly underused in this population, with fewer than 1% of PWID in one study ever having received it.[57] In practice, several important challenges related to PrEP use in this population exist including relatively low awareness about PrEP, lack of access to PrEP, and cost. Most PWID are eligible for PrEP, either because of their injection practices, sexual practices, or both, and a significant percentage report that they would be willing to take it when asked[58]; however, as many as two-thirds of those surveyed in one study had never heard of it.[59] Factors impacting access to PrEP are varied and include limited engagement with the health system, lack of insurance, as well as provider and/or patient reluctance to discuss PrEP, often owing to embarrassment, fear, or concerns about partner disclosure.[58,59] Although studies on the cost effectiveness of PrEP in PWID have been conflicting,[60,61] it seems that PrEP may be most effective when combined with other interventions, when IDU is a significant driver of the local HIV epidemic, and when PrEP is targeted toward those PWID at highest risk.[62,63] Taken together, these data underscore the need for clinicians to use open, nonjudgmental language with their patients (see video link elsewhere in this article), and to discuss PrEP as a potential option in the HIV prevention toolkit.

Syringe Service Programs

SSPs (also referred to as needle exchange programs) are an effective way of decreasing needle and other drug use-related equipment sharing. Evidence that such programs reduce HIV prevention to date is modest but growing,[64–66] and the Centers for Disease Control and Prevention recently urged local health departments to expand SSP access to combat the threat of HIV, viral hepatitis, and other infectious complications of IDU.[67]

Where local SSP programs are not available, many states allow individuals to buy needles and syringes through a pharmacy without a prescription, and this practice is specifically prohibited in only 2 states (**Fig. 4**). When new needles are not available, the Harm Reduction Coalition's "Getting Off Right – A Safety Manual for Injection Drug Users" providers clear English-language instructions on safe injection practices, including the safest way to clean needles when no other options exist.[54]

Supervised Injection Facilities

Although there are no supervised injection facilities (SIFs) currently operational in the United States, largely because of legal and political obstacles, support for their use among US physicians is growing.[68,69] This support is based on a robust body of evidence from SIFs elsewhere demonstrating that they are associated with reductions in overdose-related morbidity and mortality, decreased drug-related risk behaviors, increased access to OUD treatment and health care in general, decreased public drug use, decreased discarded needles, and no change in crime in the neighborhoods where they are located.[70,71] Although many arguments are made about the potentially negative consequences of such sites (largely countered by the aforementioned data), few consider the negative consequences of not having them available, such as the evidence that public injecting is associated with higher viral loads among HIV-infected PWID.[72] Moreover, they have the potential to be highly cost saving: a recent modeling

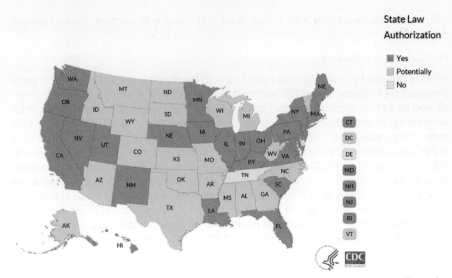

Fig. 4. July 2016 assessment of whether a state or Washington, DC, law exists that allows the retail sale of syringes and needles to a person who injects drugs. (*From* https://www.cdc.gov/hepatitis/policy/RetailSaleOfSyringes.htm; downloaded 12/23/18)

study estimated that a hypothetical SIF in Baltimore could save nearly $8 million annually through the prevention of hospitalizations for infection-related complications, new HIV and HCV infections, and overdose deaths.[73]

IMPROVING CARE FOR HUMAN IMMUNODEFICIENCY VIRUS–INFECTED AND AT-RISK PERSONS WITH SUBSTANCE USE DISORDER

Various interventions and care models have been proposed to address the HIV care cascade gaps among HIV-infected PWID, with mixed results. Such interventions include adherence counseling, patient navigation, directly observed therapy, financial incentives, and SUD treatment itself.[74] Project HOPE, one of the largest randomized controlled trials to look at the impact of 2 of these programs (patient navigation and financial incentives) showed improved viral suppression rates at 6 months, but this benefit was not sustained 6 months after the intervention was removed.[75] Not surprisingly, the intervention with the greatest benefit on ART outcomes is SUD treatment itself as detailed elsewhere in this article (**Fig. 5**). Although data on OUD treatment on mortality in HIV-infected PWID have been mixed,[17] a recent study from Vancouver demonstrated that both OUD and ART conferred significant mortality benefits, with the greatest reduction in mortality occurring among those who received both.[76]

To address this complexity, novel models of care are needed. One such model that is gaining traction is a comprehensive integrated services model, where members of the same care team are able to provide services in 4 key areas: SUD treatment, treatment of HIV and HCV, behavioral health services, and access to PrEP and additional harm reduction services such as SSP.[77] Although establishing or transitioning to such a model may seem daunting, we would point out that, for most HIV practice settings, the key missing link is SUD treatment. Ensuring that providers are licensed to prescribe buprenorphine is all that is needed to provide this integration. Additional models that are being explored to enhance and improve integration include the use of Internet- and cell phone-based technologies,[77] as well as low-threshold[78,79] and mobile SUD treatment.[80]

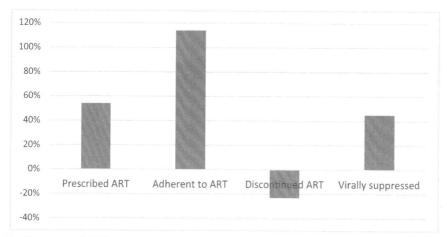

Fig. 5. Impact of OUD treatment on HIV treatment outcomes in PWID (expressed as change in likelihood of specific outcome). (*Adapted from* Low AJ, Mbaru G, Welton NJ, et al. Impact of opioid substitution therapy on antiretroviral therapy outcomes: A systematic review and meta-analysis. *CID.* 2016;63(8):1094-1104; with permission.)

CRIMINALIZATION OF DRUG USE AND OTHER STRUCTURAL FACTORS

It is difficult to estimate the exact impact that sociostructural factors such as stigma, unstable housing, and the criminalization of drug use have on overall morbidity and mortality among HIV-infected and at-risk PWID. However, a recent comprehensive review demonstrated that drug use criminalization was consistently associated with negative impact on HIV prevention and treatment.[81] The framework proposed by Parashar and colleagues[24] (**Fig. 6**) provides an elegant conceptualization of the many different such factors that must be addressed to see significant and lasting improvements in health outcomes in this population.

PHYSICIAN AS ADVOCATE

A truly effective response to the overlapping SUD and HIV syndemic will ultimately require physicians to embrace the role of advocate. Effective advocacy begins at the individual level, with physicians working with other members of the health care team to ensure that those suffering from SUD have access to available treatments and other evidence-based interventions to improve their health outcomes. The physician voice is critical in the fight to decrease the stigma against SUD in our communities, to reform clinical education and training to expand the number of qualified SUD treatment providers, and to address the ongoing criminalization of SUD and other policy barriers that currently impede an effective and coordinated response to this syndemic.[82] Toward that end, the Infectious Diseases Society of America and the HIV Medical Association have released a number of thoughtful, relevant policy statements (see **Table 3**) that we can and should use in such efforts.

RESOURCES FOR CLINICIANS

Table 3 details a variety of helpful resources for the HIV provider caring for persons suffering from SUD. These include educational resources from the American Society of Addiction Medicine, training programs to obtain the Drug Addiction Treatment Act

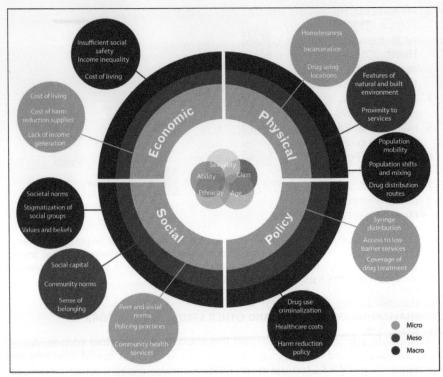

Fig. 6. Sociostructural factors impacting HIV-infected PWID. (*From* Parashar S, Collins AB, Montaner JS, Hogg RS, Milloy MJ. Reducing rates of preventable HIV/AIDS-associated mortality among people with HIV who inject drugs. *Curr Opin HIV AIDS.* 2016;11(5):507–513; with permission.)

2000 buprenorphine waiver, as well as toolkits for starting both outpatient and inpatient SUD treatment programs.

SUMMARY

The ongoing syndemic of SUD and HIV threatens progress made in preventing new infections and improving outcomes among those infected. To address this challenge effectively, HIV physicians can and must take an increased role in the screening, diagnosis, and treatment of SUDs. Such treatment decreases HIV risk behaviors and improves both HIV and SUD-related outcomes. Ultimately, however, an effective response to this syndemic will require increased access to adjuvant interventions like overdose prevention, SSPs, PrEP, and safe injection facilities as well as a radical movement away from the current stigmatization and criminalization of those suffering from SUDs. Physicians can play a key role in propelling the sociostructural changes needed to make this happen by advocating for their patients at both the individual and community levels.

REFERENCES

1. American Psychiatric Association. Diagnostic and statistical manual of mental disorders. 5th edition. Washington, DC: American Psychiatric Association; 2013.

2. Mimiaga MJ, Reisner SL, Grasso C, et al. Substance use among HIV-infected patients engaged in primary care in the United States: findings from the Centers for AIDS Research Network of Integrated Clinical Systems cohort. Am J Public Health 2013;103(8):1457–67.
3. Jacquet JM, Peyriere H, Makinson A, et al. Psychoactive substances, alcohol and tobacco consumption in HIV-infected outpatients. AIDS 2018;32(9):1165–71.
4. Klinkenberg W, Sacks S. Mental disorders and drug abuse in persons living with HIV/AIDS. AIDS Care 2004;16(suppl):22–42.
5. Halkitis PN, Parsons JT, Stirratt MJ. A double epidemic: crystal methamphetamine drug use in relation to HIV transmission. J Homosex 2001;41(2):17–25.
6. Peters PJ, Pontones P, Hoover KW, et al. HIV infection linked to injection use of oxymorphone in Indiana, 2014-2015. N Engl J Med 2016;375(3):229–39.
7. Cranston K, Alpren C, John B, et al. Notes from the field: HIV diagnoses among persons who inject drugs – northeastern Massachusetts, 2015-2018. MMWR Morb Mortal Wkly Rep 2019;68(10):253–4.
8. Evans ME, Labuda SM, Hogan V, et al. Notes from the field: HIV infection investigation in a rural area- West Virginia, 2017. MMWR Morb Mortal Wkly Rep 2018; 67(8):257–8.
9. Singer M, Bulled N, Ostrach B, et al. Syndemics and the biosocial conception of health. Lancet 2017;389(10072):941–50.
10. Goedert JJ, Neuland CY, Wallen WC, et al. Amyl nitrite may alter T lymphocytes in homosexual men. Lancet 1982;1(8269):412–6.
11. Shilts R. And the band played on: politics, people, and the AIDS epidemic. New York: St. Martin's Griffin; 1987.
12. Hari J. Chasing the scream: the first and last days of the war on drugs. New York: Bloomsbury; 2015.
13. Wejnert C, Hess KL, Hall HI, et al. Vital signs: trends in HIV diagnoses, risk behaviors, and prevention among persons who inject drugs- United States. MMWR Morb Mortal Wkly Rep 2016;65(47):1336–42.
14. Wolfe D, Carrieri MP, Shepard D. Treatment and care for injection drug users with HIV infection: a review of barriers and ways forward. Lancet 2010;376:355–66.
15. Aralis HJ, Shoptaw S, Brookmeyer R, et al. Psychiatric illness, substance use, and viral suppression among HIV-positive men of color who have sex with men in Los Angeles. AIDS Behav 2018;22:3117–29.
16. Wood E, Hogg RS, Lima VD, et al. Highly active antiretroviral therapy and survival in HIV-infected injection drug users. JAMA 2008;300(5):550–4.
17. Low AJ, Mbaru G, Welton NJ, et al. Impact of opioid substitution therapy on antiretroviral therapy outcomes: a systematic review and meta-analysis. Clin Infect Dis 2016;63(8):1094–104.
18. Feldman MB, Thomas JA, Alexy ER, et al. Crystal methamphetamine use and HIV medical outcomes among HIV-infected men who have sex with men accessing support services in New York. Drug Alcohol Depend 2015;147:266–71.
19. Carrico AW, Hunt PW, Neilands TB, et al. Stimulant use and viral suppression in the era of universal antiretroviral therapy. J Acquir Immune Defic Syndr 2018; 80(1):89–93.
20. DeLorenze GN, Weisner C, Tsai AL, et al. Excess mortality among HIV-infected patients diagnosed with substance use dependence or abuse receiving care in a fully integrated medical care program. Alcohol Clin Exp Res 2011;35(2): 203–10.
21. Suárez-García I, Sobrino-Vegas P, Dalmau D, et al. Cohort of the Spanish HIV Research Network (CoRIS). Clinical outcomes of patients infected with HIV

through use of injected drugs compared to patients infected through sexual transmission: late presentation, delayed anti-retroviral treatment and higher mortality. Addiction 2016;111(7):1235–45.

22. Young J, Psichogiou M, Meyer L, et al. CD4 cell count and the risk of AIDS or death in HIV-Infected adults on combination antiretroviral therapy with a suppressed viral load: a longitudinal cohort study from COHERE. PLoS Med 2012; 9(3):e1001194.

23. Bosh KA, Crepaz N, Dong X, et al. Opioid overdose deaths among persons with HIV infection, United States, 2011-2015. Oral abstract at: Conference on Retroviruses and Opportunistic Infections. Seattle, WA, March 4–7, 2019.

24. Parashar S, Collins AB, Montaner JS, et al. Reducing rates of preventable HIV/AIDS-associated mortality among people living with HIV who inject drugs. Curr Opin HIV AIDS 2016;11(5):507–13.

25. May MT, Justice AC, Birnie K, et al. Injection drug use and hepatitis C as risk factors for mortality in HIV-infected individuals: the Antiretroviral Therapy Cohort Collaboration. J Acquir Immune Defic Syndr 2015;69(3):348–54.

26. Grebely J, Dalgard O, Conway B, et al. Sofosbuvir and velpatasvir for hepatitis C virus infection in people with recent injection drug use (SIMPLIFY): an open-label, single-arm, phase 4, multicentre trial. Lancet Gastroenterol Hepatol 2018;3(3): 153–61.

27. Madras BK, Compton WM, Avula D, et al. Screening, brief interventions, referral to treatment (SBIRT) for illicit drug and alcohol use at multiple healthcare sites: comparison at intake and 6 months later. Drug Alcohol Depend 2009;99(1–3): 280–95.

28. Herron AJ, Brennan TK. The American Society of Addiction Medicine Essentials of addiction medicine. Riverwoods (IL): Lippincott Williams & Wilkins; 2019.

29. Roy-Byrne P, Bumgardner K, Krupski A, et al. Brief intervention for problem drug use in safety-net primary care settings: a randomized clinical trial. JAMA 2014; 312(5):492–501.

30. Saitz R, Palfai TP, Cheng DM, et al. Screening and brief intervention for drug use in primary care: the ASPIRE randomized clinical trial. JAMA 2014;312(5):502–13.

31. Bernstein SL, D'Onofrio G. Screening, treatment initiation, and referral for substance use disorders. Addict Sci Clin Pract 2017;12(1):18.

32. WHO ASSIST Working Group. The alcohol, smoking and substance involvement screening test (ASSIST): development, reliability and feasibility. Addiction 2002; 97(9):1183–94.

33. Smith PC, Schmidt SM, Allensworth-Davies D, et al. A single-question screening test for drug use in primary care. Arch Intern Med 2010;170(13):1155–60.

34. Magill M, Ray LA. Cognitive-behavioral treatment with adult alcohol and illicit drug users: a meta-analysis of randomized controlled trials. J Stud Alcohol Drugs 2009;70(4):516.

35. Scherbaum N, Kluwig J, Specka M, et al. Group psychotherapy for opiate addicts in methadone maintenance treatment- a controlled trial. Eur Addict Res 2005; 11(4):163.

36. Gossop M, Steward D, Marsden J. Attendance at narcotics anonymous and alcoholics anonymous meetings, frequency of attendance and substance use outcomes after residential treatment for drug dependence: a 5-year follow-up study. Addiction 2008;103(1):119.

37. Lee JD, Nunes EV, Novo P, et al. Comparative effectiveness of extended-release naltrexone versus buprenorphine-naloxone for opioid relapse prevention

(X:BOT): a multicenter, open-label, randomized controlled trial. Lancet 2017; 391(10118):309–18.

38. Zoorob R, Kowalchuk A, Mejia de Grubb M. Buprenorphine therapy for opioid use disorder. Am Fam Physician 2018;97(5):313–20.

39. Rosenthal RN, Goradia VV. Advances in the delivery of buprenorphine for opioid dependence. Drug Des Devel Ther 2017;11:2493–505.

40. Crits-Christoph P, Siqueland L, Blaine J, et al. Psychosocial treatments for cocaine dependence: National Institute on Drug Abuse Collaborative Cocaine Treatment Study. Arch Gen Psychiatry 1999;56(6):493.

41. Vocci FJ, Montoya ID. Psychological treatments for stimulant misuse, comparing and contrasting those for amphetamine dependence and those for cocaine dependence. Curr Opin Psychiatry 2009;22(3):263–8.

42. Johnson BA, Ait-Daoud N, Wang XQ, et al. Topiramate for the treatment of cocaine addiction. JAMA Psychiatry 2013;70(12):1338–46.

43. Mooney ME, Herin DV, Schmitz JM, et al. Effects of oral methamphetamine on cocaine use: a randomized, double-blind, placebo-controlled trial. Drug Alcohol Depend 2009;101(1–2):34.

44. Colfax GN, Santos GM, Das M, et al. Mirtazapine to reduce methamphetamine use: a randomized clinical trial. Arch Gen Psychiatry 2011;68(11):1168–75.

45. Anderson AL, Li SH, Markova D, et al. Bupropion for the treatment of methamphetamine dependence in non-daily users: a randomized, double-blind, placebo-controlled trial. Drug Alcohol Depend 2015;150:170–4.

46. Wakeman SE, Barnett ML. Primary care and the opioid-overdose crisis - buprenorphine myths and realities. N Engl J Med 2018;379(1):1–4.

47. Cicero TJ, Ellis MS, Chilcoat HD. Understanding the use of diverted buprenorphine. Drug Alcohol Depend 2018;193:117–23.

48. Provenzano AM. Caring for Ms. L.- overcoming my fear of treating opioid use disorder. N Engl J Med 2018;378(7):600–1.

49. Lee JD, Grossman E, DiRocco D, et al. Home buprenorphine/naloxone induction in primary care. J Gen Intern Med 2009;24(2):226–32.

50. Hawk M, Coulter RWS, Egan JE, et al. Harm reduction principles for healthcare settings. Harm Reduct J 2017;14(1):70.

51. National Center for Health Statistics. Drug overdose deaths in the United States, 1999–2017. NCHS Data Brief 2018;(329):1–8.

52. Substance abuse and mental health service Administration Center for the application of prevention technologies. Preventing the consequences of opioid overdose: understanding naloxone access laws. Available at: https://www.samhsa.gov/capt/sites/default/files/resources/naloxone-access-laws-tool.pdf. Accessed December 23, 2018.

53. Uyei J, Fiellin DA, Buchelli M, et al. Effects of naloxone distribution alone or in combination with addiction treatment with or without pre-exposure prophylaxis for HIV prevention in people who inject drugs: a cost-effectiveness modelling study. Lancet Public Health 2017;2(3):e133–40.

54. Harm Reduction Coalition. Getting off right- A safety manual for injection drug users 2009. Available at: https://harmreduction.org/drugs-and-drug-users/drug-tools/getting-off-right/. Accessed December 23, 2018.

55. Choopanya K, Martin M, Suntharasamai P, et al, Bangkok Tenofovir Study Group. Antiretroviral prophylaxis for HIV infection in injecting drug users in Bangkok, Thailand (the Bangkok Tenofovir Study): a randomised, double-blind, placebo-controlled phase 3 trial. Lancet 2013;381(9883):2083–90.

56. Martin M, Vanichseni S, Suntharasamai P, et al, Bangkok Tenofovir Study Group. The impact of adherence to preexposure prophylaxis on the risk of HIV infection among people who inject drugs. AIDS 2015;29(7):819–24.

57. Kuo I, Agopian A, Opoku J, et al. Assessing PrEP needs among heterosexuals and people who inject drugs, Washington, DC. Oral presentation at: Conference on Retroviruses and Opportunistic Infections. Boston, MA, March 4–7, 2018.

58. Roth AM, Aumaier BL, Felsher MA, et al. An exploration of factors impacting pre-exposure prophylaxis eligibility and access among syringe exchange users. Sex Transm Dis 2018;45(4):217–21.

59. Bazzi AR, Biancarelli DL, Childs E, et al. Limited knowledge and mixed interest in pre-exposure prophylaxis for HIV prevention among people who inject drugs. AIDS Patient Care STDs 2018;32(12):529–37.

60. Bernard CL, Owens DK, Goldhaber-Fiebert JD, et al. Estimation of the cost-effectiveness of HIV prevention portfolios for people who inject drugs in the United States: a model-based analysis. PLoS Med 2017;14(5):e1002312.

61. Bernard CL, Brandeau ML, Humphreys K, et al. Cost-effectiveness of HIV preexposure prophylaxis for people who inject drugs in the United States. Ann Intern Med 2016. https://doi.org/10.7326/M15-2634.

62. Alistar SS, Owens DK, Brandeau ML. Effectiveness and cost effectiveness of oral pre-exposure prophylaxis in a portfolio of prevention programs for injection drug users in mixed HIV epidemics. PLoS One 2014;9(1):e86584.

63. Fu R, Owens DK, Brandeau ML. Cost-effectiveness of alternative strategies for provision of HIV preexposure prophylaxis for people who inject drugs. AIDS 2018;32(5):663–72.

64. Vlahov D, Junge B. The role of needle exchange programs in HIV prevention. Public Health Rep 1998;113(Suppl 1):75–80.

65. Aspinall EJ, Nambiar D, Goldberg DJ, et al. Are needle and syringe programmes associated with a reduction in HIV transmission among people who inject drugs: a systematic review and meta-analysis. Int J Epidemiol 2014;43(1):235–48.

66. Patel MR, Foote C, Duwve J, et al. Reduction of injection-related risk behaviors after emergency implementation of a syringe services program during an HIV outbreak. J Acquir Immune Defic Syndr 2018;77(4):373–82.

67. Centers for Disease Control and Prevention. Transcript for CDC telebriefing: new vital signs report- HIV and injection drug use. Available at: https://www.cdc.gov/media/releases/2016/t1130-vital-signs-hiv-drug-use.html. Accessed November 30, 2016.

68. Gaeta JM, Racine M. New strategies are needed to stop overdose fatalities: the case for supervised injection facilities. Ann Intern Med 2018;168(9):664–5.

69. Wakeman SE. Another senseless death - the case for supervised injection facilities. N Engl J Med 2017;376(11):1011–3.

70. Potier C, Laprévote V, Dubois-Arber F, et al. Supervised injection services: what has been demonstrated? A systematic literature review. Drug Alcohol Depend 2014;145:48–68.

71. Kennedy MC, Karamouzian M, Kerr T. Public health and public order outcomes associated with supervised drug consumption facilities: a systematic review. Curr HIV/AIDS Rep 2017;14(5):161–83.

72. Ickowicz S, Wood E, Dong H, et al. Association between public injecting and drug-related harm among HIV-positive people who use injection drugs in a Canadian setting: a longitudinal analysis. Drug Alcohol Depend 2017;180:33–8.

73. Irwin A, Jozaghi E, Weir BW, et al. Mitigating the heroin crisis in Baltimore, MD, USA: a cost-benefit analysis of a hypothetical supervised injection facility. Harm Reduct J 2017;14(1):29.

74. Altice FL, Kamarulzaman A, Soriano VV, et al. Treatment of medical, psychiatric, and substance-use comorbidities in people infected with HIV who use drugs. Lancet 2010;376(9738):367–87.

75. Metsch LR, Feaster DJ, Gooden L, et al. Effect of patient navigation with or without financial incentives on viral suppression among hospitalized patients with HIV infection and substance use: a randomized clinical trial. JAMA 2016; 316(2):156–70.

76. Nosyk B, Min JE, Evans E, et al. The effects of opioid substitution treatment and highly active antiretroviral therapy on the cause-specific risk of mortality among HIV-positive people who inject drugs. Clin Infect Dis 2015;61(7):1157–65.

77. Rich KM, Bia J, Altice FL, et al. Integrated models of care for individuals with opioid use disorder: how do we prevent HIV and HCV? Curr HIV/AIDS Rep 2018;15(3):266–75.

78. Kourounis G, Richards BD, Kyprianou E, et al. Opioid substitution therapy: lowering the treatment thresholds. Drug Alcohol Depend 2016;161:1–8.

79. Bhatraju EP, Grossman E, Tofighi B, et al. Public sector low threshold office-based buprenorphine treatment: outcomes at year 7. Addict Sci Clin Pract 2017;12(1):7.

80. Hall G, Neighbors CJ, Iheoma J, et al. Mobile opioid agonist treatment and public funding expands treatment for disenfranchised opioid-dependent individuals. J Subst Abuse Treat 2014;46(4):511–5.

81. DeBeck K, Cheng T, Montaner JS, et al. HIV and the criminalisation of drug use among people who inject drugs: a systematic review. Lancet HIV 2017;4(8): e357–74.

82. Springer SA, Korthuis PT, Del Rio C. Integrating treatment at the intersection of opioid use disorder and infectious disease epidemics in medical settings: a call for action after a National Academies of Sciences, Engineering, and Medicine Workshop. Ann Intern Med 2018;169(5):335–6.

On the Road to a HIV Cure
Moving Beyond Berlin and London

Nikolaus Jilg, MD, PhD[a,b,1], Jonathan Z. Li, MD, MMSc[b,c,*]

KEYWORDS

- HIV • HIV persistence • HIV cure • HIV vaccine
- Broadly neutralizing antibodies (bNAbs) • Long-term remission
- Posttreatment controllers • PTC

KEY POINTS

- A reliable therapeutic approach to human immunodeficiency virus (HIV) cure is currently not available for clinical practice.
- Cure is either defined as a complete elimination of any replication-competent virus, sterilizing cure, or a functional cure characterized by long-term remission despite remaining replication-competent virus.
- The latent reservoir consisting of silent proviruses integrated into cellular DNA is the main obstacle to cure.
- Numerous strategies for the depletion of the latent reservoir have been investigated with some promising results.
- Examples of people with long-term nonprogression and HIV remission, like the case of the Berlin patient, have amplified optimism about the general feasibility of a cure.

INTRODUCTION

AIDS was first described as a new immunodeficiency syndrome in 1981.[1] The relatively short history of human immunodeficiency virus (HIV) medicine is marked by major successes and breakthroughs in research, leading to the development of specific therapies that turned a once uniformly deadly disease into a chronic carrier state and facilitates lives not affected by complications of HIV/AIDS for most people on antiretroviral therapy (ART).[2] Despite this impressive advance, there is still no strategy for HIV remission or cure that can be readily employed in clinical practice.

Disclosures: Dr J.Z. Li has consulted for Quest Diagnostics and Jan Biotech.
[a] Massachusetts General Hospital, 55 Fruit Street, Boston, MA 02114, USA; [b] Harvard Medical School, 25 Shattuck Street, Boston, MA 02115, USA; [c] Brigham and Women's Hospital, 75 Francis Street, Boston, MA 02115, USA
[1] Present address: 65 Landsdowne Street, Room 421, Cambridge, MA 02139.
* Corresponding author. 65 Landsdowne Street, Room 421, Cambridge, MA 02139.
E-mail address: jli@bwh.harvard.edu

Infect Dis Clin N Am 33 (2019) 857–868
https://doi.org/10.1016/j.idc.2019.04.007
0891-5520/19/© 2019 Elsevier Inc. All rights reserved.

id.theclinics.com

The authors discuss the relevance of HIV persistence as the major obstacle to cure. Next, they present several intriguing cases that have informed the field and have entertained hopes of long-term remission and cure, including the case of 1 single person, who is by many seen as the only example to date of a human being cured of HIV. Different methods are being studied or proposed as candidate therapies for cure and are described here.

CONTENT
Why Does HIV Persist?

Following an initial rapid decline in HIV-DNA in the first year on ART, the decay of the HIV reservoir slows down and eventually plateaus beyond year 4 of therapy.[3] Cessation of suppressive therapy at any time leads to viral rebound, typically seen within 2 to 4 weeks for most individuals.[4] What are the mechanisms behind HIV persistence?

Active viral replication

The presence of viral evolution in lymphoid tissue has been reported in participants on ART with undetectable viremia, leading to the proposal of active viral replication as a contributing factor to viral persistence.[5] This cryptic viremia might explain the abnormal immune activation and inflammation seen in people on ART.[6] Data from some treatment intensification studies provided support for this hypothesis, where the addition of an integrase inhibitor in individuals already on suppressive ART led to an increase of short-lived episomal HIV-DNA (2-LTR circles), reflecting new rounds of viral infection.[7,8] There has been controversy, as the article by Lorenzo-Redondo and colleagues[5] involved relatively few individuals, all with recent ART initiation, and concerns have been raised about the methodology.[9,10] In contrast, there was no evidence of viral replication or evolution on ART in several other studies, including those with ART intensification.[11–13] Viral replication on ART was detected in tissue compartments, such as the B cell follicles in lymph nodes, in non-human primate (NHP) elite controllers, which was explained by the absence of antiviral CD8+ cells in the B cell follicles.[14] Similarly, replication competent cells were found in lymph nodes of aviremic patients.[15,16] Low drug concentrations in B cell follicles may be a contributing factor.[5,17] HIV sanctuary sites in certain tissues may be a relevant part of the reservoir, but these are often not easily accessible for studies.[17] There was no viral replication detected on longitudinal tissue sampling of ART-suppressed individuals in 1 study.[18] Finally, suboptimal ART adherence may result in persistent low-level viral replication, even for individuals with apparent viral suppression by commercial viral load assays.[19]

Prolonged cellular survival

HIV integrates into the host genome and persists as provirus during the lifetime of the cell. Most cells die shortly after infection, either due to cytopathic effects of the virus or host immune responses, but in latency, HIV is transcriptionally/translationally silent and allows these cells to evade the immune response.[20] Identification of the small fraction of HIV-infected CD4+ cells, that form the reservoir and cause rebound when ART is stopped, has been a major focus of HIV cure research. T memory stem cells are a particularly long-lived subset of central memory T cells carrying proviral DNA in relatively high frequency.[21] The latent reservoir consists mainly of intact proviruses in quiescent cells and might have been considerably underestimated in many studies.[22] Hematopoietic stem and progenitor cells (HSPCs) that are capable of lifelong survival, self-renewal, and clonal expansion may be infected and contribute to the viral reservoir.[23]

Homeostatic or clonal proliferation

Homeostatic proliferation, the physiologic response to maintain T cell numbers, and clonal proliferation of infected cells are increasingly recognized as key mechanisms behind the maintenance and expansion of the HIV reservoir. HIV preferably integrates into regions of actively transcribed genes, particularly genes that are involved in onco-genesis or cell-cycle control.[24–26] A large fraction of the cells that carry proviruses was shown to be of clonal origin. While most of these only harbor defective provirus, some clonally expanded CD4+ T cells do indeed produce infective virus in vivo.[27] One report suggested that more than 99% of infected cells belong to clonal populations after a year of ART.[28]

Has There Been a Cure? Notable Examples and Strategies Toward Control and Elimination of Human Immunodeficiency Virus

An HIV "cure" may either refer to sterilizing cure, meaning that there is no remaining virus capable of reactivation left in the body, versus functional cure, a state of long-term remission in that intact virus or proviral sequences are still present, but are being controlled and the disease does not progress. There have indeed been several well-described examples of patients who have achieved long-term re-missions, some where prematurely considered cured by the non-scientific community.

Why should "cure" matter in the times of highly successful and well-tolerated ART? Some people are not well controlled by or do not tolerate currently available regimens due to factors such as drug resistance, limited access to ART and medical care in many areas of the world, comorbidities (eg, cardiovascular and metabolic diseases), pill fatigue, and the stigma still associated with HIV infection, that are persisting challenges with current ART. Finally, life-long ART accrues a significant cumulative cost.

Stem Cell Transplantation

The Berlin and London patients

A 2009 case report described long-term remission of HIV infection reviving optimism regarding feasibility of a cure: the so-called Berlin patient had been HIV positive and on suppressive ART when he developed acute leukemia (unrelated to HIV) requiring a myeloablative allogeneic hematopoietic stem cell transplant (HSCT).[29] After HSCT from a matching donor who was additionally selected for homozygosity of CCR5 Δ32, a 32-base-pair deletion in the CCR5 gene that renders the host cells resistant to viral entry, the Berlin patient has remained off combined ART without evidence of residual virus so far (>10 years) despite an extensive search.[30] Hence, most experts consider him the first documented example of a sterilizing HIV cure, although negative tests cannot completely exclude the presence of intact virus everywhere in the pa-tient's body.[30] In a recently published report, there is hope that a second patient may now be free of HIV. This individual, known as "the London patient", received an allo-HSCT for Hodgkin's lymphoma from a donor homozygous for the CCR5Δ32 mutation. This patient has been in HIV remission for 18 months after ART discontinuation with undetectable plasma viral load by an ultrasensitive assay and undetectable HIV DNA in peripheral CD4 T cells.[31] As the authors point out, the duration off ART for this individual is far shorter than that of the Berlin patient and it is premature to conclude that this patient has been cured. In contrast to the Berlin patient, the London patient received only one transplant that included a reduced intensity conditioning regimen without whole body irradiation, suggesting that a less intensive approach may be sufficient to induce HIV remission.

The Boston patients and other examples of allogenous hematopoietic stem cell transplantation in people with HIV infection

In addition to administration of donor cells homozygous for the CCR5 Δ32 mutation, the Berlin patient's treatment also included chemotherapy, whole-body irradiation, and a second transplantation from the same donor after a relapse of his leukemia. Two men with HIV infection and hematologic malignancies in Boston received allogeneic HSCT from donors who did not have the CCR5 Δ32 mutation, leaving the donor T cells susceptible to HIV infection. While there was a significant reduction of the viral reservoirs, both patients eventually rebounded, albeit with a significant delay of 12 and 32 weeks after cessation of ART.[32,33] Another patient who underwent allogeneic HSCT with donor cells harboring wild-type *CCR5* experienced rebound after more than 9 months.[34] These results point to a pivotal role of the CCR5 Δ32 allele in preventing the resurgence of infection, although the rarity of the homozygous genotype in the donor pool and the toxicity of allo-HSCT have made it challenging to replicate the Berlin patient's experience.[35–37] The ICiStem consortium (International Collaboration to guide and investigate the potential for HIV cure by Stem Cell Transplantation) found a profound reduction in the HIV reservoirs after allogeneic HSCT in 6 individuals.[38] Finally, autologous stem cell transplantation or cytoreductive chemotherapy in the absence of HSCT led only to a transient reduction of the reservoir followed by recovery and even expansion of reservoir size.[39]

Allogeneic hematopoietic stem cell transplantation as a strategy

Current allogeneic bone marrow transplantation is fraught with high morbidity and mortality prohibiting its use for HIV infection other than in patients with an accepted medical indication for HSCT. Further attempts with hematopoietic stem cells (HSCs) from CCR5 Δ32 homozygous donors led to reduction of the reservoir and transient viral control, but were limited by high mortality.[35,40,41] Of note, routine screening for CCR5 Δ32 has recently been established in several cord blood and bone marrow banks and facilitates identification of HLA identical donors that are also homozygous for CCR5 Δ32, increasing the chance for a respective match to 20%-25% for patients with Central European ancestry.[42] One patient experienced viral escape after HSCT from a CCR5 Δ32 positive donor which was caused by the emergence of CXCR4 tropic virus, while pre-interventional HIV testing had shown CCR5 tropism.[40,41] Moreover, CCR5 Δ32 homozygous individuals with HIV have been identified, illustrating once more that the mutation does not confer complete resistance to infection.[43]

Gene Therapy

Host gene modification

Molecular approaches to altering host factors, offer the prospect of reproducing the Berlin patient's experience while avoiding the morbidity of allogeneic HSCTs. Zinc-finger nucleases (ZNF) have been used to knockout *CCR5* in both CD4$^+$ T cells and CD34$^+$ hematopoietic stem and progenitor cells (HSPCs). *CCR5* editing in autologous cells of HIV$^+$ subjects was safe in a phase 1 trial, and several subsequent early phase trials have used the technique.[44,45] More recently developed gene editing tools like TALEN and CRISPR-Cas9 will probably be preferred going forward because of their relative ease of use and improved specificity. These techniques still bear the risk of off-target effects leading to insertions, deletions, and point mutations, including some that may only manifest after long periods of time, which currently prohibits their routine use in humans.[46] Knocking out both coreceptors may provide broad protection from viral entry. While a specific, systemic CCR5 knockdown may be well tolerated as suggested by the naturally occurring CCR5 Δ32 mutation, CXCR4 has important functions in bone-marrow mobilization, and systemic knockdown may not be safe. There are, however, promising results by Didigu and colleagues,[47] who used ZFNs to knock out both coreceptors in CD4$^+$ T cells ex vivo and infused them into humanized HIV+ mice, which did not cause any apparent functional immune defects. T cell proliferation is expected to amplify effects of genetically altered T cells because these HIV-resistant populations are expected to replace HIV-susceptible host T cells that are depleted in the setting of active infection.

Proviral inactivation

Besides their use for targeting host factors, ZNFs, TALENs, and CRISPR-Cas9 have been used to directly disrupt proviral DNA: an HIV-specific CRISPR-Cas9 with a lentiviral vector suppressed viral replication in humanized mice after engraftment of patient-derived peripheral blood mononuclear cells (PBMCs).[48] Based on the Cre/loxP system, Karpinski and colleagues[49] have created a recombinase (Brec1), which site specifically recognizes a highly conserved 34-bp sequence in the long terminal repeats (LTRs) allowing for precise excision of proviral DNA. The strategy led to elimination of provirus from patient-derived infected cells in ex vivo experiments and achieved HIV eradication in a humanized mouse model. Off-target effects were not detected. Efficient, reliable, and safe delivery of the relevant molecules to humans has been the hurdle to using these molecular technologies in clinical studies.

Early Therapy for Cure and Posttreatment Control

The Mississippi baby and the role of very early treatment

A girl who had perinatally contracted HIV and was started on ART 30 hours after birth, then had stopped ART after 18 months when she was lost to follow-up. She found to be aviremic when reestablishing care after 12 months off therapy.[50] This case nurtured hopes that very early treatment initiation might prevent establishment of latency. The child eventually relapsed after 27 months off ART.[51] While disappointing, the prolonged period of HIV remission in this case further supported the hypothesis that early treatment restricts the seeding of the viral reservoir and may increase the chances of sustained HIV remission, at least in infants. Other treatment interruption studies of adults who had initiated ART during the very early stages of infection (Fiebig I and Fiebig II, ie, before specific HIV-antibodies are detectable) failed to demonstrate that early treatment prevented the establishment of HIV infection.[52,53] As discussed later, early initiation of ART may, however, increase the chances of sustained HIV remission.[54–56]

The VISCONTI cohort and early capture studies

ART-free remission, that is, functional cure, following early treatment initiation, like in the case of the Mississippi baby, was also studied in the VISCONTI cohort (Viro-Immunological Control after Treatment Interruption). Sáez-Cirión and colleagues[55] identified 14 patients from a large database that began ART during primary infection, who controlled viremia and preserved CD4$^+$ T cell counts for several years after ART interruption. Of note, these individuals started therapy within 2 months of infection, but considerably later than in the examples above, that is, during Fiebig stage III to V for almost all participants, when HIV-specific antibodies are already reliably detectable. Individuals that display HIV control *after*, but not before ART, like the participants of the VISCONTI cohort, were termed posttreatment controllers (PTCs).

Early capture cohorts aim to systematically and prospectively study the effects and outcomes of early treatment initiation by continuously screening at-risk populations in highly endemic areas (eg, South Africa, East Africa, Thailand) and start treatment as soon as participants turn positive, which may further shed light on PTC frequency amongst patients treated within a narrow, early timeframe.[57,58]

Further posttreatment controllers studies

A central question is how ART facilitates viral control by the immune system after treatment cessation.[59] Several observations support a lower reservoir size during therapy in PTCs versus noncontrollers.[60–62] Namazi and colleagues[56] have recently identified and characterized 67 PTCs from existing trials. There was a significantly higher probability of achieving PTC status in the participants with treatment starting during early versus chronic infection (13% vs 4%; P<.001).

Latency Modifying Agents

"Shock and kill" or "kick and kill" has been proposed as a strategy well suited to overcome the specific obstacles of latency.[63] It involves the seemingly at first counterintuitive activation of the reservoir which results in viremia and is important for 2 reasons: first, latently infected cells are, per definition, not making any viral molecules and therefore remain invisible to the immune system; second, non-replicating proviruses do not provide any targets for specific antiviral drugs. Hence, forcing these long-lived cells out of latency is a way to uncover them. Once activated, mean survival of infected CD4$^+$ T cells would hypothetically be quite short, due to both the cytopathic effect of the virus and the unfolding immune response, but there is evidence that the immune system actually has trouble clearing these cells efficiently.[64–66] The "kick" by latency reversing agents (LRAs) is followed by interventions that promote killing of infected cells, typically while measures like ART would protect from new rounds of infection. Purging the body from latently infected cells would diminish or eliminate the reservoir. A number of drugs that are already in clinical use were identified as LRAs, which expedites human trials in HIV infection. These drugs include valproic acid, disulfiram, histone deacetylase inhibitors (HDACi), protein kinase C agonists, and Toll-like receptor (TLR) agonists.[67] Despite significant increases of viral transcription and replication in multiple trials, there has been no relevant reduction in the viral reservoir dampening the initial excitement about the strategy.[68] A potential explanation for this finding is that many LRAs may not reach high enough levels to activate the cells in the relevant compartments or may only be capable of activating a small fraction of proviruses.[69] Another concern regarding these agents are off-target effects, such as activation of uninfected T cells, which may render them susceptible to HIV, and unwanted activation of additional cell types that may, for example, cause reactivation of other latent viruses, like the herpes family viruses or human T cell lymphotropic virus (HTLV). "Block and lock" or "soothe and snooze" is an approach that would eventually cause a state of deep viral hibernation by means of latency securing agents, ideally lowering the risk of proviral reactivation to 0. Didehydrocortistatin A, a specific inhibitor of the HIV protein Tat (transactivator of transcription), has been studied for this purpose.[70] Tat is crucial for HIV reactivation and is therefore an attractive target for proviral silencing strategies. Short hairpin RNA (shRNA) targeting the HIV promoter region in the long terminal repeats (LTRs) was cloned into lentiviral vectors and protected against reactivation by LRAs in cell culture models.[71] The proteasome is a key contributor to viral latency, which at least partially is achieved by breaking Tat down, and thereby blocking viral transcription. Thus, proteasome inhibition reverses latency, whereas inactivating Tat promotes it.[72]

Antibody Therapy

In virology, no antibody (Ab) responses have been as extensively studied as those to HIV.[73] Ab-based therapies have been explored for HIV prevention and control, and applications aiming for cure may involve a delivery system of Ab genes to humans facilitating sustained in vivo Ab production. Broadly neutralizing antibodies (bNAbs) that target highly conserved regions of the envelope protein (Env) occur naturally in a minority of HIV-infected individuals. A limited number of highly selected candidate monoclonal antibodies have been studied: in a humanized mouse model, therapy with a specific bNAb not only led to viral neutralization but also led to enhanced clearance of HIV-infected cells.[74] Several groups have tested bNAbs in the simian-human immunodeficiency virus (SHIV) infection model in non-human primates (NHP) and have demonstrated that specific bNAbs protect from new infection, reduce plasma viral loads, extend time to viral rebound, and reduce PBMC and lymph node proviral DNA levels.[75–79] Treatment with a single monoclonal Ab appears prone to resistance, but combination therapy likely obviates resistance mutations.[80–82] In a 2018 proof-of-principle paper, a bioengineered trispecific Ab combining specificities to 3 independent HIV envelope determinants conferred complete immunity against SHIV infection in monkeys.[83] Several monoclonal bNAbs have been shown to reduce viremia in HIV-positive, untreated individuals, and delay time to rebound in ART-treated subjects after analytical treatment interruption.[81,84] Widespread tissue penetrance may be one of the advantages of Ab therapy, because ART may not reach adequate drug levels in all relevant compartments.[85] Borducchi and colleagues[86] have recently outlined a promising strategy to deplete the viral reservoir by using a combination of ART, a TLR7 agonist (vesatolimod), and a bNAb (PGT121) in SHIV-infected monkeys: TLR7 acts as an antiviral through type I interferon-dependent activation of immune cells, but moreover, it has LRA properties, potentially due to the induction of $CD4^+$ T cell activation. NHPs on ART that had been treated with both vesatolimod and PGT121 experienced diminished viral rebound kinetics after treatment cessation compared with the sham or monotherapy groups.

Therapeutic Vaccination

Preventative HIV vaccine trials have generally been disappointing, and only 1 clinical study has demonstrated a modest protective effect from new infection (31%) when given to HIV-negative individuals. After some of these study subjects acquired HIV, but there was no noticeable effect on degree of viremia or $CD4^+$ T cell numbers induced by the vaccine.[87] As noted above, there is evidence that reversal of HIV latency may not necessarily lead to clearance of reactivated cells, and a number of therapeutic vaccine strategies have been tested.[64–66] While the overall track record of therapeutic vaccines has been disappointing, there may be a modest effect of immunization on viral set point.[88–90] In view of the encouraging results from work with bNAbs (discussed above), a vaccine that could trigger production of highly effective bNAbs would theoretically be a powerful therapeutic. It remains unclear to which degree neutralizing, or nonneutralizing antibodies, T cell, NK cell, or other specific immune responses are necessary for an adequate immune response to HIV.[91]

SUMMARY

Two well documented cases of HIV long-term remission - and possible cure - have raised the hope that curative treatments may one day be available in clinical practice to replace ART. There are many promising leads for targeting the viral reservoir, including therapeutic latency reversal, molecular host factor modification, silencing or excision of the provirus, administration of monoclonal broadly neutralizing antibodies, and therapeutic immunizations. It is likely that a combination of strategies will be required for cure. The Berlin and London patients remain a living testament to the feasibility of HIV remission in the absence of ART. The remaining challenge is how to develop reliable and safe curative therapies to make them available to people living with HIV.

ACKNOWLEDGMENT

Dr. Jilg was supported by the National Institutes of Health Multidisciplinary AIDS Training grant (AI007387, PI: Dr. D. Kuritzkes). Dr. Li was supported by the Harvard University Center for AIDS Research (CFAR) (National Institute of Allergy and Infectious Diseases grant number 5P30AI060354-08) and a subcontract from UM1 AI106701 to the Harvard Virology Specialty Laboratory.

REFERENCES

1. Gottlieb MS, Schroff R, Schanker HM, et al. Pneumocystis carinii pneumonia and mucosal candidiasis in previously healthy homosexual men: evidence of a new acquired cellular immunodeficiency. N Engl J Med 1981;305(24):1425–31.
2. Barre-Sinoussi F, Ross AL, Delfraissy JF. Past, present and future: 30 years of HIV research. Nat Rev Microbiol 2013;11(12):877–83.
3. Besson GJ, Lalama CM, Bosch RJ, et al. HIV-1 DNA decay dynamics in blood during more than a decade of suppressive antiretroviral therapy. Clin Infect Dis 2014;59(9):1312–21.
4. Li JZ, Etemad B, Ahmed H, et al. The size of the expressed HIV reservoir predicts timing of viral rebound after treatment interruption. AIDS 2016;30(3):343–53.
5. Lorenzo-Redondo R, Fryer HR, Bedford T, et al. Persistent HIV-1 replication maintains the tissue reservoir during therapy. Nature 2016;530(7588):51–6.
6. Martinez-Picado J, Zurakowski R, Buzon MJ, et al. Episomal HIV-1 DNA and its relationship to other markers of HIV-1 persistence. Retrovirology 2018;15(1):15.
7. Buzon MJ, Massanella M, Llibre JM, et al. HIV-1 replication and immune dynamics are affected by raltegravir intensification of HAART-suppressed subjects. Nat Med 2010;16(4):460–5.
8. Hatano H, Strain MC, Scherzer R, et al. Increase in 2-long terminal repeat circles and decrease in D-dimer after raltegravir intensification in patients with treated HIV infection: a randomized, placebo-controlled trial. J Infect Dis 2013;208(9): 1436–42.
9. Kearney MF, Wiegand A, Shao W, et al. Ongoing HIV replication during ART reconsidered. Open Forum Infect Dis 2017;4(3):ofx173.
10. Rosenbloom DIS, Hill AL, Laskey SB, et al. Re-evaluating evolution in the HIV reservoir. Nature 2017;551(7681):E6–9.
11. Josefsson L, von Stockenstrom S, Faria NR, et al. The HIV-1 reservoir in eight patients on long-term suppressive antiretroviral therapy is stable with few genetic changes over time. Proc Natl Acad Sci U S A 2013;110(51):E4987–96.
12. Kearney MF, Spindler J, Shao W, et al. Lack of detectable HIV-1 molecular evolution during suppressive antiretroviral therapy. PLoS Pathog 2014;10(3): e1004010.
13. Rasmussen TA, McMahon JH, Chang JJ, et al. The effect of antiretroviral intensification with dolutegravir on residual virus replication in HIV-infected individuals: a randomised, placebo-controlled, double-blind trial. Lancet HIV 2018;5(5): e221–30.
14. Fukazawa Y, Lum R, Okoye AA, et al. B cell follicle sanctuary permits persistent productive simian immunodeficiency virus infection in elite controllers. Nat Med 2015;21(2):132–9.

15. Banga R, Procopio FA, Noto A, et al. PD-1(+) and follicular helper T cells are responsible for persistent HIV-1 transcription in treated aviremic individuals. Nat Med 2016;22(7):754–61.

16. Boritz EA, Darko S, Swaszek L, et al. Multiple origins of virus persistence during natural control of HIV infection. Cell 2016;166(4):1004–15.

17. Fletcher CV, Staskus K, Wietgrefe SW, et al. Persistent HIV-1 replication is associated with lower antiretroviral drug concentrations in lymphatic tissues. Proc Natl Acad Sci U S A 2014;111(6):2307–12.

18. Van Zyl GU, Katusiime MG, Wiegand A, et al. No evidence of HIV replication in children on antiretroviral therapy. J Clin Invest 2017;127(10):3827–34.

19. Li JZ, Gallien S, Ribaudo H, et al. Incomplete adherence to antiretroviral therapy is associated with higher levels of residual HIV-1 viremia. AIDS 2014;28(2):181–6.

20. Finzi D, Blankson J, Siliciano JD, et al. Latent infection of CD4+ T cells provides a mechanism for lifelong persistence of HIV-1, even in patients on effective combination therapy. Nat Med 1999;5(5):512–7.

21. Buzon MJ, Sun H, Li C, et al. HIV-1 persistence in CD4+ T cells with stem cell-like properties. Nat Med 2014;20(2):139–42.

22. Ho YC, Shan L, Hosmane NN, et al. Replication-competent noninduced proviruses in the latent reservoir increase barrier to HIV-1 cure. Cell 2013;155(3):540–51.

23. Zaikos TD, Terry VH, Sebastian Kettinger NT, et al. Hematopoietic stem and progenitor cells are a distinct HIV reservoir that contributes to persistent viremia in suppressed patients. Cell Rep 2018;25(13):3759–73.e9.

24. Anderson EM, Maldarelli F. The role of integration and clonal expansion in HIV infection: live long and prosper. Retrovirology 2018;15(1):71.

25. Wagner TA, McLaughlin S, Garg K, et al. HIV latency. Proliferation of cells with HIV integrated into cancer genes contributes to persistent infection. Science 2014;345(6196):570–3.

26. Maldarelli F, Wu X, Su L, et al. HIV latency. Specific HIV integration sites are linked to clonal expansion and persistence of infected cells. Science 2014;345(6193):179–83.

27. Simonetti FR, Sobolewski MD, Fyne E, et al. Clonally expanded CD4+ T cells can produce infectious HIV-1 in vivo. Proc Natl Acad Sci U S A 2016;113(7):1883–8.

28. Reeves DB, Duke ER, Wagner TA, et al. A majority of HIV persistence during antiretroviral therapy is due to infected cell proliferation. Nat Commun 2018;9(1):4811.

29. Hutter G, Nowak D, Mossner M, et al. Long-term control of HIV by CCR5 Delta32/Delta32 stem-cell transplantation. N Engl J Med 2009;360(7):692–8.

30. Lederman MM, Pike E. Ten years HIV free: an interview with "the Berlin patient," Timothy Ray Brown. Pathog Immun 2017;2(3):422–30.

31. Gupta RK, Abdul-Jawad S, McCoy LE, et al. HIV-1 remission following CCR5Δ32/Δ32 haematopoietic stem-cell transplantation. Nature 2019;568(7751):244–8.

32. Henrich TJ, Hu Z, Li JZ, et al. Long-term reduction in peripheral blood HIV type 1 reservoirs following reduced-intensity conditioning allogeneic stem cell transplantation. J Infect Dis 2013;207(11):1694–702.

33. Henrich TJ, Hanhauser E, Marty FM, et al. Antiretroviral-free HIV-1 remission and viral rebound after allogeneic stem cell transplantation: report of 2 cases. Ann Intern Med 2014;161(5):319–27.

34. Cummins NW, Rizza S, Litzow MR, et al. Extensive virologic and immunologic characterization in an HIV-infected individual following allogeneic stem cell

transplant and analytic cessation of antiretroviral therapy: a case study. PLoS Med 2017;14(11):e1002461.

35. Duarte RF, Salgado M, Sanchez-Ortega I, et al. CCR5 Delta32 homozygous cord blood allogeneic transplantation in a patient with HIV: a case report. Lancet HIV 2015;2(6):e236–42.

36. Rothenberger M, Wagner JE, Haase A, et al. Transplantation of CCR532 homozygous umbilical cord blood in a child with acute lymphoblastic leukemia and perinatally acquired HIV infection. Open Forum Infect Dis 2018;5(5):ofy090.

37. Verheyen J, Thielen A, Lubke N, et al. Rapid rebound of a preexisting CXCR4-tropic human immunodeficiency virus variant after allogeneic transplantation with CCR5 Delta32 homozygous stem cells. Clin Infect Dis 2019;68(4):684–7.

38. Salgado M, Kwon M, Galvez C, et al. Mechanisms that contribute to a profound reduction of the HIV-1 reservoir after allogeneic stem cell transplant. Ann Intern Med 2018;169(10):674–83.

39. Henrich TJ, Hobbs KS, Hanhauser E, et al. Human immunodeficiency virus type 1 persistence following systemic chemotherapy for malignancy. J Infect Dis 2017; 216(2):254–62.

40. Hutter G. More on shift of HIV tropism in stem-cell transplantation with CCR5 delta32/delta32 mutation. N Engl J Med 2014;371(25):2437–8.

41. Kordelas L, Verheyen J, Beelen DW, et al. Shift of HIV tropism in stem-cell transplantation with CCR5 Delta32 mutation. N Engl J Med 2014;371(9):880–2.

42. Hutter G. The cure of Timothy Brown. How is his condition now and has this case been repeated? MMW Fortschr Med 2018;160(Suppl 2):27–30 [in German].

43. Smolen-Dzirba J, Rosinska M, Janiec J, et al. HIV-1 infection in persons homozygous for CCR5-Delta32 allele: the next case and the review. AIDS Rev 2017; 19(4):219–30.

44. Huyghe J, Magdalena S, Vandekerckhove L. Fight fire with fire: gene therapy strategies to cure HIV. Expert Rev Anti Infect Ther 2017;15(8):747–58.

45. Tebas P, Stein D, Tang WW, et al. Gene editing of CCR5 in autologous CD4 T cells of persons infected with HIV. N Engl J Med 2014;370(10):901–10.

46. Cradick TJ, Fine EJ, Antico CJ, et al. CRISPR/Cas9 systems targeting beta-globin and CCR5 genes have substantial off-target activity. Nucleic Acids Res 2013; 41(20):9584–92.

47. Didigu CA, Wilen CB, Wang J, et al. Simultaneous zinc-finger nuclease editing of the HIV coreceptors ccr5 and cxcr4 protects CD4+ T cells from HIV-1 infection. Blood 2014;123(1):61–9.

48. Bella R, Kaminski R, Mancuso P, et al. Removal of HIV DNA by CRISPR from patient blood engrafts in humanized mice. Mol Ther Nucleic Acids 2018;12:275–82.

49. Karpinski J, Hauber I, Chemnitz J, et al. Directed evolution of a recombinase that excises the provirus of most HIV-1 primary isolates with high specificity. Nat Biotechnol 2016;34(4):401–9.

50. Persaud D, Gay H, Ziemniak C, et al. Absence of detectable HIV-1 viremia after treatment cessation in an infant. N Engl J Med 2013;369(19):1828–35.

51. Luzuriaga K, Gay H, Ziemniak C, et al. Viremic relapse after HIV-1 remission in a perinatally infected child. N Engl J Med 2015;372(8):786–8.

52. Colby DJ, Trautmann L, Pinyakorn S, et al. Rapid HIV RNA rebound after antiretroviral treatment interruption in persons durably suppressed in Fiebig I acute HIV infection. Nat Med 2018;24(7):923–6.

53. Henrich TJ, Hatano H, Bacon O, et al. HIV-1 persistence following extremely early initiation of antiretroviral therapy (ART) during acute HIV-1 infection: an observational study. PLoS Med 2017;14(11):e1002417.

54. Whitney JB, Lim S-Y, Osuna CE, et al. Prevention of SIVmac251 reservoir seeding in rhesus monkeys by early antiretroviral therapy. Nat Commun 2018;9(1):5429.

55. Sáez-Cirión A, Bacchus C, Hocqueloux L, et al. Post-treatment HIV-1 controllers with a long-term virological remission after the interruption of early initiated antiretroviral therapy ANRS VISCONTI Study. PLoS Pathog 2013;9(3):e1003211.

56. Namazi G, Fajnzylber JM, Aga E, et al. The control of HIV after antiretroviral medication pause (CHAMP) study: posttreatment controllers identified from 14 clinical studies. J Infect Dis 2018;218(12):1954–63.

57. Dong KL, Moodley A, Kwon DS, et al. Detection and treatment of Fiebig stage I HIV-1 infection in young at-risk women in South Africa: a prospective cohort study. Lancet HIV 2018;5(1):e35–44.

58. Robb ML, Eller LA, Kibuuka H, et al. Prospective study of acute HIV-1 infection in adults in East Africa and Thailand. N Engl J Med 2016;374(22):2120–30.

59. Goulder P, Deeks SG. HIV control: is getting there the same as staying there? PLoS Pathog 2018;14(11):e1007222.

60. Assoumou L, Weiss L, Piketty C, et al. A low HIV-DNA level in peripheral blood mononuclear cells at antiretroviral treatment interruption predicts a higher probability of maintaining viral control. AIDS 2015;29(15):2003–7.

61. Goujard C, Girault I, Rouzioux C, et al. HIV-1 control after transient antiretroviral treatment initiated in primary infection: role of patient characteristics and effect of therapy. Antivir Ther 2012;17(6):1001–9.

62. Sharaf R, Lee GQ, Sun X, et al. HIV-1 proviral landscapes distinguish posttreatment controllers from noncontrollers. J Clin Invest 2018;128(9):4074–85.

63. Darcis G, Van Driessche B, Van Lint C. HIV latency: should we shock or lock? Trends Immunol 2017;38(3):217–28.

64. Deng K, Pertea M, Rongvaux A, et al. Broad CTL response is required to clear latent HIV-1 due to dominance of escape mutations. Nature 2015;517(7534): 381–5.

65. Huang SH, Ren Y, Thomas AS, et al. Latent HIV reservoirs exhibit inherent resistance to elimination by CD8+ T cells. J Clin Invest 2018;128(2):876–89.

66. Jones RB, O'Connor R, Mueller S, et al. Histone deacetylase inhibitors impair the elimination of HIV-infected cells by cytotoxic T-lymphocytes. PLoS Pathog 2014; 10(8):e1004287.

67. Kim Y, Anderson JL, Lewin SR. Getting the "kill" into "shock and kill": strategies to eliminate latent HIV. Cell Host Microbe 2018;23(1):14–26.

68. Gallo RC. Shock and kill with caution. Science 2016;354(6309):177–8.

69. Battivelli E, Dahabieh MS, Abdel-Mohsen M, et al. Distinct chromatin functional states correlate with HIV latency reactivation in infected primary CD4(+) T cells. Elife 2018;7 [pii:e34655].

70. Mediouni S, Chinthalapudi K, Ekka MK, et al. Didehydro-cortistatin A inhibits HIV-1 by specifically binding to the unstructured basic region of Tat. MBio 2019;10(1) [pii:e02662-18].

71. Mendez C, Ledger S, Petoumenos K, et al. RNA-induced epigenetic silencing inhibits HIV-1 reactivation from latency. Retrovirology 2018;15(1):67.

72. Li Z, Wu J, Chavez L, et al. Reiterative Enrichment and Authentication of CRISPRi Targets (REACT) identifies the proteasome as a key contributor to HIV-1 latency. PLoS Pathog 2019;15(1):e1007498.

73. Sok D, Burton DR. Recent progress in broadly neutralizing antibodies to HIV. Nat Immunol 2018;19(11):1179–88.

74. Lu CL, Murakowski DK, Bournazos S, et al. Enhanced clearance of HIV-1-infected cells by broadly neutralizing antibodies against HIV-1 in vivo. Science 2016; 352(6288):1001–4.

75. Julg B, Liu PT, Wagh K, et al. Protection against a mixed SHIV challenge by a broadly neutralizing antibody cocktail. Sci Transl Med 2017;9(408) [pii: eaao4235].

76. Julg B, Pegu A, Abbink P, et al. Virological control by the CD4-binding site antibody n6 in simian-human immunodeficiency virus-infected rhesus monkeys. J Virol 2017;91(16) [pii:e00498-17].

77. Julg B, Sok D, Schmidt SD, et al. Protective efficacy of broadly neutralizing antibodies with incomplete neutralization activity against simian-human immunodeficiency virus in rhesus monkeys. J Virol 2017;91(20) [pii:e01187-17].

78. Barouch DH, Whitney JB, Moldt B, et al. Therapeutic efficacy of potent neutralizing HIV-1-specific monoclonal antibodies in SHIV-infected rhesus monkeys. Nature 2013;503(7475):224–8.

79. Shingai M, Nishimura Y, Klein F, et al. Antibody-mediated immunotherapy of macaques chronically infected with SHIV suppresses viraemia. Nature 2013; 503(7475):277–80.

80. Klein F, Halper-Stromberg A, Horwitz JA, et al. HIV therapy by a combination of broadly neutralizing antibodies in humanized mice. Nature 2012;492(7427): 118–22.

81. Scheid JF, Horwitz JA, Bar-On Y, et al. HIV-1 antibody 3BNC117 suppresses viral rebound in humans during treatment interruption. Nature 2016;535(7613): 556–60.

82. Mendoza P, Gruell H, Nogueira L, et al. Combination therapy with anti-HIV-1 antibodies maintains viral suppression. Nature 2018;561(7724):479–84.

83. Xu L, Pegu A, Rao E, et al. Trispecific broadly neutralizing HIV antibodies mediate potent SHIV protection in macaques. Science 2017;358(6359):85–90.

84. Caskey M, Klein F, Lorenzi JC, et al. Viraemia suppressed in HIV-1-infected humans by broadly neutralizing antibody 3BNC117. Nature 2015;522(7557): 487–91.

85. Halper-Stromberg A, Nussenzweig MC. Towards HIV-1 remission: potential roles for broadly neutralizing antibodies. J Clin Invest 2016;126(2):415–23.

86. Borducchi EN, Liu J, Nkolola JP, et al. Antibody and TLR7 agonist delay viral rebound in SHIV-infected monkeys. Nature 2018;563(7731):360–4.

87. Rerks-Ngarm S, Pitisuttithum P, Nitayaphan S, et al. Vaccination with ALVAC and AIDSVAX to prevent HIV-1 infection in Thailand. N Engl J Med 2009;361(23): 2209–20.

88. Pantaleo G, Levy Y. Therapeutic vaccines and immunological intervention in HIV infection: a paradigm change. Curr Opin HIV AIDS 2016;11(6):576–84.

89. Schooley RT, Spritzler J, Wang H, et al. AIDS clinical trials group 5197: a placebo-controlled trial of immunization of HIV-1-infected persons with a replication-deficient adenovirus type 5 vaccine expressing the HIV-1 core protein. J Infect Dis 2010;202(5):705–16.

90. Pollard RB, Rockstroh JK, Pantaleo G, et al. Safety and efficacy of the peptide-based therapeutic vaccine for HIV-1, Vacc-4x: a phase 2 randomised, double-blind, placebo-controlled trial. Lancet Infect Dis 2014;14(4):291–300.

91. Alter G, Barouch D. Immune correlate-guided HIV vaccine design. Cell Host Microbe 2018;24(1):25–33.

Printed and bound by CPI Group (UK) Ltd, Croydon, CR0 4YY

08/05/2025

01864746-0005